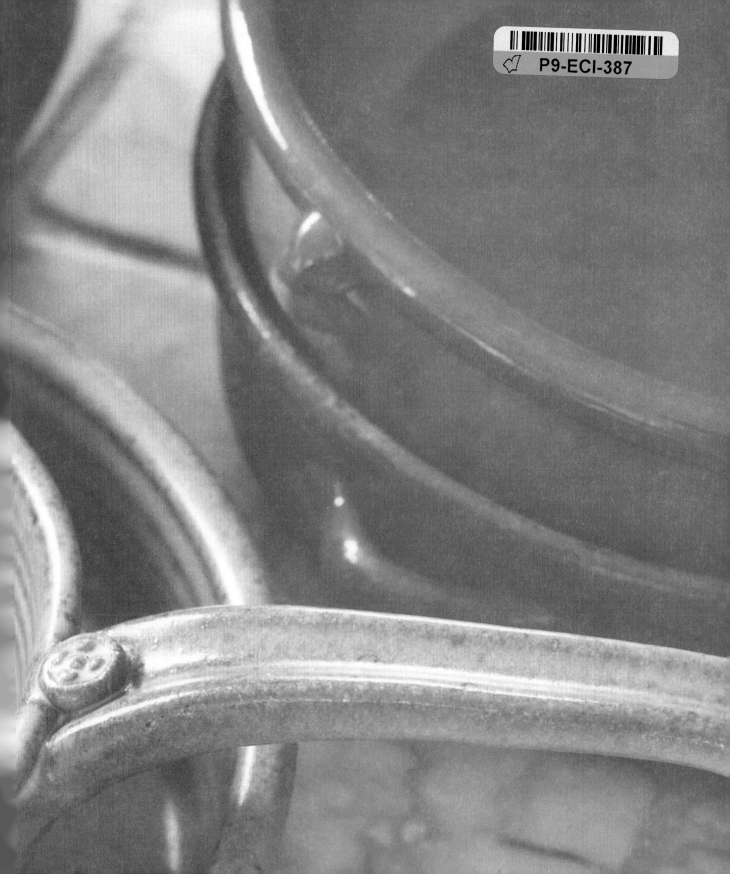

Mediterranean
Clay Pot Cooking

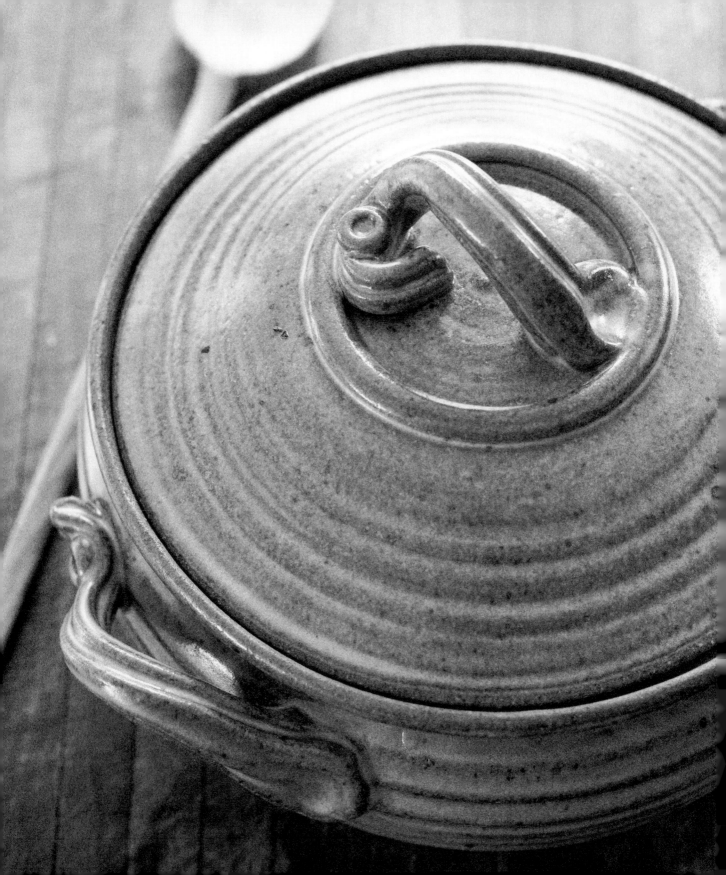

Mediterranean Clay Pot Cooking

Traditional and Modern Recipes
to Savor and Share

PAULA WOLFERT

WILEY

John Wiley and Sons, Inc.

Photo Copyright © Ed Anderson

Interior design by Joel Avirom and Jason Snyder

Published by John Wiley & Sons, Inc., Hoboken, New Jersey

Published simultaneously in Canada

Portions of this book have appeared in somewhat different form in *The Pleasures of Cooking, Food & Wine* magazine, *Metropolitan Home,* and *Saveur* magazine.

For general information on our other products and services or for technical support, please contact our Customer Care Department within the United States at (800) 762–2974, outside the United States at (317) 572–3993 or fax (317) 572–4002.

Wiley also publishes its books in a variety of electronic formats. Some content that appears in print may not be available in electronic books. For more information about Wiley products, visit our web site at www.wiley.com.

Library of Congress Cataloging-in-Publication Data

Wolfert, Paula.
    Mediterranean clay pot cooking / Paula Wolfert.
        p. cm.
    Includes index.
    ISBN 978–0–7645–7633–1 (cloth)
    1. Clay pot cookery. 2. Cookery, Mediterranean. I. Title.
    TX825.5.W65 2009
    641.59182'2—dc22   2008055912

Printed in the United States of America

10 9 8 7 6 5 4 3 2 1

For Leila, Nicholas Bato, and Bill

Contents

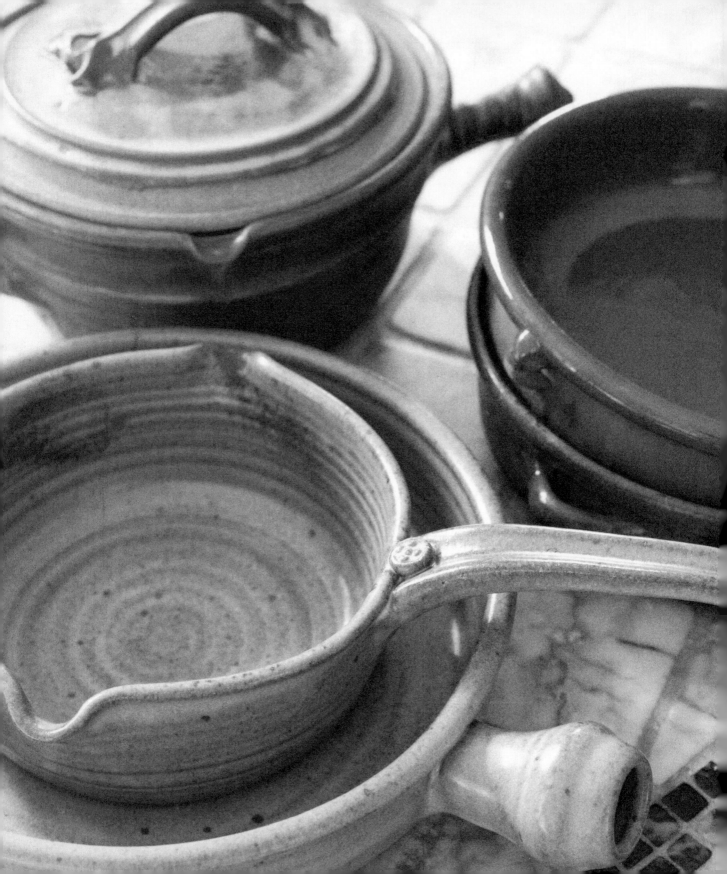

Introduction

I'm not quite sure how it happened that I became a clay pot "junkie." At age nineteen I bought my first clay pot, a beautiful, potbellied *tripière,* used for cooking tripe. I had as yet no idea what tripe was and chose the vessel solely for its looks. Thus began a collection that grew exponentially through the years—enlarged by my travels and culinary adventures. Perhaps it was the different shapes and sizes, the colors and glazes, the myriad variations on primal shapes that attracted me. Or perhaps it was just that earthenware produced such great-tasting food.

And that's where I begin this book, by asserting a simple truth: Most food—and Mediterranean food in particular—tastes better cooked in clay. Since taste is largely subjective, it's hard to prove my claim scientifically, but plenty of evidence abounds. Ever since I started studying Mediterranean cuisines fifty years ago, I heard cooks from the south of France to Morocco sing the praises of clay pots and how they enhanced the local food. Furthermore, whenever I conduct a comparison in my classes of slow-cooked dishes prepared in clay and in metal of any sort, clay wins out.

This is true for many reasons, some obvious, others not. Think of the difference in taste between organically grown fruits and vegetables and typical supermarket agribusiness produce. The former always taste better. Similarly, unglazed clay vessels are organic since clay is a form of earth. Food cooked in them acquires a natural taste. When I taste heirloom beans cooked in a clay pot on top of the stove, I find a special sweetness in them. Just as food cooked in a wood-fired oven acquires the taste and aroma of wood, so food cooked in an unglazed clay pot acquires a taste and aroma I define as "earthy."

There's also the accumulation of flavors that build when a particular dish is cooked over and over in the same porous, unglazed clay pot. I have discovered that the more I use such a dedicated pot, the deeper and more delicious the food cooked in it tastes.

I use the term *clay pot* to refer to any ceramic cooking vessel, including all earthenware, stoneware, and flameware. These come in myriad shapes, each designed for a different dish: tall pots for cooking beans, soups, and stews; round earthenware vessels for cooking rice and sauces; deep-flaring terra-cotta and glazed casseroles for dishes such as cassoulets and tians; shallow, round dishes for baking pies and gratins; stovetop skillets made of ceramic for cooking eggs and sautéing vegetables; shallow glazed rounds for oven baking custards and flans; and clay forms for baking bread.

Ceramic cooking pots speak to me of soothing and nurturing grandmother-style dishes. Each of my vessels has a story to tell—where I learned a wonderful new recipe, or the special smile of the woman who taught it to me; or as a souvenir of a remote Italian mountain village or Greek island town, the way a certain pot caught the light on a particular day when I passed by. Each piece evokes a gastronomical moment frozen in my memory, reminding me of the mysterious process by which raw products are transformed into magnificent food. In the morning, I may glance at a pot and decide to cook a dish special to it that night. Or I may come home from the market with a bag of groceries and search for just the proper pot.

My kitchen overflows with clay. Mediterranean pots line the walls: Spanish *cazuelas,* Italian *tiellas,* Moroccan tagines, Provençal tians and *daubières,* and Turkish *guvecs.* Many vessels are not just for cooking. One of my favorites is a stoneware colander, which in addition to its prime function serves beautifully as the top portion of an improvised *couscousier.* There are also pots for storing flour, dried herbs, preserved butter; pitchers for water; and crocks for vinegar, olive oil, and confits.

All Mediterranean food used to be cooked in clay. Neolithic artifacts from this region abound in clay vessel shards. Some of these early pots were used for storage, some to carry water, others for cooking. It is thought that these early unglazed pots were used primarily for cooking tough cuts of meat, as they are today. In this book I present Mediterranean recipes that are still cooked primarily in clay vessels.

Eventually different cultures developed specialized clay pots designed for the foods of their region. Cooks had their needs; potters listened. Deep vessels were created for cooking beans, wide-bellied pots with narrow necks for simmering meat, heat-resistant clay pans for standing up to direct heat. The Italians cook beans in narrow-necked pots called *pignatas,* which encourage the circulation of moist heat. The French simmer stews in earthenware *daubières,* with water containers built into their tops to help recirculate steam from the food simmering below. The Moroccans created special flat-bottomed pots, called *tagras,* for oven baking fish, and convex earthenware tagines for sitting over a bowl of embers.

While not everyone cooks the old way, these pots are treasured because they make such a noticeable difference in the food. Friends who live around the Mediterranean tell me that lately there's been a clay pot resurgence. A Lebanese friend wrote to me that many Beirut restaurant menus now include a *fakhar,* or clay, section, comprising dishes that are baked in clay and then served in the same vessels. I know of restaurants in Turkey that specialize in clay pot dishes, and lately San Francisco chef Loretta Keller has opened a restaurant, The Moss Room in the new California Academy of Sciences, that features dishes cooked in Columbian black clay.

Italian-American chef Walter Potenza of Walter's in Providence, Rhode Island, has been called "the master of clay" not only because he cooks mainly in clay pots, but he also sells a custom line of terra-cotta cookware, which he designs. "Each clay pot has its own voice," he told me to explain the many shapes and sizes he produces. "And the flavor imparted by these pots is unique and healthy. One uses less fat, and clay-cooked food has more character. I believe most any recipe can be adapted to clay pot cookery. During my research I was struck by the fact that most of the pots sold in Italy at the turn of the century carried the slogan *la salute a nella cotta,* which means 'health is in terra-cotta.'"

These vessels also speak of the potter's skill. For eons these craftsmen have been essential partners to cooks. Art historian Bernard Duplessy describes potters in his book *From The French Country Table: Pottery & Faience of Provence:* "Gods of clay who work the elements—earth, water, fire, and air—to create platters, stew pots, plates, and skillets." There's something very special about cooking in pots that bear traces of what craftspeople call "the maker's hand."

While researching this book, I interviewed numerous potters. One of my favorite potters is Philippe Beltrando of Aubagne, a village near Marseilles, France, whose beautiful, hefty work is perfect for preparing Provençal dishes. I have several of Philippe's daubières, each in a different bold color—green and deep red. I also have one of his mortars, perfect for making aïoli, several of his *poêlons* for stovetop stewing, and a number of other pieces including tart pans and pitchers.

A tall, lanky, and gracious man with beautiful tender eyes and hair flowing to his shoulders, Philippe is an avid gastronome, who studies old texts so as to better create the traditional cooking pots of his native Provence. Over lunch, I asked him why he thought food tastes better when cooked in clay. His answer was both moving and mystical.

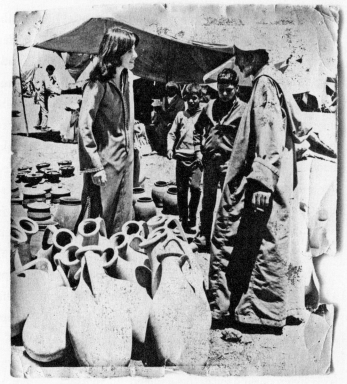

"Maybe someday scientists will come up with an explanation," he told me. "It most likely has to do with the even diffusion of heat, soft heat that creates great alchemy in the kitchen. Think of bubbles rising slowly from within a stew, hatching slowly on the surface to the rhythm of a slowly ticking clock. Personally," he added, "I believe something I was told by my grandmother, who was an extraordinary cook. She insisted that the best daubes were cooked in her oldest casseroles, because, she told me, pottery has a kind of 'memory' of the food it held, and only a clay pot can keep the memory of the love the cook put into it when preparing the dish."

Potter Tom Wirt runs the wonderful Clay Coyote Pottery in Hutchinson, Minnesota, with his wife,

Betsy Price. They specialize in oven- and microwave-safe classic-looking pottery at affordable prices, or, as they put it, "high-fired, hand-thrown functional pottery for everyday use." I have many of their superb pieces: stoneware casseroles, baking dishes, colanders, vinegar crocks, couscous cookers. Recently they have begun a flameproof ceramic cookware line, which includes ceramic skillets and casseroles that can be set over direct heat. Massachusetts potter Bill Sax helped them develop their formulas and introduced me to flameproof ceramic cookware through his gorgeous custom-made pots.

When I asked Tom Wirt the same question I posed to Philippe—why food cooked in clay tastes better—he initially came up with a similar explanation: "Clay heats up more slowly and then becomes uniformly hot, cooking food more evenly. Also, the heat of the clay is softer, causing the flavors to blend differently, without burning the way food often does in metal. And because clay cookware can also be used to serve in, it ties the kitchen to the table and vice versa."

Then he added something interesting: "One thing I've wondered about is whether it's just the clay pot or the fact it's hand-made that makes the greater difference. As cooks, do we get the same response from a machine-made pot that we get from one formed by an artisan? True, it's the clay that makes the basic difference, but I also feel that this completes the cycle of hand-grown food products and hand-cooked food by virtue of the way it touches our humanity. Food sustains us, and there is much love in the whole process. Add to that the emotion inherent in the creation of clay cooking vessels, and you have a chain of caring that is never broken."

Finally, I can't resist quoting from nineteenth-century French novelist Marcelle Tinayre, who wrote in the anthology *La France à Table,* about the dish "Cèpes in the Old Style of the Perigord":

"Take an earthenware casserole that we call in the Perigord a *poêlon.* If you don't have one, use a thick copper casserole. But frankly nothing is as good as clay for all sorts of slow simmered dishes. The clay maintains even heat and doesn't brutalize all the good things you entrust to it. Never cook in iron, enamel or aluminum. These are the work of the devil!"

On that delicious note, I rest my case!

which keeps the food moist, and then, when all the moisture has evaporated, it acts as a dry roaster.

These clay bakers come in many sizes, and are labeled according to the number of pounds of food they can hold. I especially like them for roasting chickens and stuffed breast of lamb and for tenderizing tough cuts of meats efficiently in moist heat. I also use them for bread baking.

Romertopfs are easy to clean, but sooner or later they will develop clogged pores. To remedy, combine ¼ cup of distilled white vinegar with two quarts of water, pour into the pot, and let soak overnight. The next day, rinse well and use a plastic brush to scour the insides of both the pot and the lid with baking soda and water if necessary; drain and dry well before storing.

Chinese Sandpot

A Chinese sandpot is a lidded round pot, similar in shape to a bean pot or deep casserole with round sides. While it is glazed on the inside, the outside is unglazed and bound with metal wire, which encourages even heat distribution. This Asian wonder is a great all-purpose pot, an inexpensive substitute for a French *marmite,* Italian *coccio,* or any number of other small-scale Mediterranean earthenware cooking vessels.

These pots are efficient, inexpensive, and easily available. They come in many sizes; I use a three-quart sandpot to cook many Mediterranean dishes, such as stews, soups, beans, and rice dishes, featured in this book. The sandpot is also an excellent choice for waterless cooking of vegetables such as potatoes, carrots, turnips, and beets, because it allows them to steam in their own natural moisture and thus develop deep, rich flavors. For example, an eggplant tucked into a dry sandpot and then covered and steamed on top of the stove will emerge with an extraordinary texture and aroma.

When newly bought, I prep these pots by soaking them in water for a whole day before first use. And each time I put them in the oven, I usually soak them in water for five minutes just beforehand.

Chinese sandpots sometimes develop hairline cracks. I've had great luck filling these cracks by simmering them in milk. (Milk contains casein, a protein that is insoluble in water and thus works like glue.)

Clay Casseroles

You will need at least one deep earthenware or flameware casserole with a cover to use for cooking soups, daubes, stews, beans, and other slow-cooked dishes on top of the stove or in the oven. Gentle and even cooking preserves the flavors and binds them brilliantly. There is less of a tendency for food to burn, and cleanup is effortless. There are beautiful casseroles available online from North America, France, Italy, Spain, Egypt, Turkey, Colombia, and Chile.

Micaceous Cooking Pots

Pots made of micaceous clay have a lovely glittery surface and are thus always left unglazed. One inexpensive line I particularly like, La Chamba, is imported from Colombia. These pots make superb clay cooking vessels that stand up to direct heat and retain heat beautifully. They are strong and particularly good for cooking slow-simmered soups, sauces, vegetables, beans, and stews. They come in the form of skillets, baking pans, and casseroles. The La Chamba shallow baking dish is particularly useful for cooking flat breads, scrambled eggs, and gratins.

La Chamba pots are porous, so don't leave liquid in them for long periods off the heat. To season the pot, add about one inch of milk to cover the bottom, simmer for 30 minutes, remove from the heat, and allow it to cool before draining. Rinse and dry well. Or follow the manufacturer's instructions.

Because micaceous clay can scratch, use only with wooden or plastic utensils.

La Chamba–ware is oven safe to 450°F. And although they are also dishwasher safe, I wash the pots by hand to maintain their appearance and wipe them down with oil from time to time to enhance their sheen.

Moroccan Tagine

Tagines have become very popular lately, and with good reason. Tagines cook food beautifully, and they are relatively inexpensive. The high conical—or dome-shaped—cover, which fits into the shallow base, acts as a kind of closed chimney. Since the heat on a stovetop comes from below, the top of the cover remains cooler than the rest of the pot, which causes steam to condense and drip back onto the stew, preventing the food from drying out.

There are three basic types of earthenware tagines: fully glazed, elaborately decorated vessels, which are used only for serving, and the simply glazed and unglazed earthenware tagines, which are used for cooking as well as serving. My personal favorite is a mica-rich unglazed tagine from southern Morocco. And like a Scotsman's clay pipe or a

Japanese teapot, it has become seasoned through use, acquiring a lovely patina.

According to some, long-used tagines also acquire an uncanny ability to express flavor. Sami Samir, an importer of Moroccan goods, explained to me why such used pots are greatly coveted:

"After years of use a little saffron gets trapped in the pores of the top cone. Then come layers of cumin, cardamom, and our Moroccan spice mixture, *ras el hanout*. We have a joke—if you prepare food in a pot like this, eventually you won't need to add any seasonings, because they're already trapped in the clay, just waiting to be released when you cook."

I've heard similar sentiments expressed about old family clay cooking pots from one end of the Mediterranean to the other. Many matriarchs insist their best dishes must be cooked in their oldest pots. I've heard tales of daughters vying to inherit their mother's and grandmother's favorite old casseroles.

To season a new unglazed tagine: Fill the shallow bottom dish with water or milk, place it in a cold oven, and set the temperature to 350°F. Bake the pot for thirty minutes, turn off the heat, and let it cool in the slowly receding heat. Then drain off the liquid, wash the pot, dry it well, and rub with olive oil.

If you'd like to simulate the patina of an antique tagine, you can burnish the pot by rubbing the clay inside and out with a mixture of ½ cup olive oil and ¾ cup wood ash from the fireplace. Place in a cold oven, set the temperature to 250°F, and bake for two to three hours. Turn off the heat and let the pot cool in the oven. Repeat for deeper browning.

To season a new partially glazed tagine: Soak

the bottom dish in water to cover for twelve hours. Drain the dish, wipe it dry, and rub with a cut clove of garlic. Then fill the dish again with water to half an inch below the rim and add a third of a cup of vinegar. Set on a heat diffuser over low heat and slowly bring the liquid to a boil. Cook until only about half a cup liquid remains. Remove from the heat and let cool; then rinse and dry.

For more information on the pots featured in photos in this book, please see page 321.

TIPS FOR USING YOUR CLAY POTS SUCCESSFULLY

Not all clay pots should be seasoned, though some will greatly profit from it. But don't think that every clay pot needs a soaking; I've seen soaked pots break apart in the sink within a few hours. Sometimes this is the potter's fault, and sometimes it's because certain types of clay require different types of curing. My best advice is always to follow the manufacturer's directions.

When cooking in clay on a stovetop or in the oven, start at a lower temperature than you ordinarily would with metal pots; then slowly raise the heat as necessary. To put it another way: Avoid thermal shock—sudden changes in temperature—which can cause cracking. Once the heat has permeated the pot, which can take a relatively long time because clay is such a good insulator, the pot will hold the heat evenly for a long time.

When removing a hot pot or its lid from the stove or oven, use thick potholders and *always* place it on a cloth pad, folded kitchen towel, or wooden board. If you place a hot pot on a cold surface such as a marble or granite counter, it may crack. By the same token, never place a refrigerated pot in a preheated oven. Instead, bring to room temperature, then turn on the heat. Also, never place a hot pot in cold water and avoid adding cold food or liquid to a hot clay pot. (Note: Flameware is an exception to this rule.)

Food cooked in clay pots will remain moist and hot, enabling you to cook with less liquid and less fat than would ordinarily be the case.

After washing, if your earthenware pot is water-logged, turn it upside down and let it air dry thoroughly overnight.

Because unglazed earthenware is porous and thus tends to hold tastes and aromas, it's best to dedicate an unglazed earthenware pot for cooking fish, and keep another to use with meat and poultry.

Clay Safety

One concern that people have about cooking in ceramic pots is that a glaze may contain lead and/or cadmium that could possibly leach into foods if the glaze was improperly formulated, applied, or fired. There's even a theory that the Roman Empire fell due to lead poisoning from city water pipes and citizen's cooking pots.

You needn't worry about new glazed cooking pots imported or domestically produced as its manufacture is regulated. All pottery sold for cooking must be tested and certified as safe by the U.S. Food and Drug Administration. And nearly all small American production potters use lead-free glazes.

If you purchase a pot abroad and want to be certain it's safe, you can do a simple, inexpensive lead test at home. (I recommend Lead Check, which is sold at hardware stores or through www.leadcheck. com). Note that the swabs in the kits can test only for surface lead. If a pot is damaged, be sure to test it again before continuing to use it in food preparation.

Antique pots, made before lead glazes were regulated, look great on the shelf; but they should not be used for cooking or food storage.

There are no proven undesirable health effects from clean, unglazed clay pots such as Romertopf, La Chamba, Pomaireware, and Turkish guvecs.

Mold is another problem that can develop with clay. To prevent mold, wet porous earthenware pots should be allowed to dry out thoroughly. If you see any evidence of mold, simply wash the pot with vinegar and scrub with a paste of salt or baking soda. If you're concerned about bacterial growth, use the French country cook's method: rub your earthenware pot with garlic before each use; many claim this confers natural antimicrobial protection.

CLAY OVEN ENVIRONMENTS

If you want to cook restaurant-quality roast chickens, bake breads and pizzas like a pro, brown gratins with marvelous glazes, you must create a clay environment in your home oven to simulate an old-fashioned brick oven. This is done by outfitting an ordinary electric or gas oven with some sort of unglazed heat-absorbing ceramic. There are several ways to accomplish this, ranging from relatively expensive to quite cheap. However you do it, there is a major trade-off: energy.

Baking in a simulated clay oven will take from thirty to sixty minutes longer than normal to achieve the desired oven heat. On the other end, you can often turn off the heat sooner and let the dish finish cooking in the receding heat concentrated in the tiles, akin to the old way of cooking gratins and long-cooked stews that were transported to a local baker's oven and then moved about in the receding heat until, in the case of gratins, they became beautifully glazed or, in the case of stews, cooked till rich and thick.

You can use pizza stones or a pair of FibraMent slabs on your top and bottom oven racks. Another adaptation is to line your oven with thick, food-safe quarry tiles or fire bricks available at your home improvement store. If you go this route, be sure to wash the tile or bricks, allow them to dry *completely*, and, when lining your oven, leave a one-inch gap between walls and bricks. The first time you use it, heat your dry tile-lined oven slowly to prevent cracking. A final alternative is to use a La Cloche stoneware domed baker, thus simulating a small Mediterranean beehive-style oven. This works especially well for breads, small roasts, and tians.

Hints for using your clay oven adaptation:

* Always preheat the oven and the stone at the same time. Do not heat the oven and then insert the stones later.

* Check the temperature of the tiles or stone rather than the oven air before roasting or baking.

* For gratins, always use a flat-bottomed dish so heat distributes evenly and transfers directly into the gratin.

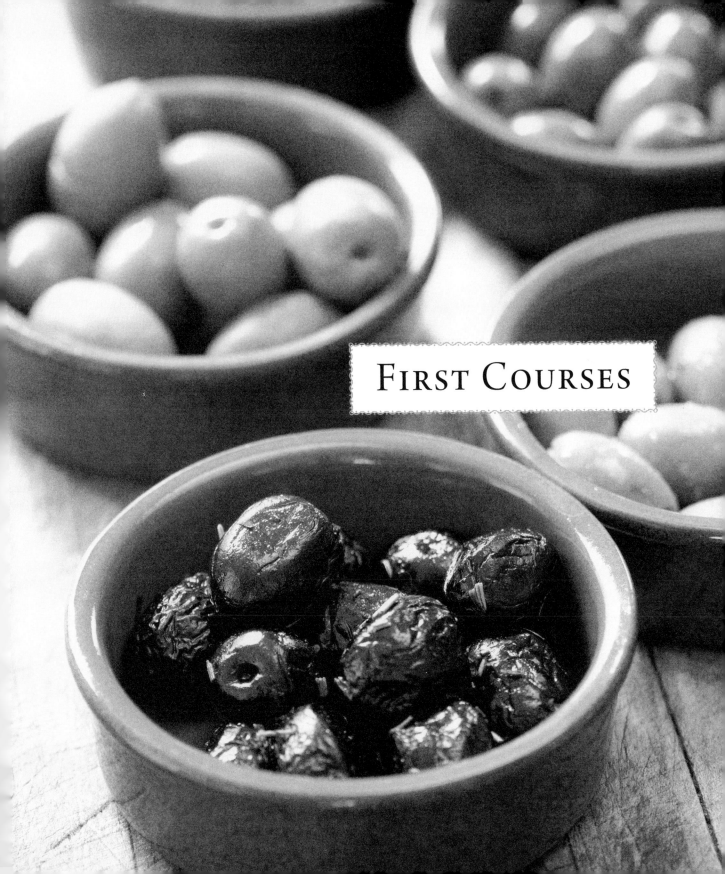

FIRST COURSES

Roman Artichokes Braised with Garlic and Mint

SERVES 6 TO 8

Food and travel writer David Downie was kind enough to teach me some of his Italian mother's recipes for artichokes. One of them is my all-time favorite, especially successful when cooked in clay as presented here. It is inspired by the recipe for Roman-style artichokes in his superb *Cooking the Roman Way*.

> **PREFERRED CLAY POT:**
>
> A 3-quart glazed earthenware saucepan or casserole about 10 inches in diameter
>
> If using an electric or ceramic stovetop, be sure to use a heat diffuser with the clay pot.

2 lemons, halved

6 to 8 tender young globe artichokes, preferably with long stems

5 garlic cloves, crushed

Coarse salt and freshly ground black pepper

½ cup extra-virgin olive oil

⅓ cup minced fresh spearmint

⅓ cup minced fresh flat-leaf parsley

1½ cups Italian dry white wine, preferably Frascati or Marino

1 Prepare the artichokes: Squeeze the juice of 1 lemon into a bowl of water large enough to hold all the artichokes. Working one by one, cut off the top third of the artichokes. Snap off the tough outer leaves near the base. Use a stainless-steel knife to cut off the stem; if the stems are tender, drop them into the bowl of acidulated water. Remove the hairy choke in the center of the artichoke with a melon scoop; then scrape along the inside wall of the artichoke bottom until smooth. Squeeze a little lemon juice into the center. After cleaning the inside, remove the remaining outer tough leaves by bending them backward and snapping them off where they break. Trim the outside of the artichoke to remove any tough dark green skin with a small paring knife or a swivel-bladed vegetable peeler. Rub the artichoke all over with a piece of cut lemon as you work. Drop the cleaned artichoke into the bowl. When all are cleaned, peel the stems and return them to the acidulated water.

2 In a small bowl, mash the crushed garlic with 1 teaspoon salt and a pinch of pepper. Work in 3 tablespoons of the olive oil, the mint, parsley, and ¼ teaspoon pepper to a make a thick paste.

3 Remove the artichokes from the water and drain them well. Stuff the center of each with 2 to 3 teaspoons of the herbed garlic paste. Stand the artichokes side by side in the earthenware saucepan. Slip the peeled stems in between the artichokes. Sprinkle the artichokes with salt and pepper and drizzle on the remaining olive oil. Pour in the wine and 1 cup cold water.

4 Slowly bring to a boil over medium heat; cover with a sheet of parchment paper and the lid. Reduce the heat to low and cook until the artichokes are tender when poked with a fork, 30 to 40 minutes. Transfer the casserole to a wood surface or folded kitchen towel to prevent cracking. Serve warm or at room temperature with a fresh sprinkling of salt and pepper.

Sautéed Asparagus with Brown Butter and Parmigiano-Reggiano Cheese

SERVES 2

This great asparagus preparation is a popular starter in northern Italy, where in many recipes butter—and not olive oil—is the fat of choice. Clarified butter is the key to this dish: When it hits the hot cazuela, it turns golden brown, intensifying the flavor and giving off a hazelnut-like aroma. Yes, you can make this dish with olive oil, but it really won't be the same.

To make a French variation, substitute either shredded Cantal cheese or crumbled bleu d'Auvergne for the grated Parmigiano-Reggiano cheese.

> **PREFERRED CLAY POT:**
>
> A 9-or 10- or 11-inch Spanish cazuela or a straight-sided flameware or La Chamba skillet
>
> If using an electric or ceramic stovetop, be sure to use a heat diffuser with the clay pot.

12 fat green asparagus spears

½ teaspoon salt

4 tablespoons (½ stick) unsalted butter, clarified (see Note)

3 to 4 tablespoons freshly grated Parmigiano-Reggiano cheese (1½ ounces)

1 Preheat the oven to 400°F. Line up the asparagus and trim off about 3 inches from the bottom of the spears. Peel the stalks from the base toward the top, stopping just before the tips.

2 Fill the cazuela with 1 inch of warm water. Set the pan over medium heat, add the salt, and bring to a boil. Arrange the asparagus in the cazuela in a single layer and cook, uncovered, until just tender, 5 to 7 minutes.

3 Drain off the water and return the cazuela to the stovetop. Immediately add half of the clarified butter to the hot pan and gently roll and toss the asparagus spears to coat them. Slowly allow the butter to turn golden brown over low heat; as soon as it does, stop the cooking by adding 1 teaspoon of lukewarm water. Sprinkle the cheese over the asparagus and transfer to the oven.

4 Bake for 5 to 7 minutes, until the cheese bubbles and a light crust forms. Set the cazuela on a wooden surface or folded kitchen towel to prevent cracking and serve right from the pan.

NOTE TO THE COOK: To clarify butter: Place 6 tablespoons sweet butter in a small saucepan. Set over very low heat. Allow the butter to melt slowly without stirring and without browning. Remove foam as it appears on the surface. When the butter is golden and clear, remove it from the heat and leave to cool. Carefully pour off the clear butter, leaving the sediment in the saucepan.

Asparagus and Truffled Ramps

SERVES 8

*H*ere's a delicious starter that evokes springtime as well as any dish I know, pairing thin early asparagus with ramps, or wild leeks, which appear as one of the first greens in the forest.

Ramps and wild leeks are as close as sisters. In the Appalachians, where they grow wild, they're called *ramps*. Around the Great Lakes, where they're picked a little later, with a somewhat larger bulb and a slightly milder flavor, they're known as *wild leeks*. In the Bordeaux region of France, where they grow wild and are foraged in the vineyards, they're called *baragnes*. Yes, ramps are difficult to find, but you can substitute green garlic or baby cultivated leeks with fine results.

Truffles, of course, aren't really a springtime ingredient, so I use black truffle oil and then, to enhance the springtime effect, scatter a few sunflower sprouts on top just before serving—a distinctly California touch.

PREFERRED CLAY POT:

A 3-quart glazed or unglazed earthenware or flameware casserole or Chinese sandpot

If using an electric or ceramic stovetop, be sure to use a heat diffuser with the clay pot.

2 pounds ramps (about 5 dozen) or 1½ pounds green garlic or baby leeks

4 tablespoons (½ stick) unsalted butter

4 pounds thin asparagus, ends trimmed, cut into 2-inch pieces

¼ cup crème fraîche or heavy cream

4 ounces Serrano ham, coarsely chopped

Salt and freshly ground black pepper

¾ teaspoon black truffle oil

1 tablespoon sherry vinegar

3 tablespoons walnut oil

4 ounces tender sweet salad greens, such as baby spinach, young chard, pea shoots, orache, or lamb's-quarters, rinsed and dried

1 cup loosely packed sunflower sprouts (optional)

1 Clean the ramps: Cut off the green leaves and purplish stems. Trim the roots and peel the white bulb under cold running water to remove all traces of soil. Pat dry.

2 Place the clay casserole over low heat. Add the ramps and butter, cover with a sheet of crumpled wet parchment, and slowly raise the heat to medium until the ramps are sizzling softly. Cook, shaking the pan gently once or twice, until the ramps soften, 5 to 10 minutes.

3 Lift off the parchment and add the asparagus, cream, and ham. Season with ¾ teaspoon salt and ¼ teaspoon pepper. Toss gently, cover with the same parchment paper and the lid, and cook for 5 to 10 minutes longer, until the asparagus and ramps are tender. Drizzle on ½ teaspoon of the truffle oil and toss gently to combine. Transfer the casserole to a wooden surface or folded kitchen towel to prevent cracking.

4 With a slotted spoon, divide the asparagus, ramps, and ham among 8 plates. Continue to cook the creamy sauce until it is reduced to 2 to 3 tablespoons, about 2 minutes. Meanwhile, whisk together the vinegar, oil, and remaining ¼ teaspoon truffle oil. Whisk in the reduced creamy liquid and season the vinaigrette with salt and pepper to taste.

5 In a mixing bowl, toss half the vinaigrette with the baby greens. Drizzle the remaining vinaigrette over the ramps and asparagus on the plates. Garnish each serving with a bit of salad and top with a sprinkling of sunflower sprouts.

NOTE TO THE COOK: Ramps or wild leeks can be found regionally in early spring at farmers' markets or online at www.earthydelights.com.

Clay Pot–Roasted Eggplant with Cheese

SERVES 4

Here's a modern interpretation of an old Catalan dish. The combination of sweetened eggplant and cheese may strike you as strange, but, in fact, adding honey to offset the mild bitterness of eggplant really works.

The key here is slow-roasting the eggplant to achieve a rich, distinctive flavor and aroma. You can do this over coals, under the broiler, directly over the flame of a gas stovetop, or, my new favorite method, by placing an unpeeled eggplant in a dry Chinese sandpot and cooking it on the stovetop—the way potatoes and chestnuts are traditionally cooked in western France. The result is smoky, creamy, and intensely tasty.

This dish is lovely served in individual shallow earthenware cazuelitas or ramekins.

> **PREFERRED CLAY POTS:**
>
> A 3-quart Chinese sandpot
>
> 4 individual shallow cazuelitas or small ramekins (6 ounces each)
>
> If using an electric or ceramic stovetop, be sure to use a heat diffuser with the clay pot.

(continued)

2 medium eggplants (12 ounces each), preferably organic

5 ounces sheep's milk cheese, such as Spanish Roncal or manchego, Italian ricotta salata, or Greek myzithra, grated (about 1 cup)

2 tablespoons milk

1 egg

1 egg yolk

1 scant teaspoon fine sea salt

¼ teaspoon freshly ground black pepper

⅛ teaspoon freshly grated nutmeg

2 tablespoons unsalted butter

1 tablespoon honey, preferably lavender, rosemary, or blackberry

1 Rinse the eggplants; drain, trim off the top, prick each once with a sharp fork (to keep them from exploding), and place side by side in the sandpot. Cover and set over low heat. Gradually raise the heat to medium and cook, turning every 15 minutes, until the eggplants are blackened in spots and very soft, 30 to 40 minutes.

2 Set an oven rack on the highest rung. Preheat the oven to 350°F. Meanwhile, set a colander in the sink and drop in the eggplants, slit each one, and let stand for 10 minutes, turning once, to drain off the brown juices.

3 When the eggplants are cool enough to handle, peel and place in a mixing bowl. Add two-thirds of the cheese, the milk, egg, and egg yolk; mix well, mashing the eggplant. Season with the salt, pepper, and nutmeg. Use half the butter to grease the cazuelitas or ramekins. Divide the eggplant mixture among them, flatten the tops, and sprinkle with the remaining cheese. Warm the remaining butter with the honey until fluid; drizzle over the tops.

4 Set the ramekins on a baking sheet and transfer to the oven. Immediately raise the heat to 450°F. Bake for 20 minutes, or until the eggplant custards are golden brown and puffed on top. Serve warm.

NOTE TO THE COOK: This recipe can be made up to 4 hours in advance. Keep covered in a cool place. Reheat in a preheated 300°F oven for 15 minutes.

Thanks to the late Catalan culinary expert Rudolf Grewe for translating this recipe from a medieval cookbook, Le Libre del Coch, *by Robert de Nola, published in 1520.*

Sicilian Caponatina with Olives, Pine Nuts, and Currants

MAKES 5 CUPS, SERVING 8

This recipe is inspired by one taught to me by Palermo-born Maria Sindoni, who shared her secrets with me at the kitchen stove in her restaurant Azzurro in New York back in the early eighties. While her version of this traditional dish has never bored me as others have, I must admit I've tampered with it over the years, adding a little more here, a little less there to make it my own. What I did not change, and what I found so inspiring, is Maria's method of cooking each vegetable separately to retain its natural flavor and texture.

If you follow my instructions closely in steps 1 and 5, you will not have the problem endemic to so many fried eggplant dishes: heaviness due to the vegetable's propensity to absorb large amounts of oil. By first soaking the eggplant in a water bath and then frying the vegetable in a cazuela, which keeps the temperature of the oil constant, you'll attain the lightest possible golden brown eggplant.

You can make this great appetizer spread several days in advance. It's one of those magical dishes that gets better and better as it mellows.

> **PREFERRED CLAY POT:**
>
> A 10-or 11-inch Spanish cazuela or an earthenware or straight-sided flameware skillet
>
> If using an electric or ceramic stovetop, be sure to use a heat diffuser with the clay pot.

2 large eggplants (about 1½ pounds each)

2 tablespoons plus 1 teaspoon coarse salt

½ to ¾ cup extra virgin olive oil

1 medium onion, chopped

3 cups diced tender celery heart ribs with some leaves

¾ cup canned tomato sauce

1 tablespoon finely chopped sun-dried tomatoes

3 tablespoons red wine vinegar, or more to taste

1 tablespoon sugar

12 salted capers, rinsed and drained

12 Sicilian green olives, rinsed, pitted, and drained

3 tablespoons dried currants, soaked in warm water for 5 minutes and drained

Pinch of crushed hot red pepper

¼ cup pine nuts, lightly toasted (see Note)

24 large fresh basil leaves, stemmed

1 Cut the stems off the eggplants, peel them, and cut into 1-inch cubes. Place in a large bowl along with 2 tablespoons of the coarse salt and enough cold water to cover. Set a plate on top to keep the eggplants submerged and soak for 45 minutes.

2 Meanwhile, put 3 tablespoons of the olive oil, the onion, the remaining 1 teaspoon salt, and ½ cup warm water in the cazuela and set over medium-low heat. Slowly warm the pan, raising the heat gradually, until the onion begins to cook. Continue to cook, stirring from time to time, until the water evaporates and the onion turns golden, about 15 minutes.

(continued)

3 In a medium saucepan of boiling salted water, cook the celery for 10 minutes. Drain and add to the onion in the cazuela. Stir in the tomato sauce and sun-dried tomatoes and cook, stirring often, until the mixture sizzles and thickens to a jamlike consistency, about 10 minutes. Scrape into a bowl and let cool.

4 Without rinsing the cazuela, add the vinegar and sugar and cook over medium to medium-high heat, stirring, until the sugar dissolves and the syrup is slightly reduced, about 3 minutes. Add the capers, olives, currants, and hot pepper and cook, stirring, for 5 minutes. Scrape the contents of the cazuela into the celery and tomato. Set the cazuela on a wooden surface or folded kitchen towel to prevent cracking and allow to cool down; then wash and dry.

5 Drain the eggplants, rinse under cold running water, and drain well. Squeeze to remove as much moisture as possible; then press dry with paper towels. (It doesn't matter if the eggplant cubes lose their shape.) Pour ⅓ cup of the remaining olive oil into the cazuela; carefully tilt the cazuela away from you on one side so the oil gathers on the opposite side. Slowly warm the oil over medium-low heat, raising the heat gradually to medium or medium-high, until the oil registers 340°F. Reduce the heat to maintain the temperature. Add no more than 4 eggplant cubes at a time and fry until cooked through and golden brown all over, about 2 minutes per batch. With a slotted spoon, transfer the eggplant to paper towels to drain. Repeat until all the eggplant is browned, adding a few tablespoons more oil if needed. Total frying time should be about 20 minutes.

6 When all the eggplant is cooked, pour off the oil from the cazuela. Add the tomato mixture and cook for 20 seconds, stirring. Season with salt and pepper to taste. Let cool, then pack the caponatina into a jar, cover, and refrigerate. Return caponatina to room temperature before serving, garnish with a shower of toasted pine nuts and torn basil leaves.

NOTE TO THE COOK: To toast pine nuts: place in a small dry skillet over medium-low heat, tossing often, until golden brown, about 5 minutes. Turn onto a dish to cool.

Tile-Caramelized Mushrooms

SERVES 2 TO 4

When I first started traveling in Turkey, cooking on unglazed ceramic roof tiles was a relatively obscure practice restricted to west-central Anatolia, where the tiles are made. Now, many years later, this type of peasant cooking has become all the rage throughout the country. Today lamb, steak, chicken, fish, and vegetables are baked this way. Sometimes the meat—or, in this case, mushrooms—is tossed with fresh tomatoes and peppers, which caramelize along with the main ingredient. Grated cheese is often melted on top.

The oval terra-cotta tiles are set in the oven to heat while the mushrooms are seared in oil or butter in a skillet on top of the stove. The sautéed mushrooms are then slipped onto the hot tiles to finish caramelizing. The principle is simple: Cook hot food on even hotter tiles.

Actual Turkish *kiremit* tiles are 8 or 9 inches long, 3 inches wide, and 1 inch thick—perfect for one serving. I substitute an earthenware, shallow, straight-sided skillet, such as the Colombian La Chamba, with fine results.

> **PREFERRED CLAY POT:**
>
> An 8- or 9-inch La Chamba or flameware skillet a thick, unglazed terra-cotta saucer

2 tablespoons unsalted butter

24 small brown or white mushrooms, stemmed

1 garlic clove, chopped

1 medium tomato, peeled, seeded, and diced

Salt and freshly ground black pepper

½ teaspoon fresh lemon juice

2 tablespoons mixed chopped fresh flat-leaf parsley, oregano, and mint

2 tablespoons grated firm sheep's milk cheese, such as kashkaval or kasseri

1 Place the skillet in a cold oven. Set the temperature at 400°F and heat the pan for 20 minutes.

2 Meanwhile, in a conventional medium skillet, melt 1 tablespoon of the butter over medium heat. Add the mushrooms, cover with parchment paper and a lid, and cook over low heat for 20 minutes, shaking the pan once or twice. Uncover the skillet and remove the paper. Raise the heat to medium-high and quickly boil off any moisture. Add the remaining 1 tablespoon butter and cook, shaking the pan to coat the mushrooms and brown them lightly, 1 to 2 minutes.

3 Scrape the sautéed mushroom onto the very hot clay in the oven; they should sizzle. Add the garlic and tomato. Season with salt and pepper to taste.

4 Bake for 5 minutes. Sprinkle the lemon juice and herbs over the mushrooms and top with the grated cheese. Transfer the pan to a wooden surface or folded kitchen towel to prevent cracking. Serve at once.

Grape Leaves Stuffed with Rice, Rose Petals, Currants, and Mint

SERVES 6 TO 8

*H*ere dried rose petals and both fresh and dried mint add an unusual dimension of flavor to a traditional Turkish starter. The combination of seasonings generates a haunting aroma, and cooking in clay ensures steady heat, which produces a velvety melt-in-the-mouth texture.

After cooking, the stuffed grape leaves should be chilled so the filling can set up, but they are best served at room temperature. They will keep well in the refrigerator for three or four days.

> **PREFERRED CLAY POT:**
>
> **A 4- to 5-quart glazed or unglazed earthenware or flameware casserole**
>
> **If using an electric or ceramic stovetop, be sure to use a heat diffuser with the clay pot.**

48 to 54 tender young grape leaves, freshly picked, defrosted, or packed in brine

¼ cup extra virgin olive oil

2 medium onions, finely chopped

1 cup short-grain white rice, such as Baldo or Arborio

¼ cup pine nuts

1 tablespoon tomato paste, canned or homemade (page 317)

⅓ cup finely chopped fresh mint

1 tablespoon dried currants

1 tablespoon sugar

Salt

1 tablespoon dried mint

¼ teaspoon ground allspice

¼ teaspoon ground cinnamon

⅓ cup crushed dried organic rose petals

2 cups boiling water

1 Choose young grape leaves that have not been sprayed with pesticides, and blanch in small bunches in a saucepan of lightly salted boiling water for 30 seconds. If you are using thawed frozen grape leaves, blanch for 60 seconds. If using brined, carefully separate each leaf and rinse first under water; then blanch in *unsalted* boiling water for 3 minutes, rinse under cool running water, and drain well.

2 Add the olive oil to the casserole, set over medium-low heat, and warm slowly, gradually raising the heat to medium. Add the onions and cook, uncovered, stirring occasionally, until soft and golden, 15 to 20 minutes.

3 Meanwhile, soak the rice in 2 cups very hot salted water for 10 minutes. Pour into a sieve, rinse, and drain well.

4 Stir the pine nuts and tomato paste into the golden onions and cook for a few minutes. Mix in the rice, fresh mint, currants, sugar, 1 teaspoon salt, dried mint, allspice, cinnamon, and rose petals. Add 1 cup of the boiling water and stir once. Cook, uncovered, until the water is absorbed, about 5 minutes; remove from the heat. (The rice will finish cooking later.) Transfer to a wide bowl and spread out so the rice can cool down quickly.

5 To fill the leaves, place them ribbed side up on a kitchen towel. Snip off the stems with scissors. If any of the leaves are more than 4 inches across, trim off the excess or cut the leaves in half along the spine. Save these trimmings. Put 1 heaping teaspoon of rice filling on each leaf near the base. Fold the bottom of the leaf over the filling, fold in the sides toward the center, and roll up snuggly, squeezing gently so each roll is compact and as thin as possible. (At this point the stuffed grape leaves can be wrapped and frozen.)

6 Line the bottom of the same casserole used to cook the rice with the grape leaf trimmings. Place the stuffed leaves close together, seam side down, in perpendicular layers. Season them lightly with salt. Weight the stuffed grape leaves with an upside-down heatproof plate to keep the rolls in place. Add the remaining 1 cup boiling water, cover with the lid, and cook for 30 to 60 minutes, depending on the age and tenderness of the leaves. After half an hour, check for doneness every 15 minutes; the leaves should not be mushy. Remove from the heat and let stand, covered, until cool; the rolls will continue to absorb the cooking liquid. Remove the plate and pour off any liquid in the pot. Invert the rolls onto a flat plate, cover tightly with plastic wrap, and refrigerate until chilled and set. Serve at room temperature.

With thanks to Ayfer Ünsal for sharing this recipe.

Wrinkled Potatoes with Spicy Red Mojo as Prepared on the Island of Tenerife

SERVES 4 TO 6

There's a nice story about how *papas arrugadas,* a Canary Islands tapas bar specialty, came about: Because fresh water is fairly scarce on the islands, potatoes were often cooked in seawater. A certain cook forgot her potatoes were on the stove and returned to discover all the seawater had boiled away and her potatoes were sizzling in the salt residue. She removed the potatoes from the fire, covered the pan, and shook it to loosen the stuck-on salt. When she lifted the lid, she discovered her potatoes had

developed firm, flavorful wrinkled skins enclosing soft, creamy interiors. Thus, according to the story, *papas arrugadas* were born.

Tapas bars in Tenerife serve these great-tasting potatoes hot, warm, or cold with a spicy red dipping sauce called *mojo picon,* made with cumin, hot peppers, and olive oil prepared in a clay mortar. Yes, you can make your *mojo* in a food processor or blender, but I've found it comes out smoother when pounded by hand. The sauce is also excellent with grilled fish or roast pork.

(continued)

16 to 18 small new potatoes (1½ pounds), preferably organic

1⅓ cups coarse salt mixed with ⅓ cup aromatic sea salt

3 or 4 large lettuce or cabbage leaves

Mojo Picon (recipe follows)

1   Scrub the potatoes, but do not peel them. In the deep clay pot, dissolve the salt in 2½ cups warm water. Add the potatoes. If the salted water does not reach to about 1 inch below the top of the potatoes, add a little more. The potatoes should float in the water; if they don't, add more salt. Cover with the lettuce leaves and slowly bring to a boil over medium-low heat, occasionally shaking the pot gently. Boil until the potatoes are almost tender and most of the water has evaporated, about 25 minutes.

2   Pour off any remaining water. Return the pot to the stove, cover with a kitchen towel or paper towels and a lid, and continue to cook the potatoes over the low heat for about 10 minutes, grasping the handles of the pot with both hands and shaking the pot firmly to toss the potatoes in the residual salt several times.

3   The potatoes are ready when they are dry with a light coating of salt and test tender when pierced with the tip of a knife. Serve hot, warm, or cool, smothered with Mojo Picon.

NOTE TO THE COOK: Since these are eaten as a snack, choose potatoes that are as small as possible. And for even cooking, make sure they are of equal size.

Mojo Picon

MAKES ABOUT ¾ CUP

Lola Massieu, a wonderful painter and cookbook author from Tenerife, told me that a good *mojo picon,* or "spicy sauce," should include three types of dried red peppers: one mild, one sweet, and a local hot pepper called *la pimienta de puta madre.* This last is a Canary Islands joke, Lola explained, and refers to "peppers so hot they make you cry and thus evoke an instinctive memory of your mother!"

These hot Canary Islands peppers, which are very small, are pounded into a paste once a year and stored in clay jars. Small portions are removed as needed, then diluted with water and vinegar to the consistency of a dipping sauce. Because these particular chiles are unavailable here, I substitute harissa or Turkish hot pepper paste (see Sources).

3 tablespoons stale bread crumbs

5 or 6 garlic cloves

1 teaspoon ground cumin

½ teaspoon coarse salt

1 tablespoon plus 1 teaspoon Turkish hot pepper
paste or harissa

1½ teaspoons sweet paprika, preferably Spanish

Pinch of sugar

½ cup extra virgin olive oil

1 tablespoon red wine vinegar

1 In a small bowl, soak the bread crumbs in ½ cup water until soft and swollen, 5 to 10 minutes. Drain and squeeze dry.

2 In a ceramic or marble mortar, crush the garlic, cumin, and salt to a smooth paste. Add the bread crumbs, pepper paste, paprika, and sugar, pounding until well combined.

3 Gradually work in the olive oil, little by little, stirring constantly with the pestle. Add the vinegar and enough water to make a smooth sauce. Pour into a small bowl, and let stand at room temperature for 1 to 2 hours before serving.

Wrinkled Potatoes with Cilantro Mojo

Substitute Cilantro Mojo (recipe follows) for Mojo Picon.

Cilantro Mojo

MAKES ABOUT ¾ CUP

On the island of Las Palmas, chef-owner Maria Dolores Mejias, of the Cho Zacarias in Vegueta in the Old Quarter, shared this recipe with me.

1 teaspoon cumin seeds

6 small garlic cloves

½ teaspoon coarse salt, or more to taste

1 Anaheim pepper, peeled, seeded, and chopped

½ cup packed fresh cilantro leaves

¼ cup plus 2 tablespoons extra virgin olive oil

2 to 3 tablespoons cider vinegar, rice vinegar,
or muscatel vinegar

1 In a small dry skillet, toast the cumin seeds over medium heat until lightly browned and fragrant, 1 to 2 minutes. Crush the seeds in a ceramic or marble mortar, then add the garlic and salt and grind to a paste.

2 Work in the Anaheim pepper and cilantro until smooth. Gradually add the olive oil and then the vinegar and 2 tablespoons water. Season the sauce with additional salt if needed.

3 Pour into a small bowl, and let stand at room temperature for at least 2 and up to 5 hours before serving.

Warm Green Olives with White Wine, Garlic, and Hot Red Pepper

There are many varieties of Mediterranean olives, each in various shades of green, violet, or black, depending on their stage of ripeness. After picking, olives are altered by different methods of curing and then preserved in oil, vinegar, or salt brine or simply dried. Each type has its special taste, texture, and degree of oiliness.

For this dish I'd ordinarily recommend a Greek or Spanish olive, but lately I've been pleasantly surprised by two California home-style cured olive brands, Graber and Lindsay. I've found their products top-notch, especially when baked in a clay pot, which in my view, of course, makes almost anything taste better. Rinse these domestic tree-ripened olives, then cook them in a clay pot with garlic, aromatics, and white wine, and you'll be surprised at how luscious they can be. If you decide to go with imported olives, I suggest the Spanish Farga Aragon, Italian Gaeta, or Greek Amphissa.

> **PREFERRED CLAY POT:**
>
> A 3-quart Chinese sandpot or other glazed earthenware or flameware saucepan or casserole
>
> If using an electric or ceramic stovetop, be sure to use a heat diffuser with the clay pot.

1 can (7.5 ounces) California tree-ripened olives, rinsed and drained

3 tablespoons dry white wine

1 garlic clove

1½ tablespoons extra virgin olive oil

2 teaspoons red wine vinegar

1 tablespoon chopped fresh flat-leaf parsley leaves

1 teaspoon dried Mediterranean oregano

¼ teaspoon crushed hot red pepper

1 Place the olives in the sandpot with the wine and garlic. Cover with a crumpled sheet of parchment and the lid and set over low heat. Cook for 45 minutes, shaking the pot from time to time to be sure the olives do not stick.

2 Use a slotted spoon to transfer the olives to a dish. Prick each with the tines of a fork. Remove and crush the cooked garlic clove; set aside. Boil down any juices in the pot to a glaze; add the olive oil, vinegar, parsley, oregano, and hot pepper. Return the crushed garlic to the pot and heat, stirring, for an instant. Pour the seasoned oil over the olives and let stand for 2 to 3 days in a cool place before serving. Roll them in paper towels before serving to remove excess oil.

Fonduta Valdostana

SERVES 4

*Y*ou don't need a traditional glazed fondue pot for this extraordinary northern Italian melted cheese confection enriched with egg yolks and laced with aromatic white truffle oil. A ceramic bowl set over simmering water is my clay pot version of a double boiler; it will produce just the amount of low heat to melt the cheese. (Cheese that melts too quickly can turn stringy and seize up.) I am indebted to Matt Kramer's wonderful cookbook *A Passion for Piedmont: Italy's Most Glorious Regional Table* for this useful kitchen secret: To avoid any chance of a rubbery consistency, soak the cheese in milk overnight.

Your first choice for cheese should be an Italian Alps fontina from Valle d'Aosta. Less expensive look-alikes are usually too bland. If you cannot find a good fontina, use a finely shredded French Beaufort or Comté cheese.

This *fonduta* is not served from a central pot, which would have to be kept warm on the table, but in individual porcelain, earthenware, or stoneware ramekins that have been preheated.

PREFERRED CLAY POTS:

A ceramic fondue pot or a French *poêlon* or saucepan. As a substitute, set a heatproof ceramic bowl over a pan of simmering water.

Four 8-ounce porcelain, stoneware, or earthenware ramekins

If using an electric or ceramic stovetop, be sure to use a heat diffuser with the clay pot.

---

5 ounces Italian fontina or French Beaufort or Comté cheese, finely shredded

¾ cup milk

2 tablespoons unsalted butter

2 egg yolks

4 drops white truffle oil, or more to taste

Salt and freshly ground black pepper

12 thin slices rye bread fried in butter, thin squares of grilled polenta or chunks of toasted Italian bread

1 In a bowl or container with a lid, combine the cheese and milk. Cover and refrigerate overnight.

2 The next day, place a ceramic fondue pot or a ceramic bowl over a pot of water—it should not be touching—and slowly bring the water to a boil. When the water is boiling, but the ceramic bowl is still cool to the touch, add the milk-soaked cheese and stir until melted and smooth.

3 Add the butter and whisk in the egg yolks. Cook, stirring constantly, until the fonduta is creamy and thickened, about 5 minutes. Do not let boil, or the egg yolks will curdle.

4 Stir the truffle oil into the warm fonduta. Season with a pinch each of salt and pepper. Divide among 4 warmed ramekins and serve at once with the bread or polenta for dipping.

NOTE TO THE COOK: If fresh white truffles are in season and you are lucky enough to possess one, a scant teaspoon of shavings can be used in place of the truffle oil. The effect will be sublime.

Turkish Lamb Tartare

MAKES 16 KOFTE BALLS, SERVING 8

Since this book is about Mediterranean clay pot cooking, I'd be remiss if I didn't share the method by which some home cooks in the ancient city of Antioch, known in modern times as Antakya, in southern Turkey produce a very light bulgur and raw lamb dish called *çi köfte*. Savory and earthy, it is markedly similar both to beef tartare and to Lebanese raw lamb kibbeh.

While lamb for meatball kebabs is hand chopped (see page 146), *çi köfte* is prepared by first pounding the meat to a pulp using a heavy mortar and pestle. For today's cooks, a food processor substitutes well here. Next the cook places a mixture of onions, spices, and pastes in an unglazed flat clay saucer or basin and kneads them until smooth. While the kneading continues, dry fine bulgur is added, little by little, until it blends in smoothly. Again, the food processor can be used for this step.

Finally, and this must be done by hand, the pureed lamb is added to the bulgur, and a long kneading begins during which the mixture turns light to the touch as the porous clay wicks off excess moisture. Just as it begins to stick to the clay, it's ready to be shaped into ovals and served immediately, preferably with glasses of *raki*, the anise-flavored brandy of Turkey, diluted with ice and cold water.

> **PREFERRED CLAY POT:**
>
> A large unglazed terra-cotta saucer or *comal,* or a Chilean Pomaireware wok

8 ounces very fresh boneless lamb leg, tenderloin, or rib, trimmed of all fat (see Note)

1 medium onion, peeled and quartered

1½ teaspoons Turkish sweet red pepper paste

1 tablespoon tomato paste

½ teaspoon Urfa crushed red pepper (optional but traditional)

1/8 teaspoon Turkish or Aleppo pepper

1/8 teaspoon ground allspice

1/8 teaspoon ground cinnamon

1/8 teaspoon ground cumin

1 cup fine bulgur

1 teaspoon sea salt

2 tablespoons chopped fresh flat-leaf parsley

5 scallions, white part and 1 inch of green, finely chopped

16 lettuce leaves

1 Scrub the saucer with a thin paste of baking soda mixed with warm water; rinse and let air dry. (The clay vessel can be prepared up to a day in advance.)

2 Trim the fat, sinews, and any gristle from the lamb. Cut the meat into small pieces and grind to a smooth paste in a food processor. Scrape the meat into a clean bowl, cover loosely with paper towels, and refrigerate until well chilled, at least 30 minutes.

3 Pulse the onion in the food processor—no need to rinse the bowl—until finely chopped. Add the Turkish red pepper paste, tomato paste, Urfa pepper, Aleppo pepper, allspice, cinnamon, and cumin. Pulse until evenly blended. Add ¼ cup of the bulgur and pulse to combine. Repeat 3 more times with equal amounts of bulgur, pulsing long enough to ensure that the grain is absorbing the onion-spice paste.

4 Scrape the contents of the food processor onto the clean, dry clay saucer. Knead the mixture with your fingers and palms and try to develop a feel for the mixture: it should be firm and moist, and the bulgur should not be too gritty. Add the chilled ground lamb and the salt and knead for 15 to 20 minutes, dipping your hands into cold water from time to time to keep the mixture moist to the touch. The tartare is ready when the meat is completely blended in, the bulgur is soft, and the mixture begins to stick to the clay.

5 Quickly work in the chopped parsley and scallions and season the tartare with salt and pepper to taste. With wet palms, form about 1½ tablespoons of the mixture into sausage shapes, flatten into small ovals, and serve immediately, to be wrapped in lettuce leaves.

NOTES TO THE COOK:

❋ Uncooked meat of any kind requires care. Inform your butcher you intend to eat the lamb raw. Pregnant women and people with compromised immune systems should avoid raw meat.

❋ Chef Musa Dağdeviren deals with possible bacterial growth caused by meat stuck in the pores of the clay dish. He does what his mother used to do: He scrubs the clay vessel with baking soda and water.

Orange-Glazed Pork Belly

SERVES 6

*H*ere's my very loose interpretation of a recipe created by two-star Michelin chef Joan Roca of El Celler de Can Roca in the Catalonian town of Girona. Of course, it's nearly impossible to duplicate his stunning food. To give one example: Roca obtains his pork bellies from local three-month-old pigs. For another, being an expert on *sous vide* cooking (his book *La Cocina al Vacio* is a seminal work), Joan prepares his pork bellies in a vacuum.

My approach is totally different for the home cook, yet, I think, yields excellent results. First I brine the pork belly; then I braise it in sweet muscatel wine along with lots of onions. After cooking, it is weighted overnight. The next day, I slice it and slowly glaze the slices in a cazuela along with apple slices plus a reduction made from caramelized sugar, sweet muscatel vinegar, and orange juice. Just before serving, the meat is reheated and served in the cazuela. I serve it as a first course with a lightly dressed green salad on the side. The result: updated home-style Catalan cooking at its best!

PREFERRED CLAY POTS:

A 10- or 11-inch Spanish cazuela or straight-sided flameware skillet

If using an electric or ceramic stovetop, be sure to use a heat diffuser with the clay pot.

---

3 pounds fresh skin-on pork belly, preferably organic

⅓ cup coarse kosher salt

2 tablespoons plus 2 teaspoons sugar

3 cloves

¼ teaspoon black peppercorns

1 bay leaf

2 medium onions, halved and thinly sliced

3 garlic cloves, thinly sliced

¾ cup sweet white wine, such as muscatel

2 tablespoons ultra-sweet muscatel vinegar

1½ cups fresh sweet orange juice, preferably Valencia

1 tablespoon extra virgin olive oil

3 Granny Smith apples, peeled, cored, and cut into wedges

1 Between 5 and 7 days before you plan to serve the meat, brine the pork belly: Rinse the pork in several changes of cold water; drain and pat dry. Mix together the salt, 1 tablespoon plus 2 teaspoons of the sugar, the cloves, and the peppercorns. Rub the seasonings all over the meat. Place in a deep container, add the bay leaf and enough cold water to cover (about 7 cups), and press to submerge. Refrigerate for 3 days, turning the pork belly at least once a day.

2   Drain the pork belly; rinse, drain, and pat dry. Pick off any whole spices and discard. Put the pork belly, onions, garlic, and wine in a large conventional roasting pan. Cover with a sheet of parchment paper or foil and place in a cold oven. Set the temperature at 250°F and braise for 5 hours.

3   Raise the heat to 350°F, remove the paper or foil, and roast for 30 minutes. Turn the pork belly over and continue to roast for 15 minutes longer, or until the meat is fork tender.

4   Remove the roasting pan from the oven; tilt slightly and pour the flavorful fat into a container; reserve for stews, soups, or confit if you like. Let the pork cool completely. When cooled and set, divide the pork belly into 6 equal portions. Wrap each separately in plastic wrap, pack into a storage container, gently weight with a plate, and refrigerate for at least 3 hours and up to 2 days.

5   About 1 hour before serving, remove the pork belly from the refrigerator and let stand at room temperature. Meanwhile, make the orange glaze: In a medium nonreactive saucepan, heat the remaining 1 tablespoon sugar over low heat until it melts, about 3 minutes. Continue to cook, swirling the pan without stirring, until the sugar slowly turns to a light brown caramel. Immediately remove from the heat, add the vinegar, and stir in the bits of hard browned sugar until dissolved. Add the orange juice, return to medium heat, and bring to a boil. Continue to boil until the sauce is reduced to about ½ cup, 5 to 7 minutes. Set the orange sauce aside.

6   Preheat the oven to 250°F. Unwrap the pieces of pork belly and pat them dry. Set a lightly oiled cazuela over medium-low heat and warm slowly, gradually raising the heat to medium-high. When the pan is warm to the touch, add the slices of pork belly, skin side down. Fry slowly until the skin turns golden brown and sizzles. Turn and continue to cook until browned on all sides, 3 to 5 minutes in all. Transfer the pork to a side dish. Set the hot cazuela aside on a wooden surface or folded kitchen towel to prevent cracking.

7   Add the apple wedges to the reserved orange sauce along with 3 tablespoons water. Bring to a boil, reduce the heat to medium, and poach until slightly softened, 2 to 3 minutes. Using a slotted spoon, transfer the apples to the cazuela (watch out for splatter) and slowly fry the apples, turning, until they are caramelized, about 3 minutes.

8   Meanwhile, boil the orange sauce until reduced to about ⅓ cup. Set the browned pork belly, skin-side up, on top of the apples and drizzle the orange sauce over all. Serve directly from the cazuela.

Greek Shrimp with Tomatoes and Feta Cheese

SERVES 4

This taverna specialty of the Athenian port of Piraeus is called *yiouvetsi*, the word for the deep, round clay vessels used throughout Greece to cook meat, game, fish, and poultry in wood-fired ovens. *Yiouvetsi* come in all sizes. For this dish you may substitute a two-quart earthenware saucepan, casserole, or cazuela. The thick tomato sauce studded with cubes of feta slows things down, producing in the end wonderfully sweet and tender shrimp.

> **PREFERRED CLAY POT:**
>
> A 2- quart glazed earthenware saucepan or casserole or a 10-inch Spanish cazuela
>
> If using an electric or ceramic stovetop, be sure to use a heat diffuser with the clay pot.
>
> **SUGGESTED CLAY ENVIRONMENT:**
>
> Double slabs of pizza stones or food-safe quarry tiles set on the upper and lower oven racks

⅓ cup extra virgin olive oil

1 large leek, white and pale green parts, finely chopped

2 garlic cloves, finely chopped

2 teaspoons tomato paste, preferably homemade (page 317)

4 large red ripe tomatoes, peeled, seeded, and chopped, or 1 can (14 ounces) diced tomatoes

⅓ cup dry white wine

¼ cup chopped fresh flat-leaf parsley

1 teaspoon dried Greek or Mediterranean oregano

Pinch of sugar

Pinch of crushed hot red pepper

Salt and freshly ground black pepper

1 pound extra- large shrimp in their shells (16 to 20)

2 tablespoons ouzo or Pernod

6 to 8 ounces sheep's milk feta cheese, crumbled

1 If possible, use one of the suggested clay environments in your oven. Preheat the oven to 350°F.

2 Heat half the olive oil with the leek and garlic in the saucepan, warming it slowly until hot. Cook over medium-low heat until soft and golden, about 5 minutes. Add the tomato paste and cook, stirring, until it turns shiny and smooth, about 2 minutes. Add the fresh tomatoes, wine, parsley, oregano, sugar, and hot pepper. Season the sauce with salt and pepper to taste. Simmer, stirring often, until thick, 15 to 20 minutes.

3 Heat the remaining olive oil in a large conventional skillet over high heat. Add the shrimp and sauté for 1 to 2 minutes, until they curl loosely. Remove from the heat, add the ouzo (or Pernod), and ignite carefully, averting your face. Scrape the contents of the skillet into the hot tomato sauce. Scatter the feta on top and place in the oven.

4 Bake until the cheese melts, about 25 minutes. Transfer to a wood surface or folded towels to prevent cracking; let cool for 5 to 10 minutes before serving right from the pot.

Sizzling Shrimp with Garlic and Hot Pepper

SERVES 4 TO 6

For many years I served another version of this dish, using giant prawns in their shells. Back in the late 1950s, I prepared them along with several other Spanish dishes for a party held in a Fifth Avenue apartment belonging to a pair of wealthy twins. Among the illustrious guests that night were the poet Allen Ginsberg and the beat generation novelist Jack Kerouac. Everyone liked my food, especially the garlicky prawn dish. In fact, Kerouac was so impressed that he eyed me carefully and then announced, "You've got great legs." I was such an obsessive foodie at the time that I wasn't sure if he was describing my legs or the long thin ones on the prawns!

I learned this two-minute tapas bar version of the same dish from my friend cookbook author Janet Mendel, who has lived in the Andalusian town of Mijas for thirty years. Janet insists on using smaller peeled shrimp, not prawns, and she portions out ten per person as a first course.

There are two ways to prepare this dish of *gambas al ajillo* ("shrimp with garlic"): Janet serves hers tapas bar style in individual five-inch cazuelitas, which sizzle as they are placed before each diner. My less dramatic but easier method involves cooking all the shrimp in one large cazuela. Janet says this is a "dish that is all about dunking," so be sure to pass plenty of good crusty bread to wipe up the garlicky sauce.

PREFERRED CLAY POT:

An 11-or 12-inch Spanish cazuela or straight-sided flameware skillet

If using an electric or ceramic stovetop, be sure to use a heat diffuser with the clay pot.

1 pound peeled small (about 60) or medium-large, deveined (24 to 30) shrimp

1 scant cup extra virgin olive oil, preferably Spanish

1 tablespoon finely chopped garlic

1 teaspoon mildly hot dried red pepper such as Aleppo or Marash

½ teaspoon sea salt

¼ teaspoon sweet pimentón de la Vera (smoked Spanish paprika)

4 to 6 slices chewy country bread

1 Rinse the shrimp and wipe dry with paper towels. Leave them at room temperature for 10 to 15 minutes so they are not ice cold when they hit the pan.

2 Combine the olive oil, garlic, and hot pepper in the cazuela. Set it over medium-low heat and warm the pan slowly, gradually raising the heat to medium or medium-high until the oil is hot. Continue to cook until the garlic sizzles and just turns golden, 2 to 3 minutes.

3 Immediately add all the shrimp and cook until they are firm and curled, 2 to 4 minutes, depending on their size.

4 Sprinkle with 2 tablespoons hot water and pinches of sea salt and pimentón. Serve at once right from the pot with the bread for soaking up the delicious oily sauce.

NOTE TO THE COOK: If you want to serve the shrimp in individual pots but are not up to juggling numerous cazuelitas on top of the stove, Janet Mendel suggests using a large metal skillet over high heat for cooking all the shrimp and then dividing them among individual warmed cazuelitas.

Stovetop Clay Pot Clams Charentaise

SERVES 4

This recipe is based on the traditional Charentaise method for baking potatoes or chestnuts in an unglazed potbellied earthenware vessel with a lid called a *diable* (page xiv). When cooking wet ingredients such as clams, Charentaise cooks line their unglazed casseroles with leaves (grape, sorrel, or chard) to protect the pot from absorbing shellfish odors and moisture.

I've found that a Chinese sandpot makes a great substitute, closely mimicking the *diable* cooking style. Because the pot has a thin interior glaze, no protection is necessary, but still, for extra fragrance, I line the sandpot with slices of fennel as well as sorrel leaves. I picked up this *truc* years ago from a home cook on the Ile de Ré in France. The sorrel not only adds flavor but also has a tenderizing effect on clams. In the Charentes, around La Rochelle, cooks use a variety of clams called *amandes de mer* ("almonds of the sea"), which have a slightly nutty flavor. I've had great success using American littlenecks. Serve this fine starter with the broth enriched with a little melted butter.

> **PREFERRED CLAY POT:**
>
> A 3-quart Chinese sandpot, a French *diable* (potato "devil"), or another stovetop earthenware or flameware saucepan with a tight-fitting lid
>
> If using an electric or ceramic stovetop, be sure to use a heat diffuser with the sandpot. Avoid using a French *diable* on an electric or ceramic stovetop.

2 pounds littleneck clams

1 fennel bulb

30 large sorrel leaves, stemmed

5 tablespoons unsalted butter, at room temperature

1 Rinse and pick over the clams; discard any that are already open.

2 Remove the fennel fronds and reserve a few for garnish. Trim off the top and bottom of the fennel bulb. Use a sharp knife or a mandoline to slice the fennel very thin. Line the bottom and sides of the pot with half the sorrel leaves and top with the slices of fennel. Coarsely chop the remaining sorrel leaves and spread half on top of the fennel. Pack in the clams, cover with the remaining sorrel, and top with the remaining slices of fennel.

3 Place a sheet of parchment directly on top of the pot, cover tightly, and set over low heat. Slowly raise the heat as the pot warms up. Cook for 20 to 25 minutes, or until the clams have opened, gently shaking the pot every 5 minutes.

4 Immediately transfer from the heat to a wooden surface or folded kitchen towel to prevent cracking and use a slotted spoon to transfer the clams and fennel to individual soup plates. Add the butter to the broth in the pot and stir until melted. Pour the broth over the clams, garnish each serving with a bit of fennel frond, and serve at once.

Mussel Tagine with Tomatoes and Moroccan Seasonings

SERVES 4

In my updated version of this classic recipe, I deviate from the traditional Moroccan approach to mussels, which is to overcook them, causing the shellfish to toughen, and then to cook them even further, which softens the shellfish and allows them to absorb flavorings. Instead, I slowly reduce grated frothy tomatoes with herbs and spices to the consistency of a thick jam and then add broth from some quickly steamed mussels. Once the sauce is ready and the tagine is still very hot, the shelled mussels plus a few mussels still in their shells are added and cooked just a little longer.

This dish is best made in summer, when tomatoes are at their peak and mussels are still small and briny.

PREFERRED CLAY POT:

A 10-or 11-inch glazed tagine or Spanish cazuela or straight-sided flameware skillet

If using an electric or ceramic stovetop, be sure to use a heat diffuser with the clay pot.

---

3 quarts fresh cultivated mussels (4 pounds), preferably large

1½ pounds red ripe tomatoes

¼ cup extra virgin olive oil

1 tablespoon finely chopped garlic

½ cup finely chopped fresh flat-leaf parsley

½ cup finely chopped fresh cilantro

2 teaspoons freshly ground cumin

1 teaspoon sweet paprika

¼ teaspoon crushed hot red pepper

Juice of 1 large lemon

Sea salt

1 Pick over the mussels and discard any that are cracked. Rinse the mussels under cold running water and drain. Scrub the mussels, pulling off any hairy beards that protrude from the shells. Place the mussels in a bowl and refrigerate until ready to steam.

2 Cut the tomatoes in half crosswise and gently squeeze out the seeds. Grate each tomato half by rubbing the cut sides against the coarsest side of a four-sided grater or on a flat shredder. You should be left with just the tomato skin in your hand; discard the skin.

3 Place the olive oil and tomato pulp in the tagine set over medium-low heat and cook slowly, stirring occasionally, until reduced to a thick sauce, 10 to 15 minutes. Add the garlic, parsley, cilantro, cumin, paprika, and hot pepper to the tomatoes. Cook, stirring, until the sauce is thick, about 5 minutes longer.

4 Meanwhile, steam the mussels in a covered conventional saucepan over medium-high heat until they just open, 3 to 4 minutes. Drain the mussels, reserving the broth. Strain the broth through a double layer of cheesecloth to remove any sand. Remove all but 6 of the mussels from their shells; discard the shells.

5 Add the strained hot mussel broth to the tomato sauce in the clay pot. Season with the lemon juice and a pinch of sea salt if it needs it. Bring to a boil, reduce the heat to medium, and boil, stirring often, until the sauce is reduced and thick again, about 10 minutes.

(continued)

6 Add the shelled and unshelled mussels to the sauce, cover loosely, bring to a boil, correct the seasoning, transfer the tagine to a wooden surface or folded kitchen towels to prevent cracking, and let stand for 5 minutes before serving from the pot.

NOTE TO THE COOK: Sometimes individual mussels will need an extra minute or two of steaming, but be sure to discard any that do not open within 5 minutes.

SALTED ANCHOVIES

Flat anchovy fillets packed in oil are a fine ingredient, but salted whole anchovies are definitely superior, and when soaked for 15 minutes are actually less salty than the oil-packed variety. With their meatier texture and briny flavor, they add great depth to *anchoïade* (page 26), spreads, pasta sauces, *pissaladière* (page 255), and stews.

I recommend Agostino Recca Salted Anchovies (see Sources). These come packed in salt in a 2-ounce tin or in a 2-pound 2-ounce can. Yes, the latter is way more than you'll need to execute even ten recipes, but salted anchovies keep for a long time when stored properly in a cool, dark cupboard in your kitchen. Once you open the can and remove what you need, transfer the rest, along with the salt from the can, to a glass jar with a tight-fitting cover; do not use a plastic container. I always add a little extra salt at the bottom and some more to top it off.

When you want to use some of the anchovies, extract them with a wooden or stainless-steel implement, soak them in milky water for 15 minutes, and then simply rub off the bones.

Creamy Bagna Cauda

SERVES 8

I never grow tired of the combination of salted anchovies, garlic, and olive oil that forms the base of an authentic *bagna cauda*. It's a spectacular blend. Historically, a *bagna cauda* was a poor person's dip, a way of embellishing and adding strong flavor to garden vegetables, especially peppers, celery, cauliflower, radicchio, turnips, baby lettuce, fennel, cardoons, and even breadsticks.

In this delicious variation, I suggest that you make the sauce the day before to allow the garlic and anchovies to mellow with the cream. My friend, Kittina Powers, who shared this recipe, tells me that leftovers make a great addition to scrambled eggs.

PREFERRED CLAY POT:

A glazed earthenware *caquelon*, fondue pot, or flameware saucepan

If using an electric or ceramic stovetop, be sure to use a heat diffuser with the clay pot.

5 salt-packed anchovies

¼ cup milk

2 tablespoons unsalted butter

1 teaspoon extra virgin olive oil

2 tablespoons chopped garlic

1½ cups heavy cream, heated until lukewarm

Assorted raw vegetables and slices of crusty bread for dipping

1 Using your thumbnail or a small knife, slit each anchovy down the belly and remove the spine and head, rinsing well under cold running water. In a small bowl, combine the milk with 1 cup cold water. Add the anchovy fillets and soak for 10 minutes.

2 Meanwhile, set an earthenware caquelon over low heat. Add the butter and oil and warm slowly, gradually raising the heat to medium-low. When the butter and oil are hot, add the garlic. Cook until soft but not brown, 2 to 4 minutes.

3 Remove the anchovies from their soaking liquid and add them to the pan one by one. Cook, stirring, until they dissolve, about 2 minutes. Pour in the cream and cook until thick and quite warm. Remove the bagna cauda from the heat and let stand for at least 10 minutes to allow the garlic and anchovies to mellow with the cream.

4 To serve, reheat the bagna cauda on the stovetop until quite warm; then place over a Sterno flame, electric hot plate, or candles. Serve with spears of vegetables and be sure to have plenty of bread on hand to catch the unctuous drippings.

Anchoïade with Creamer Potatoes, Fennel, and Celery

SERVES 4

A lot of people assume that *anchoïade,* the famous anchovy sauce of Provence, is created in a mortar. In fact, authentically it's made in a deep earthenware skillet set over very low fire. The cook crushes the anchovies with a wooden spoon or paddle, breaking them down so they melt in the olive oil to become a warm, creamy sauce. After the *anchoïade* has had time to cool and mellow, it is presented at table in the cooking skillet or transferred to a small warmed earthenware bowl. At this point it's perfect for dipping baby baked potatoes and raw vegetables, such as the fresh fennel suggested here.

PREFERRED CLAY POTS:

An 8-inch Spanish cazuela or other glazed earthenware or flameware saucepan

A 2-quart Chinese sandpot

If using an electric or ceramic stovetop, be sure to use a heat diffuser with the clay pots.

6 salted anchovies or 12 flat oil-packed anchovy fillets, drained

¼ cup milk

1 teaspoon crushed raw or roasted garlic

1 tablespoon white wine vinegar

½ cup extra virgin olive oil

Salt and freshly ground black pepper

8 to 12 creamer potatoes, preferably organic, scrubbed but not peeled

1 small fennel bulb, trimmed and thinly sliced

8 leafy tender celery ribs

24 cherry tomatoes

1 If using the salted anchovies, clean and fillet them as described in step 1 of the preceding recipe. In a small bowl, combine the milk with 1 cup cold water. Add the anchovy fillets (salted or oil-packed) and soak them for 10 minutes. Drain and pat dry.

2 Warm the cazuela over low heat. Add the anchovies to the dry pot and crush with a wooden spoon or pestle and cook until they are smooth and creamy. Gradually blend in the crushed garlic, vinegar, and olive oil to make an emulsified sauce. Remove from the heat and let stand at room temperature for at least 1 hour. Season the anchoïade with salt and pepper to taste.

3 Meanwhile, place the potatoes in the sandpot and cover with a round of parchment paper and a tight-fitting lid. Set over low heat, gradually raise the heat to medium, and cook, shaking the pot from time to time, for 45 to 60 minutes, or until the potatoes are tender and creamy with bits of crust developed on the skin.

4 When the potatoes are ready, line a serving platter with the sliced fennel. Arrange the potatoes and 7 of the celery ribs on top. Garnish with the tomatoes. Pass the anchovy sauce to be drizzled over the vegetables. Place the last celery rib in the cazuela and use to stir the sauce from time to time.

Variation:

If you have a clay garlic baker, you can bake a small head of garlic ahead of time, puree it, and blend it with the softened anchovies when making the sauce.

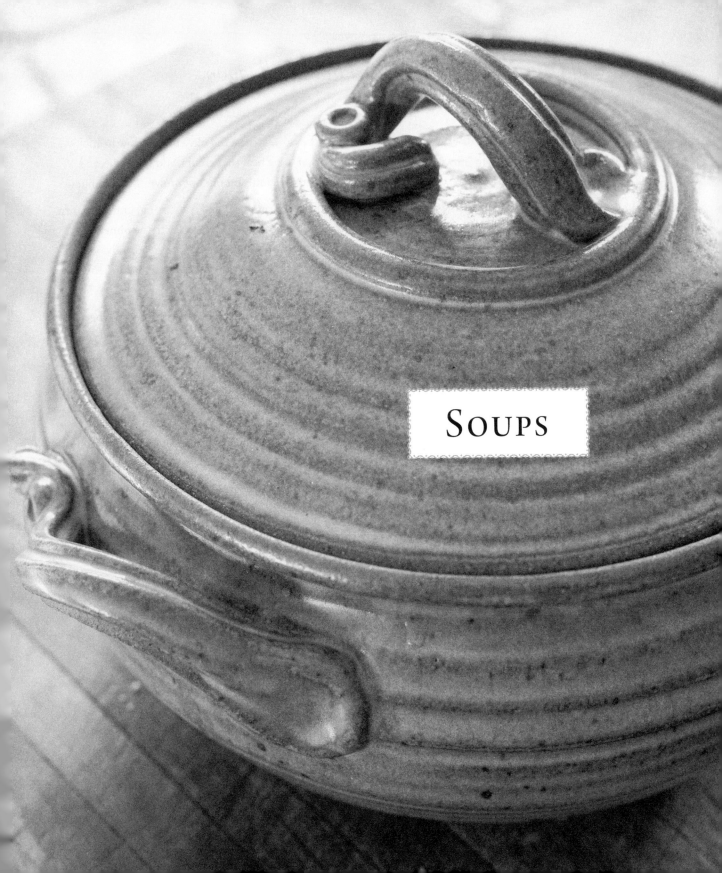

Soups

Garlic and Egg Soup as Prepared in the Aragon

SERVES 2

The nicest way to serve this famous Spanish soup is to dish out the broth into small individual earthenware bowls, add the eggs, and set them in the oven to poach until the whites are set and the yolks still runny.

> **PREFERRED CLAY POTS:**
>
> A 10- or 11-inch Spanish cazuela or straight-sided flameware skillet
>
> 2 small ovenproof ceramic soup bowls
>
> If using an electric or ceramic stovetop, be sure to use a heat diffuser with the clay pots.

3 tablespoons extra virgin olive oil

2 large garlic cloves, peeled and thinly sliced

2 slices dried bread, cubed

1 teaspoon pimentón de la Vera (smoked Spanish paprika) or sweet paprika

Salt and freshly ground black pepper

4 eggs

2 tablespoons chopped fresh flat-leaf parsley

1 In the cazuela, heat the olive oil over low heat. Slowly raise the heat to medium, add the garlic, and cook, stirring, until soft but not brown, 2 to 3 minutes.

2 Add the bread cubes and fry, stirring, until they turn golden, about 5 minutes. Season with the pimentón. Add enough hot water to cover the bread and cook slowly for 30 minutes, or until the soup is thickened. Season with salt and pepper to taste.

3 Preheat the oven to 300°F. Divide the soup between 2 individual earthenware soup bowls. Break 2 eggs into each. Tilt the bowls and spoon some of the hot liquid over the eggs.

4 Bake in the oven for about 5 minutes, until the egg whites are set but the yolks are still runny. Sprinkle with the parsley and a light dusting of salt and pepper and serve at once.

Pumpkin Soup with Creamy Roquefort

MAKES ABOUT 2 QUARTS, SERVING 4 TO 6

Roquefort, rather heady in its natural state, but mild and mellow when cooked, gives this easy-to-make soup a characteristic Southwest French flavor.

This soup can be made up to two days in advance and reheated.

> **PREFERRED CLAY POT:**
>
> A 3-quart glazed or unglazed earthenware or flameware casserole
>
> If using an electric or ceramic stovetop, be sure to use a heat diffuser with the clay pot.

2½ pounds pumpkin or butternut squash

1 tablespoon sugar

2 ounces sliced prosciutto or lean pancetta, shredded

¼ cup minced shallot

Salt and freshly ground black pepper

¼ teaspoon freshly grated nutmeg

½ cup crème fraîche or heavy cream

3 tablespoons unsalted butter

2½ ounces Roquefort cheese, crumbled

1 cup diced, crustless dense country bread, toasted in a dry skillet until golden

1 Pare the pumpkin, cut it into large chunks, and discard the seeds and fibrous centers. Cut enough of the flesh into 1-inch dice to make 5 cups or 1½ pounds cleaned pumpkin or squash. Place the pumpkin cubes and sugar in the earthenware casserole and warm over low heat. Gradually raise the heat to medium-low, cover with a sheet of parchment paper and the lid, and steam for 10 minutes.

2 Add the prosciutto and shallot and cook, covered, for 10 minutes longer, stirring occasionally. Season with salt, pepper, and nutmeg.

3 Add 3 cups hot water to the casserole, bring to a boil and cook at a simmer until everything is tender, 20 minutes. Transfer the soup in batches to a blender, and puree until smooth.

4 Add the cream, the butter, and the cheese to the last batch of soup in the blender, and puree until velvety.

5 Reheat the soup, and season with additional salt and pepper to taste. Ladle the soup into warm bowls, and top each portion with the toasted croutons.

NOTE TO THE COOK: When reheating this soup, if you notice it thickening, thin it with up to ½ cup of hot water and readjust the seasoning.

Soupe au Pistou

SERVES 6 TO 8

A well-made *soupe au pistou* makes a great summer dish. Deeply flavorful and nutritious, it may be served warm or cold. While it usually feels light on the palate and is easy to digest, I've tasted versions that are so thick a spoon will stand up in the bowl. The common element, of course, is the *pistou,* a sauce made of basil pounded with garlic, olive oil, and cheese, which is added to a vegetable and bean soup just before serving. When the cold raw sauce hits the hot soup, culinary alchemy takes place, and the flavors of each are amplified.

Along with bouillabaisse and cassoulet, *soupe au pistou* is one of the dishes over which French people love to quarrel: "My grandmother's version is the very best," they'll exclaim, and then in an undertone: "Of course, you understand. . . I can never reveal her secret." Of course not! That would be like giving away the family farm. Yet occasionally someone will lean into your ear and, in a passionate whisper, reveal one of these secrets: "Grand-mère always starts hers off with a pig's foot." "Mama adds a bit of Roquefort." "My great grandmother taught me to add some Edam with a little Parmigiano-Reggiano mixed in."

As you can see, the choice of cheese is one point at which a Provençal cook will put her signature on the dish. Most commentators recommend Parmigiano, sometimes mixed with a bit of Gruyère. My favorite cheese for this soup is waxy Mimolette, which will elevate the taste by adding a stunning butterscotch aroma and pleasing yellow-orange color. A well-aged Dutch Edam will also do nicely.

Another personal decision concerns the soup itself. Traditionally, it's made with fresh, creamy white beans; I substitute *coco* beans or Great Northern, since fresh white beans are hard to find. Also included are green beans, potatoes, and, at its base, a broth made from pork skin, according to the great Provençal food authority Guy Gedda; lamb shanks, in the opinion of the important French vintner and food writer Lulu Peyraud; or sausages or pork rind, the choice of many home cooks. Other vegetables may also be added. Patricia Wells suggests pumpkin, while Richard Olney recommends carrots. This is where you can improvise, choosing from among whatever good fresh summer vegetables are available.

As to pasta, some cooks replace shapes like elbows or shells with broken vermicelli. Chef Robert Lalleman of the famous Auberge de Noves in Avignon, France, takes a unique approach. He amplifies the richness of the soup by sautéing his pasta in butter first; he also adds lobster for a super luxurious effect.

PREFERRED CLAY POTS:

A large ceramic bean pot

A 5-quart glazed or unglazed earthenware or flameware casserole

If using an electric or ceramic stovetop, be sure to use a heat diffuser with the clay pots.

1 cup dried white beans such as coco or Great Northern, rinsed well, soaked overnight in plenty of cold water, and drained

Pancetta packet: 1-ounce slice pancetta wrapped in cheesecloth with 1 small onion, halved, 2 peeled garlic cloves, and 1 bay leaf

1 cup Pistou (page 32)

1 tablespoon extra virgin olive oil

1 small fennel bulb, trimmed and coarsely chopped

1 medium onion, coarsely chopped

2 garlic cloves, peeled and crushed

2 medium red potatoes (10 ounces), peeled and halved

12 ounces green or romano beans, cut into ½-inch pieces

3 medium tomatoes, peeled, seeded, and cut into ½-inch dice

4 small zucchini (1 pound), cut into ¼-inch dice

1 cup small pasta shells, elbows, or ditalini

1 tablespoon unsalted butter

Salt and freshly ground black pepper

Fresh basil sprigs for garnish

1 Put the drained white beans and the pancetta packet in the bean pot. Add 2 quarts plus 3 cups water, slowly heat to boiling, cover the bean pot, and simmer until the beans are tender, about 1½ hours. Discard the pancetta packet. Set the beans aside in their cooking liquid.

2 While the dried beans are cooking, prepare the Pistou (page 32). Cover and refrigerate.

3 In the casserole, heat the olive oil. Add the fennel, onion, garlic, and potatoes. Cover the pot and cook the vegetables over medium-low heat, stirring occasionally, until the vegetables are softened and lightly glazed, about 15 minutes.

4 Add 2 quarts hot water and gradually bring to a boil. Reduce the heat and simmer for 30 minutes.

5 Add the green beans to the pot and simmer for 20 minutes. Mash the potatoes against the side of the pot using a large fork; the potatoes will thicken the soup. Add the tomatoes, zucchini, and cooked white beans with their cooking liquid. Simmer for 5 to 10 minutes, until the zucchini is just tender. Remove from the heat. At this time, you can let the soup rest all day or refrigerate it overnight, which will improve the flavor significantly.

6 About 20 minutes before serving, reheat the soup to boiling. Meanwhile, in a large conventional skillet, toast the pasta shells in the butter over moderate heat, stirring until they are lightly browned, about 3 minutes. Add to the hot soup and simmer for 1 minute. Cover, remove from the heat, and let stand until the pasta is tender, about 25 minutes. Season with salt and pepper to taste.

7 Put the pistou in a soup tureen. Gradually whisk in some of the soup's liquid. Pour in the remaining soup, stirring until well blended. Add more freshly ground pepper to taste. Serve while still hot or at room temperature, garnished with basil.

NOTE TO THE COOK: This soup tastes best if the vegetable base (Steps 1 through 5) is prepared 8 to 24 hours in advance.

Pistou

MAKES ABOUT 1⅓ CUPS

In the Provençal language, the word *pistou* literally means "pestle"; so, of course, the proper way to make it is by hand. Ideally, use a wooden pestle and a ceramic mortar with a grainy textured interior, which works like an emery board. A Japanese *suribachi*, heavy mixing bowl, or Thai granite mortar is a good substitute for the French *mortier*. As a last resort, a blender or food processor may be used.

  4 or 5 garlic cloves, peeled and crushed

  1 teaspoon coarse sea salt

  4½ cups (2 ounces) fresh basil leaves, slivered

  ¼ cup extra virgin olive oil

  2 Roma or other large plum tomatoes, grated and
     drained to make about ¾ cup

  3 ounces firm, nutty-tasting cheese, such as French
     Mimolette, Dutch Edam, Swiss Appenzeller,
     Gruyère, or Italian Parmigiano-Reggiano, finely
     grated, about 1 cup

1 In a mortar or small earthenware mixing bowl, use a wooden pestle to pound the garlic and salt to a puree. Add the basil leaves by handfuls and grind them along the sides of the mortar or bowl, rather than pounding downward. The idea is to get the leaves to turn creamy and smooth.

2 Begin adding the olive oil, at first drop by drop and then by teaspoons, until it is emulsified. Then work in the grated tomato and finally the cheese.

NOTE TO THE COOK: Once the *pistou* is added, the soup must not be reheated. If it is, it will lose the very vibrancy that makes it so special.

Corsican Minestra

SERVES 6

*Y*ou can think of this delicious mix of beans, pork belly, and vegetables flavored with basil as an early fall version of *soupe au pistou*. On Corsica, it's always cooked in a tall clay pot on top of the stove, and locally the *pistou* is called *pestu*.

PREFERRED CLAY POTS:

A 3- or 4-quart ceramic bean pot

A 5-quart glazed or unglazed earthenware or flameware casserole

If using an electric or ceramic stovetop, be sure to use a heat diffuser with the clay pot.

5 ounces fresh pork belly

¾ cup dried white beans such cannellini, rinsed well, soaked overnight in plenty of cold water, and drained

1 small onion, halved, plus 1 medium onion, coarsely chopped

8 garlic cloves, peeled

1 bay leaf

½ cup plus 2 tablespoons extra virgin olive oil

1½ tablespoons tomato paste, canned or homemade (page 317)

4 medium carrots, sliced ½ inch thick

1 small fennel bulb, trimmed and coarsely chopped

2 medium red potatoes, peeled and halved

8 ounces green beans, cut into 1-inch pieces

2 cups shredded dandelion greens or escarole

1 medium zucchini, cut into ½-inch dice

4 large Swiss chard leaves, shredded

3 fresh thyme sprigs, preferably lemon thyme

1 cup small shaped pasta, such as elbow or ditalini

6 to 8 fresh basil sprigs, stemmed and shredded

Salt and freshly ground black pepper

1 In a medium conventional saucepan of boiling water, blanch the pork belly for 5 minutes. Drain and rinse. As soon as the pork belly is cool enough to handle, cut it into 1-inch chunks.

2 Put the white beans, pork belly, halved onion, 4 of the garlic cloves, and the bay leaf into the bean pot. Add 3 cups water, cover, and slowly bring to a simmer, starting on low and gradually raising the heat. Cook until the beans are tender, about 1½ hours.

3 Meanwhile, in the earthenware casserole, heat 2 tablespoons of the olive oil, beginning on low and gradually raising the temperature to medium. Add the tomato paste and fry until lightly caramelized, 3 to 5 minutes. Add the carrots, fennel, potatoes, green beans, dandelion greens, and chopped onion. Cover the pot, reduce the heat to medium-low, and cook the vegetables, stirring occasionally, until the fennel and onion are softened, about 10 minutes. Add 2 quarts hot water and gradually bring to a boil. Reduce the heat and simmer for 30 minutes.

4 Add the zucchini, chard, and thyme sprigs to the pot and simmer for 20 minutes. Mash the potatoes against the side of the pot using a large fork; the potatoes will thicken the soup.

(continued)

5 When the white beans are tender, add them along with their cooking liquid, the pork belly, and the pasta in the soup. Simmer the soup over medium heat for 10 minutes longer.

6 To make the Corsican pestu, scoop out 3 chunks of the cooked pork belly and place in a blender. Add about three-quarters of the shredded basil, the remaining 4 garlic cloves, the remaining ½ cup olive oil, and ⅓ cup of the soup liquid. Puree until smooth.

7 Put the Corsican pestu in a large soup tureen. Gradually stir in some of the liquid from the soup, then pour in the rest of the soup and stir well. Correct the seasoning with salt and pepper. Ladle the soup into bowls, garnish with the remaining basil, and serve hot or at room temperature.

Roman-Style Dried Fava Bean Soup with Pancetta and Marjoram

SERVES 6

When I lived in Morocco, I was taught this delicious, earthy fava bean soup by the late Mario Ruspoli, an old friend who frequently came down to Tangier from Paris to visit his mother. Mario was a renaissance man: a filmmaker, an expert on beetles and whaling, and a great gastronome. His mother, Princess Marta Ruspoli, was an eccentric who believed so fervently in the myth of Atlantis that she was totally snookered by her grandchildren when they cleverly seeded her garden with Indian head pennies. Finding one, she's alleged to have exclaimed, "See, the red Indians were here! This proves Atlantis existed!"

In this recipe, which is said to be older than the Lost Continent, the meaty taste of dry ham and onion complement the resinous flavor of the favas.

Dried fava beans are one of the oldest food staples of countries bordering the Mediterranean. Buy them peeled online or at your local Middle Eastern store, being sure to choose the larger split variety for this particular soup.

> **PREFERRED CLAY POT:**
> A 3- or a 4-quart glazed or unglazed earthenware casserole
> If using an electric or ceramic stovetop, be sure to use a heat diffuser with the clay pot.

3 cups dried peeled fava beans (12 ounces), rinsed
well, soaked overnight in plenty of cold water,
and drained

Coarse salt

1 slab (10 ounces) meaty pork belly or pancetta

3 ounces prosciutto, thinly sliced

2 tablespoons coarsely chopped fresh marjoram

1 tablespoon coarsely chopped fresh flat-leaf parsley

1 tablespoon extra virgin olive oil

1 medium onion, finely chopped

2 teaspoons homemade tomato paste (page 317)

Freshly ground black pepper

Grilled sliced bread

1   Remove any brown bits of skin from the soaked
beans; rinse them well and drain again.

2   In a large, heavy conventional saucepan, bring 6
cups water to a boil. Add the fava beans and a pinch of
salt; return to a boil. Reduce the heat to medium-low,
cover, and simmer for 2 hours, or until the beans are
tender. Drain the beans, discarding the cooking water.

3   Meanwhile, place the pork belly in another
saucepan, cover with cold water, and bring to a boil.
Simmer for 8 to 10 minutes. Drain into a colander, rinse,
and drain again. Cut the pork belly into 1-inch cubes.

4   Finely chop the prosciutto with the marjoram and
parsley. Set the earthenware casserole over low heat.
Add the prosciutto-herb paste and slowly warm it,
gradually raising the heat to medium or medium-high.
Add the olive oil and onion and continue to cook
slowly, reducing the heat if necessary, until the mixture
turns golden, 7 to 10 minutes. Add the tomato paste
and diced pork belly. Pour 6 cups hot water over the
mixture, add a pinch of salt, and simmer for 1 hour.

5   In a deep bowl, crush about half of the fava beans to
a puree with the back of a wooden spoon. Add to the
pot with the remaining favas and continue to cook over
medium-low heat until the soup is thick and chunky,
about 30 minutes longer. Season with plenty of pepper
and additional salt to taste. Serve hot with slices of
grilled bread.

Ribollita in the Style of Siena

SERVES 8

This famous Tuscan soup is not really a soup in the literal sense; rather, it is a thick panade, or porridge, of bread, vegetables, and beans baked under a sheet of caramelized onions. It makes a wonderful meal in a bowl.

The word *ribollita* means "reboiled" in Italian, which is just what is done in Tuscan homes with a two- or three-day-old minestrone. A good ribollita is thick with greens, such as Italian black kale (also called Tuscan kale, dinosaur kale, or lacinato kale) and spinach, mashed and whole beans, and a mix of vegetables cooked and recooked so many times that they've turned meltingly soft. The topping of thinly sliced, cooked-till-crusty caramelized onions gives this dish a lovely appearance, especially when prepared, as is proper, in a wide-mouth earthenware casserole.

A good *ribollita* is truly divine. I like it so much I skip its earlier minestrone incarnations. Rather, I make the base soup, let it sit for three days, and then go for the masterpiece! In addition, if you don't eat it all up, which wouldn't be surprising since the dish is so rich, reheat it again, and it will only get richer and thicker. It's also good served lukewarm.

> **PREFERRED CLAY POTS:**
>
> A 4- to 5-quart glazed or unglazed earthenware or flameware casserole
>
> A deep 12-inch-wide ovenproof ceramic casserole or Spanish *cazuela*
>
> If using an electric or ceramic stovetop, be sure to use a heat diffuser with the clay pots.

1½ pounds mixed greens with a predominance of Tuscan kale mixed with young Swiss chard and baby spinach (see Note)

⅔ cup extra virgin olive oil

2 medium yellow onions, chopped

⅓ cup diced celery plus a few tender celery leaves

1 cup diced carrot

3 cups cooked cannellini beans (1 cup dried)

2 teaspoons minced garlic

½ cup chopped fresh flat-leaf parsley

½ teaspoon dried thyme or Mediterranean oregano

1 bay leaf

½ cup tomato sauce or puree

1 small chunk Parmigiano-Reggiano or pecorino rind (optional)

12 slices stale country bread, torn into pieces

Salt and freshly ground black pepper

Splash of red wine vinegar

3 medium red onions, thinly sliced

1 Begin the soup 2 days in advance. Rinse the kale and other greens and strip away the hard stems. Sprinkle the leaves generously with salt and drain in a colander in the sink for 30 minutes. Rinse and squeeze dry; then coarsely chop them.

2 Meanwhile, heat half the olive oil in the 5-quart casserole over medium heat. If using earthenware, be sure to start on low and raise the heat gradually. Add the chopped yellow onions, celery, and carrot and cook until the vegetables are soft and just turning golden, about 20 minutes. Add the greens to the pot, stirring to coat them with oil.

3 Crush half the cannellini beans to a puree. Add all the beans, the garlic, parsley, thyme, bay leaf, tomato sauce, and cheese rind to the mixture and cook, stirring, for a few minutes. Pour in 3 quarts warm water and slowly bring to a boil. Cover, reduce the heat, and simmer for 30 minutes to blend the flavors. Remove from the heat, uncover, and let cool.

4 Stir the bread into the cool soup and return the pot to low heat. Raise the heat to medium-low and cook, stirring, until the bread crumbles and the soup turns creamy with small bread chunks here and there. Add water if necessary to keep the mixture smooth but always so thick a spoon can stand up in it. Let cool, cover, and refrigerate for 2 days.

5 About 3 hours before serving, remove the soup from the refrigerator. Correct the seasoning with salt, plenty of black pepper, and a splash of vinegar. Remove the cheese rind (see Note). Preheat the oven to 350°F.

6 Lightly oil the 12-inch-wide casserole and turn the ribollita into it. Top with slightly overlapping slices of red onion. Drizzle the remaining 1/3 cup olive oil over the top and bake for 2 hours. Turn off the heat and leave the dish in the oven until it cools down to warm, 35 minutes. Serve with a pepper mill and a cruet of your best Tuscan extra virgin olive oil.

NOTES TO THE COOK:

❋ I save Parmigiano-Reggiano and Romano cheese rinds in the freezer in a plastic bag, so a piece or two can be added whenever I make this soup, or any bean soup with an Italian accent. Submerged in liquid, the rind will turn soft and add depth of flavor. If you sliver a softened piece and return it to the soup, it will dissolve and impart flavor throughout.

❋ I learned a great method for preparing large volumes of greens in a soup pot from cooks on the Ligurian coast. After washing the greens, tear them up, salt lightly, and leave for 30 minutes. They will exude much of their moisture and will collapse but will retain full flavor and all their vitamins while giving up much of their bitterness. Before cooking, rinse off the salt, shred the greens even finer, and add to the soup pot.

Piedmontese Bean Soup with Spareribs

SERVES 6 TO 8

This rich and earthy Piedmontese bean soup, called *tofeja,* is made in a four-handled terracotta pot of the same name, crafted in the pottery town of Castellamonte near Turin, Italy. The handles are added so that the cook can shake rather than stir the ingredients, which would crush the beans. I substitute a one- or two-handled earthenware casserole. Though not as charming and exotic as a genuine tofeja, it will still produce a wonderful soup.

> **PREFERRED CLAY POT:**
>
> A 4- or 5- quart stovetop casserole such as: Emile Henry Fig Flame-Top Round Casserole; Le Flambadou; Italian Vulcania traditional brown pot; or a bean pot
>
> If using an electric or ceramic stovetop, be sure to use a heat diffuser with the clay pot.

1 cup dried white beans, such as cannellini, rinsed, soaked in plenty of cold water overnight, and drained

1 fresh pig's foot, preferably from the foreleg, split lengthwise (see Note)

Coarse salt and freshly ground black pepper

4 garlic cloves, peeled

1 small dried Italian hot red pepper or ½ dried New Mexican red pepper, seeded and shredded

1 cup mixed chopped fresh sage, rosemary, marjoram, basil, and flat-leaf parsley

3 tablespoons extra virgin olive oil

4 ounces fresh fatback or fatty pancetta, slivered

2 medium onions, chopped

1 bay leaf

12 ounces pork spareribs, cut into individual ribs

1 teaspoon ground cinnamon

Rind of Parmigiano-Reggiano cheese (optional)

6 to 8 slices French or Italian bread, toasted until golden brown

1 A day in advance, when you start to soak the beans, scrub the pig's foot and rub with 1 tablespoon salt. Wrap loosely with plastic wrap and refrigerate overnight.

2 The following day, in a mortar, combine 3 of the garlic cloves with 1 teaspoon salt, the shredded hot pepper, and the herbs; pound to a paste. Gradually work in the olive oil, blending until thick and smooth. (If you don't have a mortar, use a blender or a food processor.)

3 Preheat the oven to 250°F. Rinse the pig's foot, drain, and pat dry. Spread half of the herb paste on one of the cut sides. Top with the other half of the pig's foot and fasten with string.

4 Put the slivered fatback, chopped onion, remaining herbs, and bay leaf in the earthenware casserole. Set over low heat and warm slowly, gradually raising the heat until the fatback begins to sizzle. Cook slowly until the fatback turns golden, 3 to 5 minutes. Add the spareribs, cinnamon, and Parmigiano-Reggiano rind. Season lightly with salt and pepper. Cook, stirring, for a few more minutes.

5 Drain the beans. Add them along with the pig's foot to the casserole. Pour in enough hot water to cover (about 6 cups) and bring to a boil. Cover and place in the oven to cook for 4 to 5 hours, until the meat falls away from the bones and the beans are soft. From time to time, shake the pot without removing the cover.

6 Lift out the pig's foot and transfer it to a cutting board. When cool enough to handle, cut up the skin; remove and discard the bones. (Do not wait until it is cold, because then it will be very difficult to remove the bones.) Dice the skin and meat of the pig's foot and add to the pot. Remove the sparerib bones and discard; return the meat to the pot. Reheat the soup. Correct the seasoning with salt and pepper. Rub the bread with the remaining garlic clove cut in half. Place a slice in each warmed soup bowl and ladle soup over the bread. Serve hot.

NOTE TO THE COOK: The pig's foreleg is much meatier than the rear foot. You can find pig's feet at Asian, Mexican, German, or Eastern European markets.

Creamy Bean Soup with Florina Red Peppers

SERVES 6

*H*ere's a tantalizing bean soup from Greek Macedonia, garnished with sweet, aromatic, roasted Florina peppers and slivered black olives. Because earthenware keeps the heat steady and even, this soup will not scorch and will achieve a lovely smooth texture.

For this recipe, look for large white beans. I love to use Rancho Gordo runner cannellini beans, which triple in size and turn buttery when cooked. Alternatively, use the giant white Greek *fasolia gigantes* imported from Florina, Greece.

PREFERRED CLAY POT:

A 4- or 5- quart stovetop casserole such as: Emile Henry Fig Flame-Top Round Casserole; Le Flambadou; Italian Vulcania traditional brown pot; or a bean pot

If using an electric or ceramic stovetop, be sure to use a heat diffuser with the clay pot.

---

1 pound dried large white beans, such as gigantes or cannellini, rinsed, soaked overnight in plenty of cold water, and drained

4 or 5 roasted sweet red peppers, preferably Florina peppers from Greece, or 8 Spanish piquillo peppers or 3 red bell peppers

¼ cup plus 2 tablespoons extra virgin olive oil

1 tablespoon red wine vinegar

Salt and freshly ground black pepper

1 scallion, white part and 2 inches of green, sliced

2 garlic cloves, peeled

1 bay leaf

2 medium carrots, chopped

½ cup diced celery

2 medium onions, chopped

12 to 15 brine-cured black olives, such as Gaeta or kalamata, rinsed, drained, pitted, and slivered

1 A day in advance, when you start to soak the beans, cut the red peppers into ½-inch dice. In a medium bowl, whisk together 2 tablespoons of the olive oil with the vinegar and ¼ teaspoon each salt and pepper. Add the diced roasted peppers and toss to mix. Cover and marinate the peppers in the refrigerator overnight.

2 Place the drained beans in the earthenware casserole and cover with 2 quarts fresh water. Add the scallion, garlic, and bay leaf. Slowly bring to a boil, reduce the heat to low, cover, and simmer for about 1 hour, or until the beans are tender. Discard the bay leaf and garlic cloves. Season the beans with salt and pepper to taste.

3 In a large conventional skillet, sauté the carrots, celery, and onions in the remaining ¼ cup olive oil, stirring, for 1 to 2 minutes to soften slightly. Scrape into the soup and cook for 30 minutes longer, or until the beans are fully cooked.

4 Use a slotted spoon to transfer about 2 cups of the cooked beans to a food processor or blender. Add 1 cup of the liquid and puree until smooth. Stir the puree into the remaining beans and bring to a boil, stirring occasionally. The soup can be prepared ahead of time to this point. Let cool, then refrigerate.

5 Gently reheat the soup until simmering. Blot the marinated peppers dry; add them to the soup along with the olives. Season with salt and pepper to taste and serve hot.

NOTE TO THE COOK: Both Florina peppers and gigantes can be mail-ordered from www.greekolivewarehouse.com.

Lebanese Summer Wheat and Dried Corn Soup with Yogurt

SERVES 6

This terrific recipe comes from my friend Houston-based Elie Nassar, who grew up in a small village in northern Lebanon and loves to talk about the "comfort food" of his childhood:

"My grandmother, Selwa, used to make this soup, called *m'tabla,* in summer," Elie told me, "a cold version of the hot thick porridge called *amhi'ah* is prepared in winter. She would thin the soup with plain yogurt and salt along with some ice cubes so the yogurt would not curdle when mixed with the hot cooked wheat. Thinned even more, we'd drink this soup out of tall glasses. It's delicious with a sprinkling of fleur de sel."

PREFERRED CLAY POT:

A 4-quart glazed or unglazed earthenware casserole

If using an electric or ceramic stovetop, be sure to use a heat diffuser with the clay pot.

1 cup peeled or hulled wheat, or grano

½ cup dried white or yellow corn

2 to 3 cups plain yogurt, as fresh and sweet as possible

½ to 1 cup ice water

Fleur de sel

1 Place the wheat and corn in a sieve and rinse under cold running water. Soak overnight in a bowl of water to cover.

2 Drain the wheat and corn and place in the earthenware casserole with plenty of fresh cold water to cover. Slowly bring to a boil, starting on low and raising the heat gradually. Reduce the heat and simmer for about 2 hours, or until the wheat is very soft and the corn is cooked through. Add more water if it gets too dry. By the end of the process, you should have a very thick porridgelike mixture.

3 Let the mixture cool; then refrigerate. Do not mix the yogurt into the hot wheat-corn mixture, or it will curdle. When cold, dilute the yogurt with 1 cup ice-cold water and stir that into the soup. Add enough additional ice water to attain thick chowderlike consistency. Refrigerate and serve this soup very cold in a tall glass with a pinch of fleur de sel.

Moroccan Harira

SERVES 10

When we lived in Tangier, my children liked to join our housekeeper, Fatima, and her husband, Ahmed, during month-long Ramadan, when they broke their traditional daytime fast by feasting on *harira,* a rich and hearty North African soup. This culinary event took place every evening just moments after a cannon was fired in the port of Tangier to signal the official end of daylight.

Their highly aromatic *harira,* made with lamb, chickpeas, herbs, spices, and tomatoes, thickened with a slightly fermented bread starter, would have been bubbling on the stove for a good half hour before the blast. The children loved the notion that at the very moment that they were spooning up the soup, accompanied by boiled eggs, dates, and *shebakkia* (sweet fried cakes dripping with honey), nearly every person in town was devouring the same hunger-sating meal.

Each region has its unique way of making *harira,* and every family has its own recipe. Here's the version of our housekeeper, Fatima ben Lahsen Riffi, as cooked the way she did it: in a clay vessel, of course!

> **PREFERRED CLAY POTS:**
>
> A 5- to 6-quart earthenware casserole
>
> If using an electric or ceramic stovetop, be sure to use a heat diffuser with the clay pots.

1½ tablespoons bread starter or ½ teaspoon active dry yeast mixed with ¼ cup plus 2 tablespoons semolina flour and a pinch of sugar

1 cup dried chickpeas, rinsed well

¾ cup dried brown lentils

1¼ to 1½ pounds lamb shoulder with bone, trimmed of excess fat

3 medium red onions, chopped

1 cup chopped celery

2 tablespoons tomato paste, canned or homemade (page 317)

2 tablespoons smen (page 295) or butter

½ cup plus 2 tablespoons chopped fresh flat-leaf parsley

½ cup plus 2 tablespoons chopped fresh cilantro

1 tablespoon Moroccan Spice Mixture: La Kama (page 316)

⅛ teaspoon saffron threads

Salt and freshly ground black pepper

1 pound fresh tomatoes, halved, seeded, and grated

Pinch of sugar

3 tablespoons lemon juice

Lemon quarters and dates for serving

1 In a small bowl, combine the bread starter, flour, and sugar with ⅔ cup warm water. Partially cover and set in a warm place to ferment overnight.

2 Place the chickpeas in a large bowl with enough water to cover by 3 inches. Measure the water as you add it; then add 1 tablespoon kosher salt for each cup of water. Soak overnight.

3 The next day, drain the chickpeas, rinse well, and place in a small conventional saucepan. Add fresh water to cover and boil for 10 minutes. Drain and submerge the chickpeas in a bowl of cold water. Rub them between your palms or fingers to remove their skins. Return the chickpeas to the saucepan, cover again with fresh water, and simmer for 15 minutes. Meanwhile, soak the lentils in water to cover for 15 minutes; drain.

4 Finely dice the lamb meat. Place the lamb and bones in the 5- to 6-quart earthenware casserole. Warm slowly until the pot is hot; then slowly brown lamb over medium-low heat without any added fat, about 10 minutes. Add the onions, celery, and tomato paste and cook, stirring, until the onions are golden brown, 7 to 10 minutes. Add the smen, ½ cup each of the parsley and cilantro, the spice mixture, saffron, 1 tablespoon salt, and ¾ teaspoon pepper. Cover with 3 quarts hot water and bring to a boil, skimming off any scum that rises to the top.

5 When the chickpeas have cooked for 15 minutes, drain and add them to the soup, along with the grated tomatoes and the drained lentils. Cover the pot and simmer for 1½ hours. Pick out the lamb bones and discard them.

6 Stir the flour mixture and add to the simmering soup. Cook, uncovered, for 5 minutes, stirring very often, until smooth and thick. Adjust the seasoning with salt, pepper, a pinch of sugar, and lemon juice. Sprinkle with the remaining 2 tablespoons each chopped parsley and cilantro and serve very hot with lemon quarters and dates.

Italian Clay Pot Duck Soup

SERVES 4 TO 6

This is a hearty soup called *sopa coada* ("smothering soup") from the Treviso region north of Venice. It is traditionally cooked in a clay pot glazed on all sides except the bottom. Italian home cooks use pigeon, squab, or wild ducks shot in the marshes as so beautifully described in Ernest Hemingway's *Across the River and into the Trees.* I've made this dish many times with a pair of legs from a domestic duck and have always had excellent results. The soup is usually made with a pigeon that is cleaned, sautéed in butter, and stewed in a white wine–flavored broth; it is served with thick, finger-long pieces of hearty bread that have been buttered, covered with cheese, and lightly baked.

There are two ways of making this soup: the modern way, as described here, and the traditional way, which allows the soup to "brood" for five or more hours in a 250°F oven.

If you can't find good, sturdy country-style bread, you can make your own (see page 263). If you do so, be sure to bake the loaf about three to four days in advance, slice the bread, and allow it to dry partially as directed in the recipe.

PREFERRED CLAY POT:

A 10-inch-wide stovetop-safe ceramic fondue pot or a 4- to 5-quart flameware saucepan

If using an electric or ceramic stovetop, be sure to use a heat diffuser with the clay pot.

---

1 pair of large duck legs (about 1 pound), trimmed of excess fat and skin

Salt and freshly ground black pepper

5 tablespoons unsalted butter

⅓ cup finely diced celery

¼ cup finely diced carrot

¼ cup finely diced onion

2 tablespoons chopped fresh flat-leaf parsley

1½ teaspoons tomato paste, canned or homemade (page 317)

⅓ cup dry white wine

2 quarts chicken stock, heated

12 ounces slightly stale whole-wheat or whole-grain bread, cut into ½-inch thick, 3- by 1½-inch slices

2 ounces Parmigiano-Reggiano cheese, grated (about ½ cup)

1 Crack each duck leg and thigh at the joint and separate into thigh and drumstick. Season with salt and pepper. Place the fondue pot over medium-low heat. Melt 2 tablespoons of the butter in the pot. Add the celery, carrot, and onion and cook, stirring, until golden, 5 to 10 minutes.

2 Add the parsley, duck legs and thighs, tomato paste, and white wine. Cook until all the wine has evaporated; then continue to fry gently until the vegetable mixture appears thickened but still juicy, about 10 minutes. Season generously with salt and pepper. Add just enough of the hot brown chicken stock to cover the contents of the pot. Cover and cook over the lowest possible heat for 1 hour.

3 Meanwhile, preheat the oven to 250°F. Arrange the slices of bread in a single layer on a lightly buttered baking sheet. Bake for 20 minutes. Turn the slices over and bake until golden on both sides, about 20 minutes longer.

4 Remove the pieces of duck from the pot and let cool slightly. Finely shred the duck meat and skin, discarding any bones and gristle. Season generously with salt and pepper. Strain the cooking juices and reserve both vegetables and liquid.

5 Wipe out the pot, butter the inside, and arrange half the bread slices, side by side, on the bottom. Moisten with 1 cup of the remaining hot stock. Scatter half the cheese over the bread and top with the shredded duck and reserved vegetables. Lay the remaining bread slices over the duck. Scatter the remaining cheese on top.

Carefully pour the reserved liquid plus as much heated stock as necessary to cover the bread completely. Gently press down on the bread, cover with a sheet of foil, and bake for 3 hours. Reserve the rest of the stock for serving.

6 Raise the oven temperature to 350°F, uncover the pot, and dot with the remaining butter. Bake until the bread topping is swollen and golden brown, about 30 minutes. Remove from the oven and let rest for 5 minutes before serving.

7 To serve, take the soup to the table in the pot. Be sure to set it on a wooden trivet or folded kitchen towel to prevent cracking. Ladle some of the thick bread and duck and vegetables into bowls and top with some of the liquid. Offer any remaining stock in small cups on the side for each diner to moisten the soup.

Tunisian Chorba with Crushed Wheat, Lamb "Confit," and Cilantro

SERVES 4

*H*ere's a Tunisian variation on the classic meat and grain soup, *chorba,* served throughout North Africa. *Kadide,* the preserved lamb traditionally added to the dish is similar to jerky, except that after drying it's often stored in olive oil, thus my reference to confit. Very little is used, but it provides a lot of flavor and so is best thought of as a condiment or seasoning. This type of preserved meat can also be used to add depth and complexity to scrambled eggs and to lamb couscous dishes.

> **PREFERRED CLAY POT:**
>
> **A 4-quart glazed earthenware casserole**
>
> **If using an electric or ceramic stovetop, be sure to use a heat diffuser with the clay pot.**

1 cup dried mini fava beans, rinsed, soaked in plenty of cold water overnight, and drained (see Note)

Kadide or imitation Kadide (page 203)

1 cup crushed spelt, farro, or cracked wheat (not bulgur)

2 teaspoons sweet paprika

Pinch of cayenne

½ cup chopped fresh cilantro leaves

Salt and freshly ground black pepper

1 Place the soaked fava beans in a large conventional saucepan and add enough fresh water to cover them by 3 inches; bring to a boil. Reduce the heat to medium-low and simmer until tender, about 1½ hours. Drain the beans, reserving the cooking liquid.

2 Meanwhile, remove the crock of preserved meat, the kadide, from the refrigerator. Remove 10 pieces of preserved lamb. Scrape off the fat and reserve separately. Cut the meat into small pieces and set aside.

3 Place 2 tablespoons of the lamb confit fat in the earthenware casserole. Add 2 quarts water and slowly bring to a boil. Rinse the grain in a sieve under cool running water. Add the grain, paprika, and cayenne to the casserole and cook, stirring often, for 1 hour.

4 In a food processor, grind the cilantro leaves and the reserved cut-up preserved lamb to a paste. Stir the mixture into the soup, add the drained favas along with enough of the reserved bean cooking liquid to cover, and continue to cook until the soup is thick, adding more liquid if needed. Season with salt and pepper to taste and serve hot.

NOTE TO THE COOK: Dried mini fava beans are sold at Middle Eastern grocers as *ful hamam,* Egyptian brown beans, or simply *ful* beans.

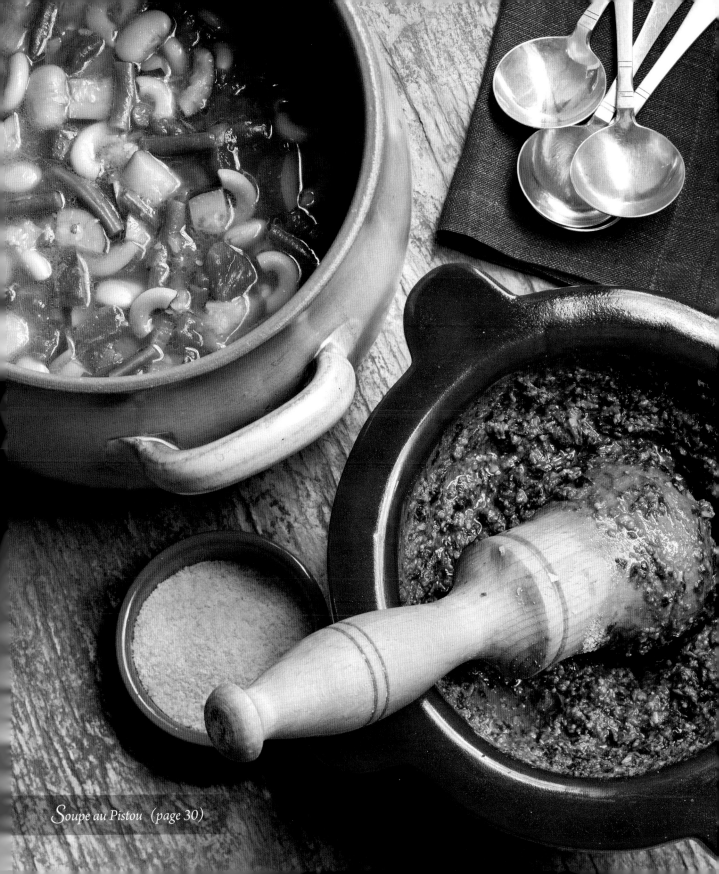

Soupe au Pistou (page 30)

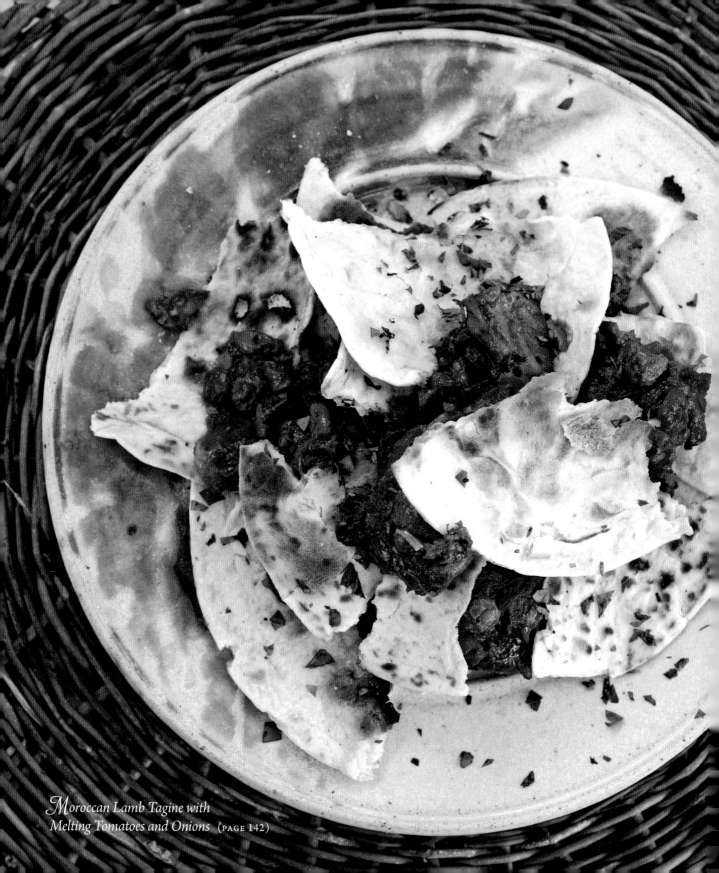

Moroccan Lamb Tagine with
Melting Tomatoes and Onions (PAGE 142)

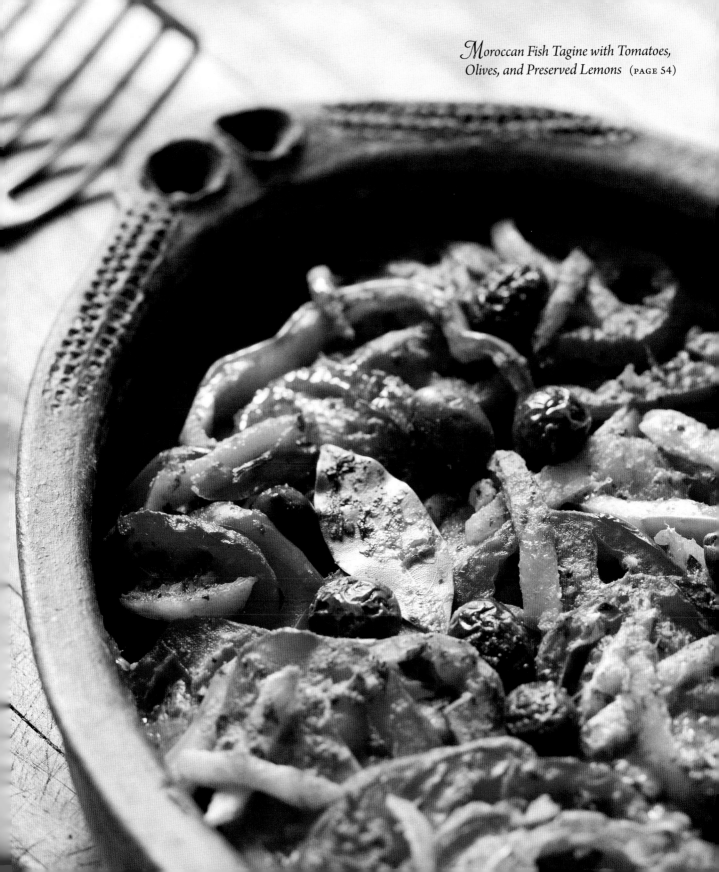

Moroccan Fish Tagine with Tomatoes, Olives, and Preserved Lemons (PAGE 54)

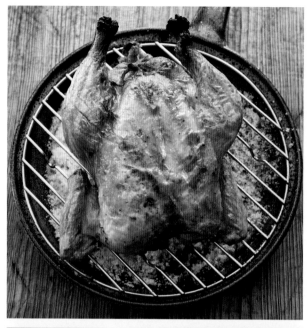

LEFT

*Chicken Stuffed with Garlic Croutons
Roasted Over a Bed of Salt* (PAGE 82)

BELOW

*Beef Paupiettes with Tomatoes
and Wild Capers* (PAGE 164)

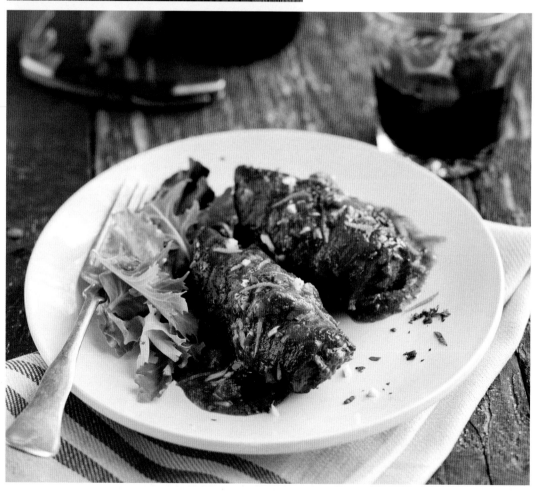

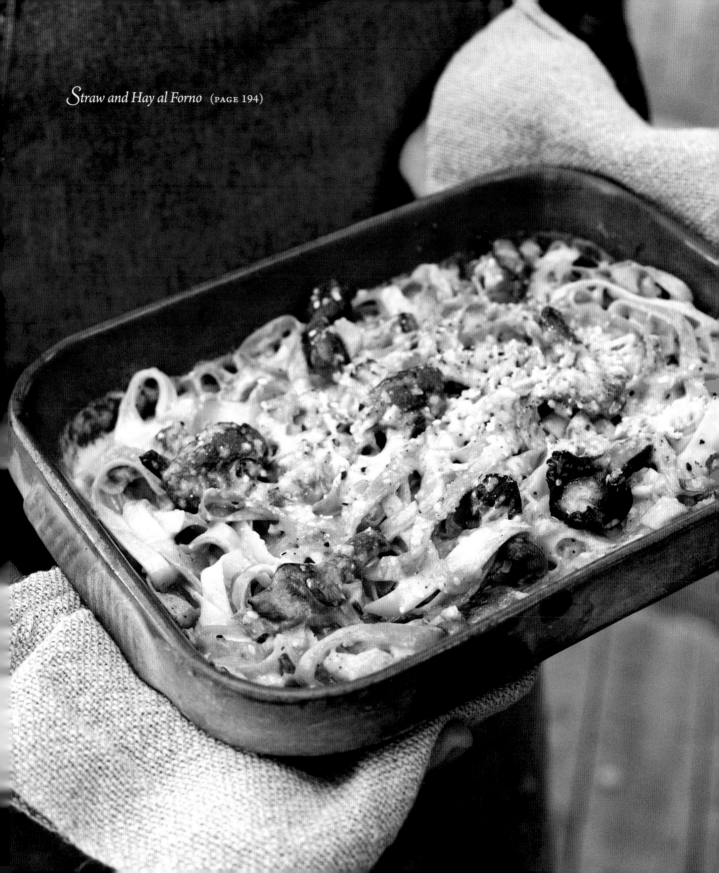

Straw and Hay al Forno (PAGE 194)

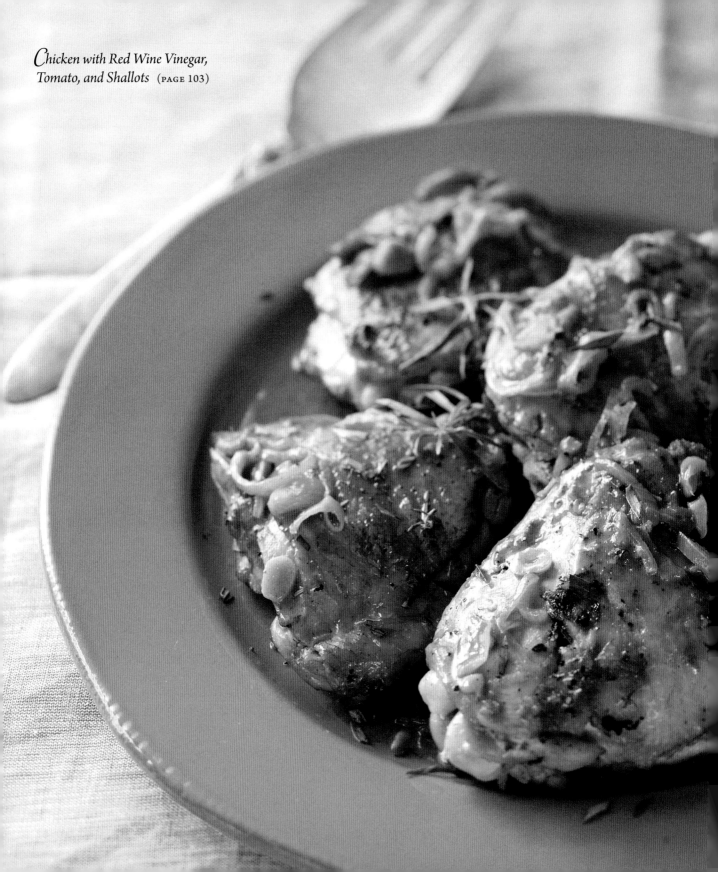

Chicken with Red Wine Vinegar,
Tomato, and Shallots (PAGE 103)

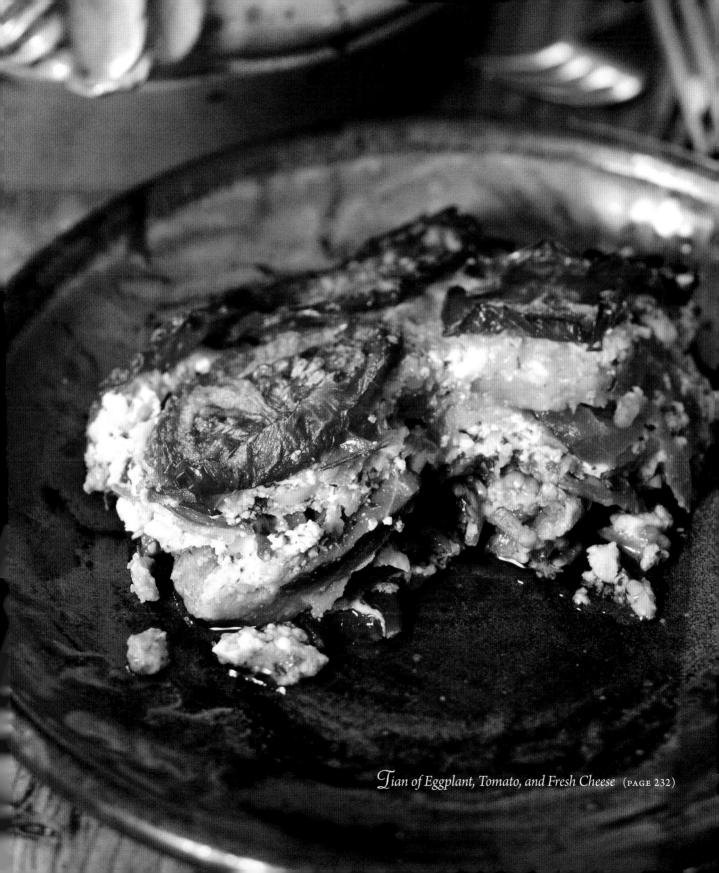

Tian of Eggplant, Tomato, and Fresh Cheese (PAGE 232)

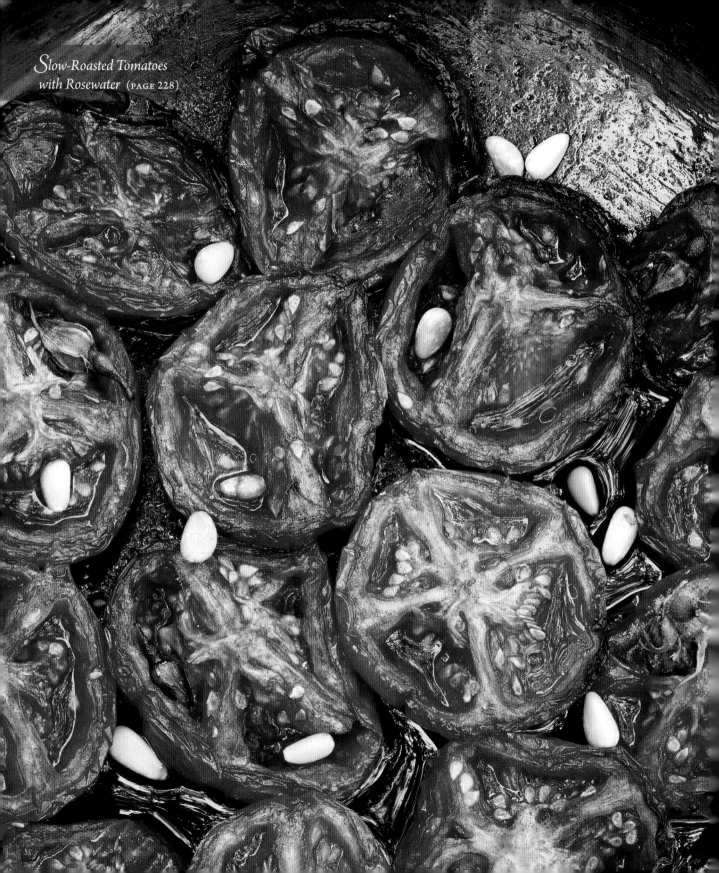

*Slow-Roasted Tomatoes
with Rosewater* (PAGE 228)

Spring Vegetable Soup with Whipped Salt Cod

SERVES 4 TO 6

This fragrant, well-balanced soup lacks a strong taste vector until the last minute, when crumbled salt cod is whisked in. The heat releases the flavor and aroma of the fish, and suddenly the soup comes alive!

> **PREFERRED CLAY POT:**
>
> A 3-quart glazed earthenware or flameware casserole
>
> If using an electric or ceramic stovetop, be sure to use a heat diffuser with the clay pot.

8 ounces boneless salt cod

1 medium leek, white and 1 inch of pale green, finely diced

1 medium waxy potato, peeled and cut into ¼-inch dice

2 small carrots, cut into ¼-inch dice

1 medium turnip, peeled and cut into ¼-inch dice

1 pound fresh fava beans

1 quart chicken stock

Freshly ground white pepper

2½ tablespoons unsalted butter

1 tablespoon chopped flat-leaf parsley

1 tablespoon chopped fresh chervil

1 tablespoon chopped fresh tarragon

1 One to two days before serving, rinse the salt cod under cool running water. Cut into 3 or 4 pieces. Place them in a large bowl and cover with cold water. Refrigerate for at least 12 and up to 36 hours, changing the water several times. Rinse the salt cod, pick out any bones, remove any skin or scales, and cut the fish into small dice. Drain on a kitchen towel–lined plate and refrigerate until ready to cook.

2 Bring a large conventional saucepan of salted water to a boil. Add the leek, potato, carrots, and turnip and blanch for 2 minutes; drain. Briefly steam the fava beans until just wilted, about 5 minutes. Rinse under cold running water. Shell the beans and peel off the skins; add to the vegetables.

3 About 20 minutes before serving, slowly bring the chicken stock to a boil in the casserole. Add the blanched and peeled vegetables, and season the soup generously with pepper. Reduce the heat to medium-low and simmer, partially covered, for 7 to 8 minutes.

4 Whisk the pieces of salt cod into the liquid while crushing some of the vegetables; then whisk in the butter. Simmer for 2 minutes. Immediately sprinkle with the parsley, chervil, and tarragon, and serve at once directly from the casserole.

With thanks to Bordeaux-based chef Francis Garcia for sharing this recipe.

Clay Pot Bourride

SERVES 4 TO 6

A bourride is a French fish soup that is a lot easier to make and just as marvelous in its homey way as a classic Mediterranean bouillabaisse. A preheated earthenware casserole is filled with layers of potatoes, leeks, onions, and cubes of fish, flooded with boiling fish stock, and then covered. The fire is turned off, allowing the fish to cook in the receding heat. Just before serving, the cooking liquid is combined with a garlicky ailloli sauce (aïoli) enriched with extra egg yolks, creating a deliciously rich fish soup.

You'll note I make this classic dish an easy way, using fish bouillon cubes in place of stock. Including several kinds of fish instead of a single variety will deepen the flavor. Avoid oily fish, like salmon, which are too strong. Instead, opt for white-fleshed fish like monkfish, halibut, cod, haddock, scrod, red snapper, or striped bass.

> **PREFERRED CLAY POT:**
>
> A deep 3- or 4-quart glazed earthenware or flameware casserole
>
> If using an electric or ceramic stovetop, be sure to use a heat diffuser with the clay pot.

2 pounds assorted lean and thick white, firm-fleshed fish fillets or steaks

Sea salt and freshly ground black pepper

1 or 2 cubes fish-flavored bouillon

1 cup dry white wine

12 ounces Yukon Gold potatoes, peeled and thinly sliced

1 small onion, finely sliced

1 large or 2 small leeks, white part only, thinly sliced crosswise

Herb bouquet: 4 to 5 each fresh flat-leaf parsley and thyme sprigs, 2 bay leaves, and 1 strip dried orange peel tied together with white kitchen string

Provençal Ailloli (see recipe below)

4 egg yolks

12 round slices of a French baguette

1 Rinse and dry the fish. Cut away any bones, gray membrane, or skin. Divide the fish into even 2-inch chunks. Season lightly with salt and pepper and set aside in a cool place.

2 In a medium conventional saucepan, bring 1 quart water and the fish bouillon cubes to a simmer. Add the wine and keep the fish broth over low heat.

3   In the earthenware casserole, toss together the potatoes, onion, and leek. Season lightly with salt and pepper. Add the hot fish broth and the bouquet garni, cover, and cook over medium heat for 10 minutes. Remove from the heat and set aside.

4   Slip the pieces of fish into the casserole, burying them in the liquid and vegetables. Bring to a boil, reduce the heat, and simmer for 2 to 3 minutes. Cover, remove from the heat, and let stand for 10 to 12 minutes, or until the fish is just cooked.

5   Meanwhile, make the ailloli as directed.

6   Transfer the fish and vegetables to a warm deep dish and cover to keep hot. Discard the bouquet garni. Reheat the soup broth in the casserole.

7   In a medium bowl, whisk together 1 cup of the ailloli with the egg yolks until well blended. Temper the mixture by carefully whisking in a few tablespoons of the hot soup. Gradually whisk up to half of the soup into the ailloli mixture in a thin stream. Scrape this liaison mixture into the remaining hot soup in the casserole, swirling to blend. Set over low heat and stir constantly until the soup thickens, but do not let boil or the egg yolks will curdle. Season with salt and pepper to taste.

8   Divide the fried bread among 4 to 6 heated soup plates. Spread the remaining ailloli over the bread. Top with the fish and vegetables and ladle the soup over all. Serve at once.

Provençal Ailloli

MAKES ABOUT 1⅓ CUPS

This garlic mayonnaise is especially made for bourride. Don't skimp on the garlic: It punches up the seafood soup. If you are careful to add the oil drop by drop, the sauce will thicken nicely.

2 tablespoons coarsely chopped garlic (about 8 cloves)

½ teaspoon sea salt

2 fresh egg yolks at room temperature

1 cup extra virgin olive oil, preferably French

¼ to ½ teaspoon fresh lemon juice

Freshly ground black pepper

1   Rinse a stone or ceramic mortar or a heavy ceramic bowl in hot water and dry thoroughly. Add the garlic and sea salt. Use a wooden pestle to pound them to a smooth paste.

2   Add the egg yolks and stir with the pestle until thick and blended. Very slowly add the olive oil, drop by drop as if you were making a mayonnaise, stirring vigorously and continually in one direction. The ailloli should be smooth and medium-thick.

3   Season liberally with up to ½ teaspoon of the lemon juice and pepper to taste.

NOTE TO THE COOK: If the ailloli breaks, place a whole raw egg in a food processor, add 2 tablespoons of the ailloli, and pulse until smooth.

Mussel Soup with Toasted Almond-Cinnamon Picada

MAKES ABOUT 6 CUPS, SERVING 4

The Catalans like to thicken their soups and stews with a *picada*—a smooth paste made of pounded nuts, garlic, and lots of aromatic flavorings—which gives a deeper and lustier taste than butter or cream.

> **PREFERRED CLAY POT:**
>
> A 10-inch Spanish cazuela or a straight-sided flameware skillet
>
> If using an electric or ceramic stovetop, be sure to use a heat diffuser with the clay pot.

1½ to 2 pounds fresh cultivated mussels, scrubbed and debearded, if necessary

Sea salt and freshly ground black pepper

1 medium onion, finely chopped

1 pound red ripe tomatoes, cored, halved, seeded, and finely chopped

Almond-Cinnamon Picada (recipe follows)

Juice of 1 lemon

Pinch of pulverized saffron threads

1½ tablespoons brandy or cognac

Pinch of cayenne

1 thin slice Serrano ham, slivered

2 tablespoons chopped fresh flat-leaf parsley

1 Swish the mussels around in a bowl of cold water, drain, and add fresh water to cover and a pinch of salt. Let soak for 45 minutes.

2 Add the onion and 2 tablespoons warm water to the cazuela. Cook over medium-low heat until softened but not browned, about 10 minutes. Add the tomatoes and cook for 15 minutes longer, stirring occasionally.

3 Make the picada as directed. Add the picada to the cazuela and cook for 5 minutes, stirring to blend. Transfer the contents of the cazuela to a deep dish. Do not rinse out the cazuela.

4 Drain the mussels and add them to the cazuela along with 1 cup hot water. Cover and steam over medium heat until the mussels open, 3 to 4 minutes. Remove the mussels with a slotted spoon, leaving the broth in the cazuela. Shell the mussels and season them lightly with salt, pepper, and a few drops of lemon juice.

5 Strain the broth into the deep bowl with the tomato picada mixture. Add a pinch of saffron and 1 cup water. In a blender or food processor, puree until smooth. Add all but 12 of the shelled mussels and puree again.

6 Wipe out the cazuela and add the puree. Pour in 3½ cups water and the brandy. Slowly bring to a boil, reduce the heat, and simmer for 5 minutes. Season with salt and cayenne to taste. Place 3 of the reserved mussels in each of 4 warmed soup plates. Ladle the hot soup over the mussels, sprinkle the slivered ham and chopped parsley on top, and serve at once.

Almond-Cinnamon Picada

MAKES ABOUT ⅓ CUP

2 tablespoons extra virgin olive oil

1 thick slice (1-inch) stale country-style bread, crust removed

12 whole blanched almonds, toasted

4 large garlic cloves, peeled and bruised

1 teaspoon salt

¼ teaspoon sweet paprika, preferably Spanish

Pinch of ground cinnamon

Pinch of sugar

1 In a medium skillet, warm the olive oil over medium heat. Add the bread and fry slowly, turning once, until golden brown on both sides, about 4 minutes. Drain on paper towels.

2 In a mortar, pound the almonds with the garlic and salt to make a smooth paste; or puree in a blender or food processor. Add the fried bread, paprika, cinnamon, and sugar and pound or puree to blend well.

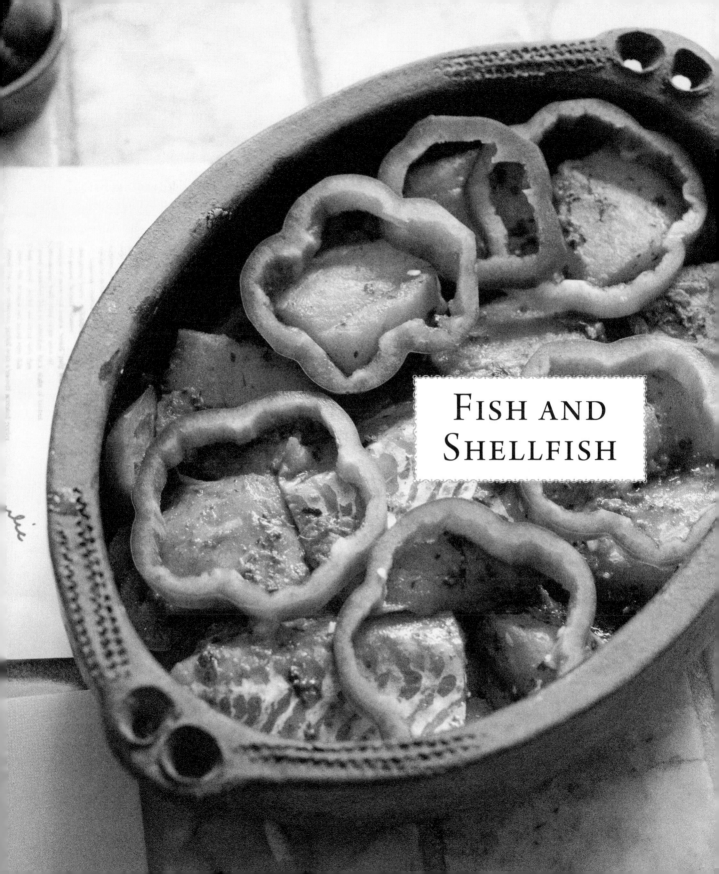

FISH AND
SHELLFISH

Moroccan Fish Tagine with Tomatoes, Olives, and Preserved Lemons

SERVES 6

Fish baked in a clay pot takes beautifully to long, slow simmering in the famous complex Moroccan herb-and- spice sauce called *charmoula*. Ingredients that include garlic, cumin, cilantro, hot pepper, and preserved lemon permeate the flesh of most any type of fish. Add time to the equation and you have a dish that is bright, savory, and exciting to eat. Serve the fish at table directly from the clay baking dish.

> **PREFERRED CLAY POT:**
>
> An 11- or 12-inch Moroccan tagine, or *tagra* or Spanish cazuela, or 3-quart flameware or La Chamba shallow baking dish

2 teaspoons cumin seeds

3 garlic cloves

1 teaspoon coarse salt

1 tablespoon sweet paprika

1½ teaspoons crushed hot red pepper

2 tablespoons coarsely chopped flat-leaf parsley

2 tablespoons chopped fresh cilantro

4 wedges preserved lemon, rinsed, pulp and peel separated

3 tablespoons fruity extra virgin olive oil

1 pound monkfish fillet or thick slabs of halibut

1 large carrot, very thinly sliced

2 celery ribs, stringed and very thinly sliced

1 pound red ripe tomatoes, peeled with a swivel serrated peeler and sliced into thin rounds

1 small green bell pepper, sliced into very thin rounds

2 dozen Moroccan red (see Note) or picholine olives, rinsed and pitted

2 imported bay leaves

Fresh cilantro sprigs for garnish

1 Early in the day, or a day in advance, toast the cumin seeds by tossing them in a hot, dry conventional skillet over medium heat for about 1 minute. Grind to a powder and set aside. Make the charmoula: In a mortar or blender, combine the garlic, cumin, salt, paprika, parsley, cilantro, the pulp of the preserved lemon, and the olive oil. Puree to a smooth sauce.

2 Rinse the fish and pat dry with paper towels. If using monkfish, cut away the gray membrane and divide the fish into 4 even chunks. Rub half of the charmoula all over the fish, and let stand for 1 hour at room temperature, or up to 24 hours in the refrigerator. Add ½ cup water to the remaining charmoula, cover, and refrigerate separately.

3 About 1½ hours before serving, preheat the oven to 300°F. Spread 2 tablespoons of the reserved charmoula sauce over the bottom of the tagine. Scatter the carrot and celery on top. Add half of the tomatoes and bell peppers; sprinkle with a little sauce. Lay the fish over the vegetables and cover with the remaining tomatoes and peppers. Spread the remaining charmoula on top. Scatter the diced preserved lemon peel and the bay leaves around the fish. Cover the dish tightly with a sheet of foil and bake for 1 hour.

4 Pour off the liquid from the dish into a small nonreactive saucepan. Bring it to a boil over moderately high heat and boil until it is thickened and reduced to ½ cup. Pour back over the fish.

5 Meanwhile, raise the oven temperature to 500°F. Baste the fish with the pan juices and bake, uncovered, in the top third of the oven for 10 minutes, or until a nice crust has formed over the vegetables. Transfer the tagine to a wooden surface or folded kitchen towel to prevent cracking. Garnish with cilantro sprigs. Serve warm or hot.

NOTE TO THE COOK: "Moroccan red" olives aren't really red; they can be russet, tan, violet, or even purple in color. Picked when ripe but not black, they are preserved in an acidic marinade and are particularly delicious when marinated in bitter orange juice. You can find them at www.chefshop.com. Another good choice is Lindsay-canned "Green Ripe Olives," which are produced in California and available at most supermarkets.

Tangier-Style Fresh Sardines with Charmoula

SERVES 6 TO 8

Cooks in the northern Moroccan cities of Tangier and Tetuan use a locally made clay vessel called a *tagra* to cook fish over embers or in a baker's oven. This oval, porous unglazed earthenware pan, made by potters near the River Oued Laou, which empties into the Mediterranean Sea, encourages slow evaporation of moisture during cooking while providing an unusual earthy flavor to fish dishes.

In this recipe, fresh sardines are layered between beds of sliced peppers, tomatoes, potatoes, and carrots. These cut vegetables, placed around the fish to protect it during cooking, become meltingly tender just as the sardines emerge perfectly (not overly) cooked. Finally, charmoula, the popular sauce combination of paprika scented with cumin and a hint of garlic, is poured over the vegetables and the fish, tying the dish together.

I set my *tagra* over my stovetop gas lava stone grill. If you don't have one, see the note that follows for oven baking with the *tagra*.

> **PREFERRED CLAY POT:**
> A Moroccan 11-inch × 8-inch tagra, or a 10- to 11-inch Spanish cazuela, or a straight-sided flameware baking dish

(continued)

2 pounds large fresh sardines (about 12)

Sea salt and freshly ground black pepper

⅓ cup plus 2 tablespoons extra virgin olive oil

2½ teaspoons sweet paprika

2 teaspoons ground cumin

4 teaspoons chopped garlic

2½ tablespoons chopped fresh flat-leaf parsley

2½ tablespoons chopped fresh cilantro

1 pound red or Yukon Gold potatoes

12 ounces carrots

1 pound Roma tomatoes, thinly sliced

1 large red bell pepper, cored, peeled with a serrated swivel peeler, and thinly sliced

1 large organic lemon, thinly sliced

1   Cut off the head from each of the sardines. Slit the belly lengthwise and remove the backbone and any innards. Do not separate the fillets. Rinse well under cold running water; pat dry. Season the fish lightly with salt and pepper.

2   In a small bowl, combine 2 tablespoons of the olive oil, 1½ teaspoons of the paprika, 1 teaspoon of the cumin, 2 teaspoons of the garlic, 2 tablespoons each of the parsley and cilantro, 1 teaspoon salt, and ½ teaspoon pepper. Smear this marinade over the flesh of each sardine. Pile the fillets on a plate, cover, and refrigerate for 1 hour.

3   Meanwhile, peel and slice the potatoes and carrots into thin rounds. If you're using coals or lava stones, heat them to the lowest temperature now.

4   Layer a third of the tomatoes, carrots, bell pepper, and potatoes in the dry *tagra*. Arrange half the sardines, skin side down, over the vegetables. Repeat, ending with a layer of potato slices. Spread the lemon slices on top.

5   In a small bowl, mix together the remaining ⅓ cup olive oil, 1 teaspoon each paprika and cumin, 2 teaspoons garlic, and 1½ teaspoons each parsley and cilantro. Pour over the sardines in the pot; gently press down so the sauce rises to cover the potatoes.

6   Place the *tagra* over the heated coals or lava stones, cover with a sheet of foil, and cook for 30 minutes, or until the potatoes are tender. Remove from the heat and place on a wooden surface or folded kitchen towel to prevent cracking. Uncover and let stand for about 30 minutes longer before serving.

NOTE TO THE COOK: To bake this dish in the oven rather than over heated coals, set the filled *tagra* in a preheated 350°F oven for 45 minutes. Remove from the oven and let settle for 30 minutes before serving. The website www.tagines.com sells traditional Moroccan *tagras,* deep oval unglazed earthenware pans. If you buy one, be sure to season it before using with grated onion, oil, and salt; then set in a 300°F oven to heat up. When hot, raise the oven temperature to 450°F and bake until the seasoning turns black. Turn the heat off and let the pan cool slowly in the oven. When cold, wash well and let dry. Use your *tagra* for fish cookery, either over charcoal or lava stones on low temperature or in the oven. A *tagra* must be bone dry when packed with food and set over heat.

Sicilian Fresh Sardines Stuffed with Pine Nuts and Raisins

SERVES 4 TO 6

*H*ere's a very popular Sicilian dish, often served as an appetizer. It is sometimes referred to as *beccafico*, a complicated reference to a bird that not only has good taste but also takes delight in eating ripe figs—thus a dish worthy of a gourmet!

Each sardine is rolled around a wonderful moist, savory stuffing of pine nuts, anchovies, and raisins and bound with bread crumbs. The stuffed fish are arranged attractively in a cazuela or stoneware baking dish with bay leaves and thick slices of orange and then quickly roasted in a medium-hot oven. The dish is served cool or cold directly from the cooking vessel.

> **PREFERRED CLAY POT:**
> A 10-inch Spanish cazuela or a 2-quart, shallow Le Creuset stoneware baking dish

12 large fresh sardines (about 2 pounds)

Salt and freshly ground black pepper

¼ cup golden raisins

5 tablespoons olive oil

½ cup soft white bread crumbs

6 oil-packed anchovy fillets, rinsed, drained, and chopped

12 pitted green olives, rinsed and coarsely chopped

¼ cup pine nuts

1 lemon, halved

12 imported bay leaves

1 tablespoon sugar

1 navel orange, thickly sliced

1 Preheat the oven to 350°F. Cut off the head from each of the sardines. Slit the belly lengthwise and remove the backbone and any innards without separating the fillets. Rinse. Season with salt and pepper.

2 Meanwhile, soak the golden raisins in warm water to cover for 15 minutes to plump them; then drain them.

3 Heat 2 tablespoons of the olive oil in a medium conventional skillet over medium heat. Add the bread crumbs and toss in the oil until golden. In a small bowl, mix the bread crumbs with the golden raisins, anchovies, olives, and pine nuts. Season with the juice of ½ lemon and salt and pepper to taste.

4 Lay the sardines on their backs, spread about 1 tablespoon of the stuffing over the fish, and roll up so that each sardine ends up with its tail sticking up. Arrange the stuffed sardines in the earthenware baking dish. Slip a bay leaf between the stuffed sardines and lay an orange slice here and there on top. Sprinkle with the sugar, the juice of the remaining lemon half, and the remaining 3 tablespoons olive oil.

5 Bake for 15 minutes. Preheat the broiler and place the dish under the broiler, about 8 inches from the heat, until the orange slices are lightly charred, about 5 minutes watching closely so they don't burn. Transfer the dish to a wooden surface or folded kitchen towel to prevent cracking. Serve at room temperature or chilled.

Salmon Fillets Slow-Baked on Clay Tiles with Favas and Green Beans

SERVES 4

In this contemporary Turkish recipe, fresh green leaves protect salmon fillets, whether they are baked on a hot clay tile or in a shallow pan. The clay advantage is clear: unlike metal, a clay pan surface will not build up heat above the surrounding oven temperature. This is important since the cooking method here is oven steaming; the moisture from the fresh leaves releases aromatic vapors, which infuse the fish.

For me, the preferred leaves for this dish are ones picked from a walnut tree, though grape or cabbage leaves may also be used. Note that the leaves will also protect your clay tile or pan from absorbing fish odors.

Since this is a late spring dish, I like to serve it with a warm salad of fresh fava beans and green beans dressed with walnut oil vinaigrette.

> **PREFERRED CLAY POT:**
> An 8- or 9-inch unglazed Turkish *kiremit*, or an unglazed and untreated flat or shallow and curved terra-cotta tile, or a La Chamba shallow baking dish, well scrubbed and completely dried

1¼ pounds fresh unshelled fava beans

12 ounces green beans, trimmed and cut into 1-inch lengths

Sea salt

4 pieces center-cut salmon fillets (8 ounces each), preferably wild king, or Arctic char

8 fresh walnut, grape, or outer cabbage leaves

2 ounces Turkish Kashar cheese, French Cantal, or American cheddar, shredded (about ½ cup)

½ cup walnut oil

Freshly ground black pepper

3 tablespoons red wine vinegar

1 Steam the fava beans in their pods until tender, 5 to 8 minutes, depending on size. Cool under cold running water. Peel off both the pod and the outer skin of each bean. Return the water in the steamer to a boil, drop in the peeled favas, and cook for 1 to 2 minutes; drain.

2 In a large conventional saucepan, boil the green beans in salted water until tender, about 10 minutes. Scoop out the beans and add them to the favas; set aside.

3 Place the terra-cotta dish on the middle rack of the oven and preheat the oven to 350°F.

4 Rinse the salmon fillets. Use tweezers to remove any small bones and pull off the skin. Season the salmon with sea salt. Carefully transfer the hot dish from the oven to a wooden surface or folded kitchen towel to prevent cracking, line the dish with the leaves, and place the fish fillets on top. Sprinkle the cheese evenly over each fillet, patting it down to adhere. Return the dish to the oven, reduce the heat to 250°F, and bake for 12 to 15 minutes, or until the flesh just begins to flake when pressed and the texture is very juicy. Remove the tile from the oven and place on a wooden surface or folded kitchen towel again. Cover loosely with foil and keep warm.

5   Meanwhile, add 2 tablespoons of the walnut oil to the beans in the saucepan and season them with salt and pepper to taste. Toss over medium heat until hot, about 3 minutes. Quickly make a vinaigrette with the remaining walnut oil, the vinegar, and a pinch each of salt and pepper.

6   To serve, spoon the beans onto 4 plates. Top with a salmon fillet, discarding the leaves. Drizzle a few teaspoons of the vinaigrette over each piece of fish and over the beans. Serve warm.

Tuna with Sweet-and-Sour Onions

SERVES 6

Here's a perfect preparation for tuna in summer—the time of year when the fish is plump and unctuous. The recipe comes from Trapani in Sicily, where tuna fishing has been a major industry for centuries. Thin tuna steaks are fried, drenched in a sweet-and-sour-onion sauce, and refrigerated overnight or for several days, which allows the flavors to meld.

PREFERRED CLAY POT:

A 10- or 11-inch Spanish cazuela or a 3-quart straight-sided La Chamba or flameware skillet or baking dish

If using an electric or ceramic stovetop, be sure to use a heat diffuser with the clay pot.

3 medium onions, thinly sliced

Sea salt and freshly ground black pepper

¼ cup plus 2 tablespoons extra virgin olive oil

¼ cup aged red wine vinegar

2 tablespoons sugar

2 pounds fresh sushi-grade tuna, preferably cut from the stomach into slices about ¾ inch thick

¼ cup all-purpose flour

Fresh flat-leaf parsley and spearmint for garnish

1   In a cazuela set over medium-low heat, place the onions, 1 teaspoon salt, and 1½ cups water. Cook until the water has evaporated, about 30 minutes.

2   Add 2 tablespoons of the olive oil and cook slowly, stirring occasionally, until the onions turn golden, about 15 minutes. Add the vinegar and sugar, raise the heat to medium, and continue cooking until the onions are juicy, soft, and lightly caramelized, about 10 minutes.

3   Transfer the cazuela to a wooden surface or folded kitchen towel to prevent cracking. Season the onions lightly with salt and pepper to taste. Let cool to lukewarm.

4   Meanwhile, rinse the tuna and soak in cold water for 5 minutes; rinse again and pat dry. Season the flour with ½ teaspoon sea salt and ¼ teaspoon pepper. Dust the tuna with the seasoned flour; shake off the excess.

5   In a large, heavy conventional skillet, heat the remaining ¼ cup olive oil over high heat until it ripples. Add the tuna slices and sauté until crisp and brown, about 1½ minutes to a side. Immediately remove from the skillet and pat dry with paper towels.

6   Nestle the tuna in the onion sauce, spooning some of the sweet-and-sour liquid over the top. Let cool; then cover and refrigerate. Serve chilled, directly from the cazuela, with a garnish of freshly torn herbs.

Oven-Poached Fillets of Sole with Tomatoes, Mushrooms, and Chiles

SERVES 4

I admit that I was skeptical when my good friend Turkish culinary writer Ayfer Ünsal informed me we'd be dining at a huge modern restaurant in Florya, a pine-scented, upscale suburb on the Marmara Sea just across from the Istanbul airport. And I actually groaned when we pulled into a grouping of modern buildings with tourist buses parked out front.

"I know the owner," said Ayfer, flashing her mischievous smile. "He's from my hometown. Prepare to be amazed."

I was. The restaurant, Kasibeyaz (actually a complex of several restaurants), turned out to be a revelation, producing wonderful food, brilliantly cooked and superbly served. It's especially convenient if you've just arrived or are about to leave the country.

Kasibeyaz means "White Eyebrow"—a strange name for a restaurant, I thought, until I met the restaurateur, Ahmet Kasibeyaz—one of his eyebrows sports a slash of white.

Ayfer and I headed straight for the fish restaurant, where, like all the diners at Kasibeyaz, we chose our fish from a big display case. There were numerous seasonal varieties available, all incredibly fresh: line-caught bluefish, local turbot, sea bass, bonito, mackerel, fresh anchovies and sardines, red mullets, sole, and swordfish. After choosing sole, we conferred with one of the cooks, who suggested steaming or poaching the fish in milk in a clay pot. Once again, I was a little skeptical but agreed. The resulting dish was marvelous!

When, after eating, I went to the kitchen to learn the recipe, the chef emphasized the use of a clay cooking vessel. "A fish just won't taste this good unless it's poached in a clay pot," he told me.

He went on to explain that it is the gentle cooking at a low temperature in a flavorful seasoned poaching liquid that creates the magic. It can be milk, as in this recipe, or vinegar, wine, broth, or even olive oil.

> **PREFERRED CLAY POTS:**
>
> A shallow, 9- × 11-inch stoneware baking dish about 2 inches deep
>
> A 3-quart unglazed or glazed earthenware or flameware casserole
>
> If using an electric or ceramic stovetop, be sure to use a heat diffuser with the clay pots.

4 skinned fillets of sole (6 ounces each)

Sea salt and freshly ground black pepper

1 tablespoon extra virgin olive oil

2 medium juicy tomatoes, peeled and sliced

6 fresh shiitake or brown mushrooms, stemmed, caps thinly sliced

2 Anaheim peppers, cored, deribbed, and thinly sliced

2 cups milk

2 shallots, sliced

1 chunk (1 inch) carrot

1 imported bay leaf

1 thick slice lemon

2 tablespoons unsalted butter

1½ tablespoons all-purpose flour

½ cup shredded Turkish Kashar, Greek kasseri, or pecorino Romano cheese (about 2 ounces)

Generous sprinklings of Greek or Turkish oregano, finely ground black pepper, and Turkish or Aleppo pepper for garnish

1 Rinse the fish fillets. Season lightly with salt and pepper. Neatly fold each fillet in half, skinned side in, and fasten with kitchen string or a toothpick. Refrigerate.

2 Oil the 9- × 11-inch baking dish. Scatter the tomatoes, mushrooms, and peppers over the bottom, cover with foil, and place in a cold oven. Set the heat to 350°F and bake for 45 minutes. Meanwhile, heat the milk with the shallots, carrot, bay leaf, lemon slice, ¾ teaspoon salt, and ¼ teaspoon pepper in the 3-quart casserole. Slowly bring just to a boil; immediately reduce the heat to very low. Add the fish and cook *below* the simmer for 10 minutes, or until half cooked. Carefully transfer the fish to a side dish, remove the picks or string, cover with foil, and let stand while you prepare the sauce.

3 In a medium conventional saucepan, melt the butter over medium-low heat. When the butter begins to foam, stir in the flour. Cook, stirring, for 1 to 2 minutes to make a roux without allowing the flour to color. Remove from the heat. Stir a few tablespoons of the simmering milk into the roux until smooth. Pour the remaining milk through a strainer into the saucepan, return it to the heat, and bring to a boil, stirring until you have a thin, smooth sauce. Reduce the heat to low and simmer gently for 10 minutes, or until the sauce is reduced to about 1½ cups. Fold ¼ cup of the shredded cheese into the sauce.

4 Transfer the baking dish from the oven to a wooden surface or folded kitchen towel to prevent cracking. Nestle the fish in the vegetables. Coat with the sauce and sprinkle the remaining cheese on top. Return to the oven and bake for 10 minutes. If necessary, lightly brown the top under the broiler. Serve at once with a generous sprinkling of oregano and black and red pepper.

Sturgeon Poached in the Manner of the Po Valley with Roasted Zucchini

SERVES 4

Here's another slow-poached fish dish, this one from northern Italy, in which sturgeon is poached in a red wine vinegar court bouillon (stock). Really good red wine vinegar will coax flavor from farmed sturgeon, which tends to be a bit too subtle and can use a little embellishment.

Serve this poached fish with a refreshing combination of sautéed zucchini slices, fresh thyme, and salty capers in the cazuela.

> **PREFERRED CLAY POT:**
>
> A 10- or 11-inch Spanish cazuela or a flameware or La Chamba straight-sided skillet
>
> If using an electric or ceramic stovetop, be sure to use a heat diffuser with the clay pot.

1 pound wild-caught white or farmed sturgeon (see Note), cut 1 inch thick, divided into 4 pieces

Coarse sea salt

3 tablespoons red wine vinegar, preferably homemade (page 313)

1 pound (3) firm zucchini, cut into ½-inch rounds

3 tablespoons extra virgin olive oil

¾ cup fish broth or water

1 shallot, halved

1 garlic clove, thinly sliced

Herb bouquet: 2 fresh flat-leaf parsley sprigs, 1 imported bay leaf, and 2 celery leaves

Freshly ground black pepper

2 tablespoons unsalted butter

1½ teaspoons chopped fresh thyme

3 tablespoons capers, drained and rinsed

1 Sprinkle the sturgeon with salt and 1 tablespoon of the vinegar. Cover and refrigerate while you prepare the zucchini.

2 Toss the zucchini slices with salt and set them out in one layer on a baking sheet lined with a paper towel. Let them stand at room temperature for about 1 hour.

3 Preheat the oven to 375°F. Rinse and dry the zucchini slices. Toss them with 2 tablespoons of the olive oil and arrange on a large baking sheet in a single layer. Bake for 30 minutes, basting once or twice with the oil.

4 Meanwhile, combine the broth, shallot, garlic, herb bouquet, ½ teaspoon salt, and ¼ teaspoon pepper in the cazuela and bring to a boil. Reduce the heat to the lowest possible setting, add the sturgeon, cover tightly, and poach for 10 minutes. Transfer the sturgeon to a side dish and let rest. Strain the broth into a side dish, discarding the aromatics. Wipe out the cazuela.

5 Mash the butter and thyme with a fork until well blended. Season with salt and pepper to taste. Set the thyme butter aside.

6 When the zucchini is ready, transfer it to the cazuela and keep warm. Heat the remaining 1 tablespoon oil in a conventional skillet and sear the fish over medium-high heat for 1 to 2 minutes per side to brown lightly. Arrange the sturgeon over the zucchini and cover with foil to keep warm. Pour the broth into the skillet and bring to a boil, scraping up any debris sticking to the pan. Add the thyme butter and capers and swirl to form an emulsion. Spoon over the sturgeon and zucchini and serve at once.

NOTES TO THE COOK:

✳ Before sautéing, make sure the sturgeon fillets are completely dry so they will brown nicely.

✳ Use only U.S.-farmed sturgeon or Columbia River wild-caught white sturgeon.

Poached Swordfish in the Style of Izmir

SERVES 4

Here's a superb clay-vessel rendering of the Black Sea style of cooking called *bugulama*—a method of poaching fish. A rich, poaching liquor of grated tomatoes, hot pepper, and cream is the cooking medium, with fresh oregano and freshly ground pepper added at the end.

This is another recipe I found at the restaurant Kasibeyaz, yielding one of the best swordfish dishes I've ever eaten—moist, succulent, and brightly flavored. Serve in the same clay vessel in which you've cooked it, accompanied by freshly baked flat bread (page 262).

> **PREFERRED CLAY POT:**
>
> A 9-inch Spanish cazuela
>
> If using an electric or ceramic stovetop, be sure to use a heat diffuser with the clay pot.

1 pound juicy ripe tomatoes, halved

1 pound swordfish, cut 1 inch thick

4 small garlic cloves, lightly bruised

1 Anaheim pepper, seeded, deribbed and finely chopped

2 tablespoons heavy cream

1 tablespoon unsalted butter

¾ teaspoon finely ground black pepper

1 teaspoon sea salt

½ teaspoon red wine vinegar

Pinch of Greek oregano

1 Use the large holes on a 4-sided box grater to shred the tomatoes into the cazuela. Discard the skins and stem.

2 Add the swordfish, garlic, Anaheim pepper, cream, butter, half the black pepper, the salt, and about ⅔ cup water, or enough to just cover the fish. Cover the cazuela with a sheet of aluminum foil and set it over medium heat. Slowly cook for 15 to 20 minutes, or until the swordfish is just opaque in the center but still juicy.

3 Remove from the heat, place the covered cazuela on a folded cloth napkin on the table, and let stand for a few minutes. Uncover, divide the fish into 4 serving pieces, and sprinkle with the remaining black pepper, vinegar, and oregano. Serve in shallow soup bowls, making sure everyone gets some of the tasty sauce.

NOTE TO THE COOK: Many people avoid swordfish these days, because of both pollution and overfishing. If you prefer, you can substitute sea bass, in which case the fish will probably take about 5 minutes less to cook.

Halibut Steaks Poached in Olive Oil with Mushrooms, Anchovies, and Capers

SERVES 2

½ ounce dried porcini or cèpes, crumbled

2 tablespoons salted capers, preferably from the island of Pantelleria

2 cups extra virgin olive oil

2 garlic cloves, bruised

1 fresh thyme sprig

¾ to 1 pound halibut steak, cut 1 inch thick

Sea salt

1 teaspoon crushed hot red pepper

8 oil-packed anchovy fillets, rinsed, patted dry, and coarsely chopped

2 tablespoons chopped fresh flat-leaf parsley

1 tablespoon fresh lemon juice

1 Soak the dried mushrooms in 1 cup warm water to cover for 20 minutes. Drain them, reserving the liquid. Rinse the mushrooms to rid them of any sand; then chop them finely. Strain the liquid through a paper filter to remove all sand. Separately, soak the capers in water for 20 minutes and drain.

2 Meanwhile, add the olive oil, garlic, and thyme to the cazuela and heat slowly to 200°F. Quickly rinse the halibut, pat dry, and slip into the oil. (The temperature of the oil will drop to about 175°F.) Poach the fish at this temperature for 12 minutes, or until the flesh just begins to flake along the edges. Transfer the cazuela from the heat to a wooden surface or folded kitchen towel to prevent cracking. Use a wide spatula to transfer the fish to a side dish. Lightly dust the fish with sea salt. Pour the poaching oil into a jar and set aside. Return the fish to the warm cazuela and cover loosely.

3 Transfer the garlic to a small conventional saucepan. Add the hot pepper, anchovies, and mushrooms along with their soaking liquid. Quickly boil over high heat until reduced by half, crushing the garlic and anchovies to a smooth paste. Reduce the heat to medium. Add the drained capers, parsley, and lemon juice and return to a boil. Enrich the sauce with 2 tablespoons of the poaching oil. Pour the sauce over the fish and serve at once.

NOTE TO THE COOK: Note that since the oil only briefly went above 175°F, it can be used again in a fish salad or for poaching more fish. It will keep for up to a week in a covered container in the refrigerator. If for any reason you notice an off smell, discard it.

Fresh Cod Roasted on a Bed of Potatoes with Olives

SERVES 4

The brilliance of this excellent Basque fish preparation resides in the composition of the marinade, a blend of olive oil, roasted red pepper, green olives, tomatoes, parsley, and thyme, and in the last-minute sprinkling of *piment d'Espelette,* a mildly sharp Spanish paprika that brightens all the flavors.

Use the freshest sweet, firm-fleshed fish you can find, preferably wild-caught. I suggest Pacific cod or halibut. The marinating takes place while you roast the potatoes (to be used as a blotter for the delicious fish juices) in a shallow earthenware pan. Serve this dish hot, with a crisp dry white wine.

PREFERRED CLAY POT:

A 10- or 11-inch Spanish cazuela or a flameware or Le Creuset stoneware baking dish

1½ pounds fresh white Pacific lingcod or black cod fillets, cut into 4 equal pieces (about 6 ounces each)

Sea salt and freshly ground black pepper

¼ cup plus 2 tablespoons extra virgin olive oil

1½ pounds large firm potatoes such as Yukon Gold

8 large garlic cloves, lightly bruised

1 jarred roasted red pepper, drained and chopped

18 green olives, such as picholine, pitted

½ cup chopped tomato

1½ teaspoons chopped fresh flat-leaf parsley

1½ teaspoons fresh thyme leaves

¼ teaspoon piment d'Espelette (Spanish paprika)

1 lemon, cut into wedges

1 Rinse and pat the fish thoroughly dry with paper towels. Toss the cod fillets with a light sprinkling of salt and pepper and 2 tablespoons of the olive oil. Refrigerate while you prepare the potatoes.

2 Meanwhile, set a rack in the upper third of the oven. Preheat the oven to 400°F. Use 1 tablespoon of the olive oil to coat the bottom of the cazuela.

3 Peel and slice the potatoes very thinly using a mandoline or the 2-millimeter blade of a food processor. Place the potatoes in the cazuela and toss them with the remaining ¼ cup olive oil, the garlic cloves, 1 teaspoon salt, and ½ teaspoon pepper. Spread out the slices in an even layer, press down gently to make them more compact, loosely cover with foil, and bake for 15 minutes. Use a wide spatula to turn the potatoes and garlic cloves over and continue to bake, loosely covered, for another 15 minutes.

4 Remove the foil. Scatter the roasted red bell pepper, olives, tomato, parsley, and thyme over the potatoes. Return to the oven and bake, uncovered, for 10 minutes longer.

5 Arrange the fish fillets in a single layer on top of the potatoes. Baste with the oil in the cazuela. Bake, uncovered, for 15 minutes, or until the fish is just opaque in the center. Sprinkle piment d'Espelette over the dish, garnish with lemon wedges, and serve directly from the cazuela.

Black Cod Baked on a Bed of Shredded Fennel

SERVES 4

In late summer and fall, when Alaskan black cod is at its best, I make an indoor version of this classic Provençal dish. Traditionally the fish is grilled outside over dried fennel branches. Instead I bake it over a bed of shredded fresh fennel in a closed clay pot. The moisture from the fennel steams the fish beautifully, creating an incredibly succulent, flaky texture.

> **PREFERRED CLAY POT:**
>
> A Romertopf fish baker or a 10-inch flameware or Le Creuset baking dish with a tight-fitting cover

1½ pounds black cod (sablefish), cut into 4 equal pieces

Salt and freshly ground black pepper

1 medium fennel bulb

2 tablespoons extra virgin olive oil

Juice of ½ lemon

2 tablespoons dry vermouth

¼ cup finely diced green bell pepper

¼ cup finely diced red bell pepper

2 teaspoons chopped fresh tarragon or 1 teaspoon dried

Pinch of cayenne or piment d'Espelette (Spanish paprika)

1 medium tomato, sliced

1 lemon, sliced

4 fresh tarragon sprigs for garnish

1 About 45 minutes before serving, soak the Romertopf baker in lukewarm water to cover for 10 minutes. (You do not need to soak the flameware or stoneware baking dish.) Season the fish lightly with salt and pepper and let stand for 10 minutes.

2 Meanwhile, rinse and trim the fennel. Shred the bulb on the large holes of a box grater or use the grating disk in a food processor. Wrap in a paper towel and press out excess moisture. You should have about 1 cup. Immediately toss the shredded fennel with the olive oil, lemon juice, and vermouth. Fold in the bell peppers, tarragon, and cayenne. Season with salt and pepper to taste.

3 Place the fennel mixture in the clay pot. Set the slices of fish on top and cover with slices of tomato and lemon. Season lightly with salt and pepper. Cover and set in a cold oven. (If using a baking dish, wrap the fennel and fish in parchment paper and fit into the pot and cover.) Set the temperature at 475°F and bake for 30 minutes. If using the baking dish, bake in a preheated 375°F oven for 20 minutes.

4 Remove the pot from the oven and place on a wooden surface or folded kitchen towel to prevent cracking. Uncover, baste the fish with the pan juices, and decorate with tarragon sprigs. Serve at once, directly from the pot.

BASQUE SALT COD WITH SIMMERING OLIVE OIL

Early in his career, David Kinch, chef-owner of the fabulous Manresa Restaurant in Los Gatos, California, spent six months working in the Akelare restaurant in the Spanish Basque country not far from San Sebastián. He told me that from this experience he learned a lot about cooking fish in clay casseroles, which he believes to this day is one of the best uses for a clay vessel.

I was particularly intrigued by his description of simmering salt cod in olive oil (*bacalao al pil pil*—*pil pil* meaning "soft bubbling") in a special two-handled, unglazed clay vessel shaped something like a wok. David told me how he learned to swirl this vessel so that the olive oil and protein-rich gelatin exuded from the salt cod skin emulsified into a thick, creamy white sauce, similar to the way oil blends with egg in a mayonnaise.

Resolving to try his recipe, I set about to find the proper clay vessel and salt cod with its skin on, since that is an essential element for the dish. I found a two-handled, unglazed clay vessel made by Pomaireware (www.kitchendance.com) and skin-on loin of salt cod (www.latienda.com). The loin, by the way, is a particularly delicious part of the cod, which produces beautiful white flakes when cooked.

I tried the dish a few times with fairly decent results but decided not to include a detailed recipe here since I couldn't perfect it and also couldn't justify asking readers to acquire yet another single-purpose clay pot. However, your total clay pot–junkie author is now on the lookout for still another clay cooking device! Basque-born and Madrid-based chef Carlos Posada told me he makes *bacalao al pil pil* using an electric machine that continually swirls a clay vessel filled with fish and gently bubbling oil over heat, producing a magnificently thick, mayonnaiselike sauce.

Stuffed Baby Squid Lungiana Style

SERVES 4

This is one of my favorite ways to prepare small squid. The method occurred to me while I was reading a book on the cooking of Lungiana, an area near the seacoast of northern Tuscany. Here small flying squid called *totani* are stuffed with their chopped tentacles mixed with soaked bread crumbs, chopped mortadella, slivered pancetta, and some powerful fresh Mediterranean marjoram and then simmered in a deep flavorful tomato sauce.

I use small calamari from Monterey, California, which come cleaned with the tentacles on the side. My version creates extra stuffing on purpose. After filling the calamari, I form the remaining savory stuffing into little cakes, which I then quickly flour and fry in olive oil. These are added to the stuffed calamari in a shallow terra-cotta casserole and cooked slowly for about an hour. You can make the dish a few hours in advance; it reheats well.

PREFERRED CLAY POT:

An 11- or 12-inch Spanish cazuela or flameware skillet

If using an electric or ceramic stovetop, be sure to use a large heat diffuser with the clay pot.

12 baby calamari, cleaned, pouches and tentacles separated

1 cup diced fresh bread

¼ cup milk

3 ounces mortadella

3 ounces pancetta, thinly sliced

3 ounces freshly grated Parmigiano-Reggiano cheese

1 small onion, coarsely chopped

1 medium onion, chopped

2 garlic cloves, chopped

2 tablespoons coarsely chopped fresh flat-leaf parsley

2½ teaspoons coarsely chopped fresh marjoram

½ teaspoon freshly grated nutmeg

Salt and freshly ground black pepper

1 egg

¼ cup plus 3 tablespoons extra virgin olive oil

½ cup dry white wine at room temperature

4 tomatoes (about 1 pound), halved, seeded, and grated

2 to 3 tablespoons all-purpose flour

Torn leaves of fresh flat-leaf parsley and marjoram for garnish

1   Early in the day, rinse and drain the calamari. Leave the pouches whole. Place the tentacles in a food processor and pulse twice to chop coarsely. Meanwhile, moisten the diced bread with the milk. Add the bread, mortadella, pancetta, Parmigiano-Reggiano, small onion, half the garlic and parsley, 1 teaspoon of the marjoram, the nutmeg, ½ teaspoon salt, ¼ teaspoon pepper, and the egg. Pulse until all the ingredients are finely chopped and well blended but not ground to a paste. Cover and refrigerate the stuffing for 1 hour.

2   Heat ¼ cup of the olive oil in the cazuela over medium heat. Add the medium onion and the rest of the garlic and parsley and cook, stirring, until the onion is very soft, about 10 minutes. Pour in the wine and cook until it evaporates, after about 5 minutes, then add the grated tomatoes, remaining 1½ teaspoons marjoram, ¼ teaspoon salt, and a pinch of pepper. Simmer the tomato sauce for 30 minutes.

3   Meanwhile, fill each calamari pouch firmly with stuffing. Roll the remaining ground mixture into 1-inch patties. Thoroughly dry the pouches. Heat the remaining 3 tablespoons olive oil in a large metal skillet over medium-high heat. Add the stuffed calamari and sauté, turning, until golden all over, about 5 minutes. Transfer to a side dish.

4   Dust the calamari patties with flour and fry in the skillet until golden brown on both sides, about 5 minutes.

5   Add the stuffed calamari and the patties to the tomato sauce, cover, and cook until they are completely tender, about 45 minutes. Set the hot cazuela on a wooden surface or folded kitchen towel to prevent cracking. Garnish with torn parsley and marjoram and serve right from the pot.

Ligurian Shellfish Amphora

SERVES 6

An amphora is a tall oval clay pot with handles on both sides, used since ancient times as a cooking or storage vessel. Australian-based scientist and foodie Adam Balic gave me this great recipe for a Ligurian shellfish dish prepared in an amphora, which he first tasted at the harbor restaurant La Lanterna in Riomaggiore in the Italian Cinque Terre region. The dish is made with whatever shellfish happen to be available, but it contains no fish. Common ingredients are langoustines, shrimp, cuttlefish, squid, clams, and mussels.

The shellfish, seasoned with tomato, wine, and spices, are packed into a clay amphora and marinated at room temperature for an hour before the vessel is sealed with a flour and water paste and popped into a very hot oven. It bakes for twenty to thirty minutes—just long enough for the shellfish to cook through but not to stew and toughen.

The material used for this particular clay amphora is not earthenware but a harder, more vitreous material, closer to stoneware, to resist breakage at high temperature. Lacking an amphora? See suggested substitutes below and omit sealing the pot with flour and water.

> **PREFERRED CLAY POT:**
> A 3-quart flameware or Le Creuset stoneware casserole with a tight-fitting cover suitable for use in an oven heated to 450°F

8 ounces squid, cleaned

8 ounces large scallops, preferably dry diver scallops

8 ounces large or jumbo shrimp, shells on

1 pound mussels

1 pound clams

2 teaspoons Turkish or Aleppo pepper

2 teaspoons freshly ground white pepper

½ teaspoon Mediterranean oregano

Pinch of saffron threads

⅔ cup pine nuts

2 salted anchovy fillets, cleaned, rinsed, and chopped (optional)

1 cup fish stock

½ cup Pinot Grigio or other dry white wine

⅓ cup extra virgin olive oil

2 medium tomatoes, peeled, seeded, and sliced

1 teaspoon sea salt

1 Preheat the oven to 450°F. Rinse the squid, scallops, shrimp, mussels, and clams in cold water. You should have about 2 quarts of shellfish.

2 In a large bowl, toss the seafood with the red pepper, white pepper, oregano, saffron, pine nuts, anchovies, fish stock, wine, olive oil, tomatoes, and salt. Pack into the clay pot, place a sheet of parchment paper directly over the shellfish, cover with a lid, and set in the oven.

3 Bake for 25 minutes. Remove the pot from the oven and place on a wooden surface or folded kitchen towel to prevent cracking. Serve directly from the pot.

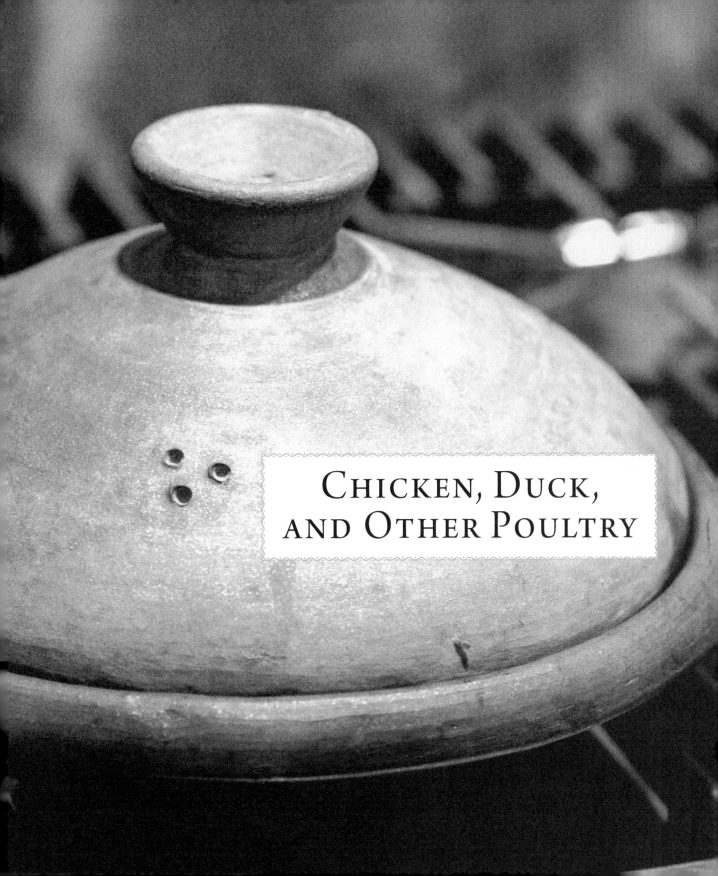

CHICKEN, DUCK, AND OTHER POULTRY

Notes on Roast Chicken

Choosing a Chicken for Roasting

The quality of a chicken is especially important when cooking in clay. Chickens are labeled so many different ways that choosing the best available can be confusing. Here are some grades and brands available at retail locations nationwide that I particularly trust: European-style air-dried or air-chilled chickens; brands such as Bell & Evans, Smart Chickens, and Maverick Ranch Chickens, as well as 100-percent certified organic and free-range chickens. (The problem with so-called "all natural" chickens is that the USDA allows up to 15 percent saltwater processing and all kinds of feed. Always check the label to ensure there's been no saltwater processing, which dilutes flavor and adds weight to the bird.) Kosher chicken is a good safe choice, but remember not to salt it as it has already been subjected to a mild salt brine.

Preparing a Chicken for Roasting

Except when I'm using a kosher chicken, I use the presalting technique espoused by Chef Judy Rodgers of the Zuni Café in San Francisco: Pat the bird dry all over. Salt the chicken inside and out using 1 teaspoon coarse salt for every 1½ pounds of chicken. Refrigerate uncovered on a paper towel–lined rack for at least one and up to two days.

Please note: Large roaster chickens (as opposed to broiler-fryers) require less seasoning, because they have naturally developed deeper, richer flavors due to age and feed.

Carlo Middione's Gypsy-Style Clay-Wrapped Chicken

SERVES 4

My friends Barbara and Jon Beckmann described a chicken wrapped in clay that they ate in the 1960s in a Madrid, Spain restaurant: "It was an upscale place on Plaza Mayor, and it was pure theater." Jon told me, "They brought this mass of baked clay out to the table, gave Barbara a silver mallet, and told her to break it open. Soon as she did we were hit by the wonderful aroma of chicken, truffles, foie gras, thyme, and cognac. The chicken was moist, skinless, and superb."

I've often baked a chicken encrusted in salt, a method that produces beautifully moist and intensely flavored chicken flesh. But ever since I heard this story I've wanted to learn how to cook a chicken encased in clay. So I consulted my friend Terrie Chrones, a culinary historian and writer from Oregon, who demonstrates the process in her children's hands-on ceramics classes.

"I use low-fire clay," Terrie confirmed, "which I have the kids roll out into half-inch slabs. We line one slab with romaine, place a chicken breast on it, cover with another romaine leaf, and top that with another slab. Then we seal the clay and place it in a 350°F oven. Cooking time varies depending on the thickness of the meat and the amount of moisture in the clay. It always works, and the kids adore it!"

Were those my choices—an haute-cuisine truffled chicken cooked in clay as at a fancy Madrid restaurant or one cooked by kids in a ceramics workshop? I was pondering this when I ran into an old friend, San Francisco restaurateur and cookbook author Carlo Middione. Learning of my interest, he offered to come to my house and demonstrate a gypsy-style recipe for wrapping and roasting an entire chicken in raw clay.

He arrived with rolling pin, bag of clay, and packets of seasoning. As expected, these were very Italian: crushed juniper berries, sage, pancetta, garlic, and heavenly fragrant olive oil. When Carlo finished seasoning and wrapping the chicken, separated from the clay by a barrier of butcher's paper, he sculpted out a chicken head and tail and added them to the ends—a nice whimsical touch.

When the roasting was finished and he cracked open the clay wrap, the aroma was wonderful. Because the chicken had steamed inside the clay, its flesh was incredibly well flavored and smooth as cream. Even though the skin wasn't crisp, it was one of the best roast chickens I had ever eaten.

Here is Carlo's version of *pollo alla zingara*, highly recommended to you "gypsies" out there like me, for whom even a delicious clay vessel–roasted chicken is not sufficient. Do try it; go all the way with clay!

(continued)

1 whole frying chicken (about 3 pounds), preferably organic

2 large garlic cloves, peeled

2 tablespoons juniper berries

4 large branches fresh sage leaves

1 large bay leaf, crumbled

1 teaspoon coarse sea salt

½ teaspoon freshly ground black pepper

3 tablespoons extra virgin olive oil

3 ounces thinly sliced pancetta, shredded

1 whole lemon, pierced all over with the tip of a knife

1 Bring the chicken to room temperature. Crush together the garlic, juniper berries, sage, bay leaf, salt, and pepper with a mortar and pestle, or use an electric spice grinder. Add the olive oil and two-thirds of the pancetta and mash to blend well. Rub half of this seasoning paste all over the bird. Slip the rest into the cavity along with the remaining pancetta and the pierced lemon. If you want a compact shape, truss the bird with white kitchen string. Wrap the chicken in 2 sheets of parchment. Bring up the long sides of the paper to meet at the top, then press together and fold down snug to the top of the breast. If the bird is too large to fit easily, bring up the short ends. Just be sure the entire chicken is enclosed in the paper. Fold and tuck the ends to make a tight and secure closure. Set the chicken aside.

2 With a heavy rolling pin, roll out the moist ceramic clay between 2 sheets of parchment or brown butcher's paper into an oval shape about ½ inch thick and wide enough to completely encase the chicken. Alternatively, you can make 2 smaller sheets of clay, one for the top and one for the bottom of the bird; but if you do so, be sure you seal them together completely. Poke one small hole somewhere in the top or top third of the clay to prevent possible cracking or breaking. It also makes a good test site for checking the internal temperature. Use more clay, if you like, to fashion a decorative chicken head and tail on the outside. Set the clay chicken on a sheet pan to support it and contain any juices that might leak out.

3 Set the chicken in the bottom third of a cold oven. Set the temperature at 450°F. Bake for 1½ to 2 hours, or until the internal temperature of the chicken registers 165°F. Remove from the oven and let stand for 15 minutes.

4 Gently crack open the clay with a hammer or other blunt instrument. Carefully remove as much clay as possible to expose the parchment-wrapped chicken. Unwrap the chicken to expose it completely; then transfer it to a cutting board or platter. Carve and serve hot, spooning any juices from the paper or carving board over the chicken.

NOTES TO THE COOK:

❋ A barrier between clay and chicken is important, since direct contact is messy when the clay wrap is broken open. I prefer parchment or butcher's paper, but some cooks have had good results with grape leaves and romaine.

❋ Carlo suggests starting the chicken in a cold oven to keep the clay from splitting.

CARLO'S CHICKEN ROASTED IN A ROMAN POT

Credit is given to both the Etruscans and the Romans for inventing the type of clay cooking vessel called a "Roman Pot," re-created for use by contemporary cooks in the form of a wonderfully useful, fitted, unglazed, earthenware top-and-bottom set sold under the trademarked name Romertopf.

Use the same ingredients as for Carlo Middione's Gypsy-Style Clay-Wrapped Chicken on page 73, but you won't need the special equipment. You will need for a 3½- or 4-pound chicken and a Romertopf baker, 3 to 5 pounds. This porous pot (top and bottom) must first be soaked in water and then drained before each use The chicken is placed in the baker, breast side up. Then the pot is closed and set in a cold oven. The general rule for roasting a medium-size chicken in a Roman Pot is to raise the oven temperature by 100°F and to decrease the cooking time by about 15 minutes. Set the temperature at 475°F and bake for 1 hour. Remove the cover and continue to bake the chicken until the skin is crisp and golden brown and the internal temperature is 165°F, 10 minutes longer.

Transfer the clay pot to a wooden surface. Lift out the chicken and tilt to drain the juices into a saucepan. Let the chicken rest for 5 to 10 minutes before carving. Meanwhile, skim as much fat as possible from the top of the juices and boil them down to a syrupy sauce. Carve the chicken, sprinkle lightly with salt and pepper, and serve with the reduced sauce.

Romertopf Clay-Baked Chicken Stuffed with Serrano Ham and Olives

SERVES 4

Slivers of cured country ham and chopped mildly pungent Manzanilla olives are a popular combination in Spanish recipes. Here the blend makes a wonderful stuffing for a chicken baked in a Romertopf pot, the combined flavors steaming and infusing the chicken as it roasts. As in the previous recipe, remove the cover of the Romertopf in the final stage of baking to obtain a crispy skin.

> **PREFERRED CLAY POT:**
>
> **A Romertopf clay baker, 3 to 5 pounds**

1 frying chicken with liver (3½ to 4 pounds), preferably organic

Salt and freshly ground black pepper

2 teaspoons chopped garlic

3 tablespoons extra virgin olive oil

1 medium onion, chopped

⅓ cup pitted and chopped green olives, preferably Manzanilla

3 ounces sliced Serrano ham, slivered

1 cup cubed stale bread without crust

¼ cup chopped fresh flat-leaf parsley

Pinch of freshly grated nutmeg

1 egg

2 celery ribs, sliced

1 carrot, sliced

1 leek, sliced

1 tablespoon brandy

1 tablespoon sherry vinegar

1 One to 2 days before you plan to roast the chicken, rinse it well inside and out and pat dry with paper towels. Cut off the wing tips and neck and chop them into small pieces. Slip your fingers under the skin of the thighs and breasts and gently separate from the meat to create an air pocket without tearing the skin. Combine pinches of salt and pepper with half of the chopped garlic and 1 tablespoon of the olive oil and insert into these pockets, massaging the seasonings into the flesh. Season the cavity and skin with more salt and pepper. Wrap the chicken in paper towels and refrigerate, uncovered, along with the chopped wing tips and neck, overnight.

2 Also in advance, rinse the chicken liver, pat dry, and coarsely chop. Heat the remaining 2 tablespoons olive oil in a medium conventional skillet. Add the onion and remaining garlic and cook over medium heat, stirring, until soft and golden, about 7 minutes. Add the liver, olives, and ham and cook for 3 minutes longer. Stir in the bread, parsley, nutmeg, and ½ teaspoon pepper, and cook until the bread is partially crisp here and there, about 3 minutes longer. Remove from the heat and let cool completely. Add the egg and blend well. Cover the stuffing and refrigerate.

3 Bring the chicken and stuffing to room temperature. About 2 hours before serving, soak the unglazed clay pot bottom and lid in cold water to cover for 15 minutes. Meanwhile, stuff the chicken. Drain the clay pot. Put the chopped neck and wing tips, the celery, carrot, and leek in the bottom of the clay pot. Lay the chicken, breast side up, on top. Season with salt and pepper. Sprinkle the brandy, vinegar, and 2 tablespoons water over the chicken. Cover the pot and place in a cold oven. Set the temperature at 475°F and bake for 1 hour.

4 Remove the pot from the oven and place on a wooden surface or folded kitchen towel to prevent cracking. Put the lid on another kitchen towel. Transfer the chicken to a work surface. Strain the juices into a conventional skillet, skim off the fat, and boil down to a syrupy sauce. Meanwhile, place a wire cake rack over the bottom of the pot, place the chicken on the rack, and return it uncovered, to the oven to finish roasting, until an instant-read thermometer registers 165°F and the skin is nicely browned, about 10 minutes.

5 Transfer the baker to a wooden surface or folded kitchen towel to prevent cracking. Let the chicken rest for 10 minutes; then transfer it to a carving board and cut into serving pieces. Be sure to include some of the stuffing and a spoonful of the reduced sauce with each portion.

Romertopf Clay-Baked Chicken with Fromage Blanc, Tarragon, and Tomatoes

SERVES 4

Generations of Provençal cooks have employed the combination of cheese, tarragon, and tomatoes to flavor chicken. The trick is to choose a type of moist cheese that will generate sufficient steam from the cavity to drive the tarragon and tomato flavors into the meat. I generally use a French-style skim-milk cheese called *fromage blanc,* which is moist, flavorful, and low in fat. You can substitute well-drained thickened yogurt, low-fat ricotta, or good-quality cream cheese.

PREFERRED CLAY POT:

A Romertopf clay baker, 3 to 5 pounds

1 frying chicken with liver (3 to 3½ pounds), preferably organic

Salt and freshly ground black pepper

1 teaspoon chopped garlic

3 tablespoons unsalted butter at room temperature

4 ounces fromage blanc or other French-style skim-milk cheese

1 tablespoon chopped fresh tarragon

1 tablespoon tomato paste, canned or homemade (page 317)

(continued)

1 Rinse the chicken inside and out and dry with paper towels. Reserve the liver for the stuffing; save the neck and giblets for stock or some other use. Slip your fingers under the skin of the thighs and breasts and gently separate from the meat to create an air pocket without tearing the skin. Combine pinches of salt and pepper and the chopped garlic with 1 tablespoon of the butter. Insert pinches of this mixture under the skin and massage into the flesh. Season the cavity and the skin with salt and pepper, wrap the chicken in paper towels, and refrigerate. Chop the chicken liver. Mash it with the cheese; then blend with salt and pepper, half the chopped tarragon, and the tomato paste. Set aside until ready to stuff the chicken.

2 About 2 hours before serving, soak the top and bottom of a medium clay baker in water for 15 minutes. Stuff the chicken with the mixture and close the opening with white kitchen string. Rub the outside of the chicken with the remaining 2 tablespoons butter and season generously with salt and pepper. Place the chicken, breast side up, in the baker, cover, and set in a cold oven. Turn the temperature to 475°F and bake until the chicken is almost tender, about 1 hour.

3 Remove the clay pot from the oven and place on a wooden surface or folded kitchen towel to prevent cracking. Put the lid on another kitchen towel. Tilt the pot and strain the pan juices into a medium skillet. Skim the fat off the top and reserve the juices.

4 Set a wire cake rack over the bottom of the clay pot, place the chicken on top, and return to the oven to finish roasting, uncovered, until an instant-read thermometer registers 165°F and the skin is nicely browned, 10 to 15 minutes. Transfer the clay baker to a wooden surface or folded kitchen towel to prevent cracking and let rest for 10 minutes.

5 Remove the cheese stuffing from the chicken and add it to the juices in the skillet, whisking to blend. Bring to a boil and continue to cook until the sauce is reduced by half. Add the remaining tarragon and season with salt and pepper to taste. Cook, stirring, for 1 minute longer. Carve the chicken, arrange on a serving platter, and pour the sauce over the chicken pieces.

Stoneware Beer Can–Chicken Baked with an Italian Rub

SERVES 4

Tom Wirt of Clay Coyote Potters makes a great, beautifully glazed ceramic "beer can" roaster—his clay, oven-proof, takeoff on the popular method of cooking a chicken over an open half-filled beer can is, in my opinion, far superior. In this recipe, the large quantity of juniper berries used to rub the chicken adds a complex flavor.

> **PREFERRED CLAY POT:**
>
> **A stoneware beer can–style chicken roaster**

1 frying chicken (3½ to 4 pounds), preferably organic

3 garlic cloves

1 tablespoon juniper berries

2 teaspoons coarse salt

1 teaspoon dried oregano

½ teaspoon black peppercorns

2 cloves

2 bay leaves

3 tablespoons extra virgin olive oil, rendered duck fat, or clarified butter

1 small lemon, sliced

1 Rinse the chicken inside and out and pat dry with paper towels. Place on a rack over paper towels and refrigerate, uncovered.

2 Use a heavy pestle to pound the garlic, juniper berries, salt, oregano, peppercorns, cloves, and bay leaves to a paste in a mortar. Or blend to a puree in an electric grinder. Blend in the olive oil. Slip your fingers under the skin of the thighs and breasts and gently separate from the meat to create an air pocket without tearing the skin. Insert pinches of this mixture under the skin of the chicken and massage into the flesh. Use the remaining mixture to season the cavity and the skin. Slip the lemon slices into the cavity.

3 Preheat the oven to 350°F. Bring the chicken to room temperature. Fill the "beer can" about two-thirds full with water and the juice of 1 lemon. Seat the chicken so its legs straddle the "beer can." Bake, uncovered, for about 1½ hours.

4 To remove the chicken, carefully lift the bird off its stand so the juices in the cavity run into the bowl. Transfer the chicken to a cutting board and let rest for 5 to 10 minutes before carving. Meanwhile, degrease the juices in the bowl, pour them into a conventional skillet, and quickly boil them down until reduced by half. Correct the seasoning and serve with the carved bird.

Chicken Roasted on a Clay Cone with Vanilla Mustard Sauce

SERVES 4

Cooking a small chicken on a slowly revolving spit will, if basted regularly, produce an evenly roasted bird with moist, velvety flesh and wonderfully crisp skin. But there are a number of other ways to obtain the same result, especially with clay. One way is to roast the chicken in an upright position so it will self-baste as the fat flows downward. There are a number of excellent devices for doing this, including various metal cones, though I think these carry heat too quickly to the cavity of these small birds, searing in both chicken juices (good) and fat (bad).

The ceramic cones I use carry heat gently and efficiently into the cavity. Thus they become heating elements that encourage the chicken to exude fat for self-basting while slowly sealing the cavity walls, allowing the bird's juices to circulate throughout the flesh. Some of these devices have bottom plates attached to catch the drippings; those that don't can be set in a shallow baking dish filled with a small amount of water or coarse salt, which will greatly reduce spattering in a hot oven by attracting the fat.

Among the standing chicken ceramic cone vertical roasters that I favor are the Romertopf stoneware chicken roaster; the Early Morning Pottery CeramiCooker, and the French earthenware cone called a Cocorico, popularized by Napa Valley chef Michael Chiarello. Michael suggests roasting your chicken upside down, an unusual technique based on the notion that since chicken legs takes longer to cook

than the breast and since heat rises in a home oven, you can take advantage of the rising hot air to obtain a more evenly cooked bird. Even though an upside-down chicken looks kind of silly, I like Michael's method. When I roast a fryer chicken that way, I can more easily add extra flavor enhancers, such as quartered lemons, garlic, and herbs, to the cavity.

I like to serve a strong-flavored sauce, such as Provençal Vanilla Mustard Sauce (page 81), with roasted fryer chickens.

> **PREFERRED CLAY POT:**
>
> A stoneware vertical cooker, such as Early Morning Pottery CeramiCooker, Romertopf stoneware chicken roaster, or NapaStyle Cocorico

1 frying chicken (3 to 3½ pounds), preferably organic

Coarse salt and freshly ground black pepper

1 teaspoon chopped garlic plus 4 to 5 whole garlic cloves, peeled

2 tablespoons olive oil, duck fat, or clarified butter

1 small lemon, quartered

Vanilla Mustard Sauce (recipe follows)

1 Bring the chicken to room temperature. Rinse it inside and out and pat dry with paper towels. Slip your fingers under the skin of the thighs and breasts and gently separate from the meat to create an air pocket without tearing the skin. Combine ½ teaspoon coarse salt and ¼ teaspoon pepper and the chopped garlic with 1 tablespoon of the olive oil. Insert pinches of this mixture under the skin of the chicken and massage into the flesh. Season the cavity with more salt and pepper. Pull back the skin on the upper back and cut out about 1½ inches of the neck bone. Cut off the wings at the first joint. Reserve the neck, backbones, and wing tips for the sauce.

2   Stand the chicken up (or upside down) on a ceramic roasting cone; it doesn't need to be pushed too far down, but be sure to leave some space between the breast of the chicken and the surrounding mat. Stuff the cavity with the lemon quarters and whole garlic cloves tossed with a little of the remaining olive oil. Thoroughly dry the skin with paper towels. Rub the outside with the rest of the fat and sprinkle with 1 teaspoon coarse salt.

3   With a rack positioned on the lowest rung, preheat the oven to 400°F. Place the chicken in the oven and roast until an instant-read thermometer set deep into the inner thigh reaches 165°F, 45 to 60 minutes. Or follow the directions that come with the ceramic cone you are using.

4   Transfer the chicken on the cone to a double layer of kitchen towels and let rest for a few minutes before moving the chicken to a carving board. Let stand for 5 to 10 minutes longer before carving. Serve with the Vanilla Mustard Sauce.

Vanilla Mustard Sauce

MAKES ABOUT 1½ CUPS

Prepare the sauce while the chicken is roasting in the oven.

2 cups chopped wings, neck, and trimmed bones reserved from the chicken

Salt and freshly ground black pepper

2 tablespoons unsalted butter

1 cup dry white wine, preferably fumé blanc

¼ vanilla bean, split

½ cup rich chicken stock or 1 cup chicken stock reduced to ½ cup

1 tablespoon grainy Dijon mustard

1 teaspoon cornstarch

1   Thoroughly dry the chopped chicken parts and season with salt and pepper. In a medium nonreactive conventional skillet or shallow saucepan, slowly melt 1 tablespoon of the butter over medium-low heat until it turns light brown. Immediately add the chicken and cook, stirring until lightly browned, about 4 minutes. Add the wine and vanilla bean and bring to a boil. Reduce the heat to low and simmer until the wine is reduced by two-thirds, about 20 minutes.

2   Add the stock, bring to a boil, reduce the heat slightly, and simmer until reduced by half. Strain and discard the chicken parts and vanilla bean. Return the stock to the saucepan. Whisk in the mustard and simmer for 10 minutes. Strain again, pressing down on the mustard grains. Let cool. (The sauce can be prepared to this point up to 30 minutes in advance. Cover and set aside; then skim off the butter that rises to the top of the sauce.)

3   To thicken the sauce, combine the remaining 1 tablespoon butter with the cornstarch. Add to the sauce and return to a boil, stirring constantly. The sauce should be shiny and thick enough to coat a spoon lightly. Correct the seasoning with salt and pepper.

NOTE TO THE COOK: I use Edmund Fallot's mustards. Pommery is another good choice. Both have a rounder, cleaner flavor than most brands.

Chicken Stuffed with Garlic Croutons Roasted over a Bed of Salt

SERVES 4

*H*ere's my method for high-temperature roasted chicken. Unlike the previous two recipes, in which the chicken is cooked standing up on a clay insert in an ordinary oven at medium-high temperature, this procedure roasts the chicken in a hot clay oven environment. A common problem with high-temperature chicken cookery is fat spattering, obviated here by roasting over a bed of salt, which attracts the fat and makes cleaning up a cinch. I recommend a heavy-duty metal roasting pan with a metal rack, since high heat may crack a clay vessel. However, if you have a stoneware or flameware baking dish suitable for use in an oven heated up to 500°F, by all means use it.

Here the clay oven environment heats up for an hour, steadies and evens out the heat, providing wonderful crispy skin and delectable juicy flesh. The results are similar to what happens in a hearth oven. A custom brick oven is costly, but you can use two FibraMent baking stones or, even less expensive, two stoneware pizza slabs. The most economical route is to use thick, unglazed quarry tiles or food-safe fire bricks. Whether using slabs, stones, or bricks, place one on the top rack of the oven and the other on the bottom rack for even heat.

> **SUGGESTED CLAY ENVIRONMENT:**
> **Double slabs of pizza stones or food-safe quarry tiles set on the upper and lower oven racks**

1 frying chicken (3½ to 4 pounds), preferably organic and free-range or air-chilled

Coarse sea salt

2 cups kosher salt

¼ teaspoon freshly ground black pepper

1 tablespoon rendered duck fat or extra-virgin olive oil or 2 tablespoons unsalted butter

3 to 4 slices country-style bread, cut ¼ inch thick, crusts removed

½ teaspoon chopped garlic

1 Preferably a day or two before roasting, rinse the chicken and pat dry with paper towels. Remove and discard any large chunks of fat. Reserve the giblets and neck for some other purpose. Liberally season the chicken with about 1 tablespoon coarse sea salt. Place the chicken on a cake rack or V-rack over paper towels and refrigerate, uncovered, for up to 2 days.

2 About 2 hours before you plan to serve, take the chicken on the rack from the refrigerator. Make a bed of kosher salt in a shallow conventional roasting pan. Set a lightly oiled cake rack on top and place in the oven. Set the temperature at 500°F.

3 Slip your fingers under the skin of the thighs and breasts and gently separate from the meat to create an air pocket without tearing the skin. Combine ½ teaspoon sea salt with the pepper and duck fat. Insert this mixture into the pockets under the skin of the chicken breast and rub into the flesh. Let the chicken come to room temperature. Meanwhile, prepare the stuffing.

4   Tear the bread into small pieces; mix with the chopped garlic. Slip the garlic and bread into the cavity of the chicken. Sew up the opening, but do not tie the legs together. Gently press down on the breasts with the heels of your hands to flatten it a little. Fold the wings under the chicken. Pat the skin dry with paper towels. Do not apply any fat to the skin.

5   About 1 hour before serving, slide the chicken, breast side down, onto the heated rack and roast for 20 minutes. Turn the chicken over and continue to roast until the chicken is golden brown and crisp and the internal temperature reaches 165°F, 20 to 25 minutes longer.

6   Transfer the chicken to a carving board and let rest for 10 minutes. Then scoop out the stuffing, carve the chicken, and arrange both on a platter. Drizzle any juices from the cavity of the chicken over the meat. Serve at once.

NOTE TO THE COOK: Barbara Kafka, author of the splendid *Roasting: A Simple Art,* provides a really helpful tip for lifting and handling a roast chicken filled with good chicken juices. She writes: "Remove the chicken to a platter by placing a large wooden spoon into the tail end and balancing the chicken with a kitchen spoon pressed against the crop end. As you lift the chicken, tilt it over the roasting pan so that all the juices run out of the cavity and into the pan." In this recipe, simply set a saucepan next to the roasting pan in order to catch the juices.

Special thanks to food writer Sam Gugino, who suggested using a salt bed to control excessive fat splattering when roasting a chicken at a high temperature.

Chicken Thighs Roasted on a Bed of Salt in the Style of the French Alps

SERVES 2 TO 4

In this recipe, which I adapted from *Cuisine et Fêtes dans Les Alpes du Sud* by Jean-Jacques de Corcelles, chicken thighs are seasoned with pepper and a pinch of salt, rolled in chopped wild thyme, wrapped separately in a thin round of pancetta, tied up with string, and then roasted in a shallow flameware or ovenproof stoneware dish. The result is delicious silky, moist chicken thighs. Half-pound chicken thighs will roast in about 20 minutes.

PREFERRED CLAY POT:

An 11-inch flameware skillet or a 9½-inch Le Creuset stoneware oval baking dish suitable for use in an oven heated to 500°F

---

2 to 2½ cups kosher salt

4 large chicken thighs (2 pounds), preferably organic

½ teaspoon salt

¼ teaspoon freshly ground black pepper

1 tablespoon fresh thyme leaves

2 ounces pancetta, sliced paper thin

1 Make a bed of the kosher salt in the skillet. Set a lightly oiled cake rack on top and place in the oven on the upper middle rack. Set the temperature at 500°F and allow the oven to preheat.

2 Meanwhile, season the chicken thighs with the salt, pepper, and thyme. Wrap them in the pancetta slices and tie with white kitchen string.

3 Remove the hot skillet from the oven and place on a wooden surface or folded kitchen towel. Arrange the chicken thighs, side by side, on the hot rack and quickly return the skillet to the oven for 10 minutes.

4 Turn each thigh over and continue roasting for another 10 minutes. Serve at once.

Hearth-Roasted Chicken with Moroccan Flavors

SERVES 4

*M*oroccan chickens are often spit roasted or sent to the local community oven to be baked at higher temperatures than a home oven could provide. The greater heat imparts better flavor, texture, and juiciness. You can provide almost the same atmosphere by rigging your own clay environment. This recipe employs a typical seasoning from northern Morocco. What makes this dish taste special is the addition of *smen,* North African preserved butter.

> **SUGGESTED CLAY ENVIRONMENT:**
> Double layer of pizza stones or food-safe quarry tiles set on the upper and lower oven racks

1 frying chicken (3½ to 4 pounds), preferably organic

2 garlic cloves

Coarse salt

1½ to 2 tablespoons clarified butter

1 tablespoon smen (page 295) or 1 more tablespoon clarified butter

1 or 2 scallions (white and 2 inches of green), finely chopped

1 teaspoon ground coriander

1 teaspoon sweet paprika

1 teaspoon freshly ground black pepper

Pinch of saffron threads

Pinch of cayenne

2 tablespoons chopped fresh flat-leaf parsley

1 lemon, quartered

1 Fit the oven with the clay environment and preheat the oven to 450°F for 1 hour.

2 Rinse the chicken inside and out; pat dry with paper towels. Remove all the fat from the cavity. Crush the garlic with 1 teaspoon coarse salt. Gently heat the clarified butter and *smen* in a small conventional saucepan over low heat. Add the scallions, crushed garlic, coriander, paprika, black pepper, saffron, cayenne, parsley, and an extra pinch of salt. Remove from the heat and mix well with a wooden spoon. Coat the chicken inside and out with this seasoned butter. Slip the lemon quarters into the cavity and let the chicken stand for 30 minutes, or just long enough to firm up the butter coating.

3 Place the chicken in a shallow roasting pan and set in the oven with the legs pointing to the rear. Roast for 30 minutes.

4 Turn off the oven and let the chicken continue to cook in the receding heat until an instant-read thermometer registers 165°F, about 15 minutes longer.

5 Remove the chicken from the oven and let rest for 10 minutes before carving. Squeeze the juice from the lemon quarters in the cavity over the chicken and serve at once.

Fried Spatchcocked Chicken

SERVES 2

A perfect example of how good food tastes when cooked in contact with clay is this ancient Etruscan recipe for a boned and flattened (i.e., butterflied) chicken cooked Tuscan style. It is called *pollo mattone,* in reference to the equipment used to cook it: a pair of heavy clay disks, the bottom one a glazed shallow rimmed saucer and the top unglazed and fitted with a handy knob. The top weighs the chicken down, which evens out the cooking, allowing the thighs and legs to finish at the same time as the breast. Furthermore, the weight drives the juices to the center of the flattened bird, sealing them inside rather than leaching them into the frying oil.

Some cooks use a cast-iron skillet and a foil-covered brick to prepare this recipe, but the chicken comes out nowhere near as crisp, juicy, or flavorful as it should. That's because a foil-covered brick does not wick off excess moisture or allow the chicken to "breathe" while it is shallow fried, as a clay *mattone* does.

This recipe comes from the Tuscan town of Lucca. All the fine points were given to me by Italian cooking expert Lynne Rossetto Kasper, whose grandmother fried her "brick chicken" on an unglazed, heavy, and shallow clay pan set atop the stove, gently pressing it down with a second unglazed clay brick. When I make this dish, I use a genuine *mattone,* which can be ordered from www.surlatable.com. If you choose not to acquire the disks, you can employ a shallow cazuela or tagine bottom as the bottom portion and an unglazed clay flowerpot saucer slightly smaller than the cazuela as the top. Set weights on top to simulate the 5½ pounds of pressure you need to properly press the chicken down against the cooking surface.

Note: If you buy a *mattone,* be sure to soak it in water to cover for two hours before using it the first time.

> **PREFERRED CLAY POT:**
>
> An Italian *mattone* or a 10- or 11-inch Spanish cazuela and a 9- or 10-inch unglazed terra-cotta saucer
>
> If using an electric or ceramic stovetop, be sure to use a heat diffuser with the clay pots.

1 frying chicken (2½ pounds), preferably organic, backbone removed

1 tablespoon finely chopped garlic

1 teaspoon coarse sea salt

1 teaspoon freshly ground black pepper

Leaves from 2 fresh rosemary sprigs, chopped, or 1 teaspoon dried

¾ teaspoon crushed hot red pepper

Juice of ½ lemon

⅓ cup extra virgin olive oil

Lemon wedges for garnish

1 Dry the chicken thoroughly with paper towels. Use a mallet or heavy rolling pin to gently pound on the chicken breast and the leg-thigh joints, flattening the chicken as evenly as possible. Make a small slit on each side of the lower breast to allow the legs to move freely and pull them up toward the back of the chicken, forming a compact, roundish shape. Twist each wing back up over the neck and fasten the legs, wings, and neck in a line with a long bamboo skewer.

2 In a wide, shallow bowl, combine the garlic, salt, black pepper, rosemary, hot pepper, lemon juice, and 2 tablespoons of the olive oil. Spread over both sides of the chicken and marinate at room temperature for at least 30 minutes or in the refrigerator for up to a day.

3 About 1 hour and 15 minutes before serving, place the bottom of the mattone and 1 tablespoon of the remaining olive oil over low heat. At the same time, slowly heat the top, flat side down, over a second burner over very low heat. Heat both parts for about 30 minutes, gradually raising the heat under each to medium-high.

4 Add the remaining olive oil to the hot clay dish, and let it sizzle before adding the chicken, breast side down. Use a pair of tongs to quickly coat the breast with the hot oil, then turn the chicken over so it is skin side up. Immediately place the heated lid on top of the chicken and press down firmly to flatten the chicken for even cooking. Fry the chicken for 8 to 10 minutes over medium-high heat. Carefully uncover and set the top on a wooden board or a folded kitchen towel to avoid cracking the hot clay. Use tongs to turn the chicken over. Insert an instant-read thermometer sideways in the thigh so it sticks out of the pan and you don't need to uncover the chicken to check it. Replace the lid and fry for 8 to 10 minutes longer over medium-high heat, or until the internal temperature registers 165°F.

Transfer the hot lid to a wooden surface or folded towel. The chicken should be a deep golden brown and crisp on both sides. There should be only oil— no juices—in the pan. Transfer the chicken to a wooden board. Turn off the heat and let the clay pan bottom and top cool before cleaning with warm water and baking soda to remove the grease.

5 Blot the chicken dry with paper towels and let rest for 5 to 10 minutes. Carve the chicken into 8 to 10 pieces and serve warm or at room temperature, sprinkled with salt and pepper and garnished with lemon wedges.

Notes to the Cook:

* Be sure to heat the *mattone,* or whatever pieces of clay you are using, slowly until very hot. If you are timid, you'll need to cook the chicken for 5 minutes longer.

* Do not try to use a *mattone* in an oven. If you do, the chicken will not brown.

* There's no need to press down hard on the *mattone* top. Heat coming from the clay top and bottom will crisp both sides.

* You can grill the chicken over live embers or heated lava stones using only the *mattone* top to weight the chicken.

* You can use your mattone to cook quail, squab, Rock Cornish hen, large chicken halves, even baby artichokes. To cook artichokes *al mattone:* Gently crush baby artichokes with the flat side of a large knife or cleaver to flatten slightly. Marinate them in a mixture of equal parts lemon juice and olive oil seasoned with garlic, fresh thyme, salt, and pepper for a few hours or overnight. Cook in the same manner as the chicken, using only 1 tablespoon olive oil for the frying. They will take about 6 minutes per side.

Chicken Guvec with Red Peppers and Sumac Syrup

SERVES 6

The brilliant Istanbul chef Musa Dağdeviren made this mouthwatering dish for me, using several ingredients hard to find here in the United States, including a strange husky-flavored berry called menengic, which comes from the terebinth tree, a member of the pistachio family. As a result I feared I'd never be able to reproduce the dish.

Then one of Musa's disciples, a young chef, Burak Epir, who owns a terrific Turkish restaurant called Pilita in the town of San Carlos in Santa Clara County, California, came to the rescue. Burak helped me develop this domestic version, substituting juniper berries for the hard-to-find menengic, with fine results.

Whether it's called a *guvec, duvech, yiouvetsi,* or any of a dozen similar-sounding names, the dish is cooked in the same type of vessel: a large, deep casserole made of partially glazed or unglazed earthenware beloved for its ability to impart a great earthy taste and aroma to food. This dish, and the one that follows, is prepared by packing chicken and other ingredients into a pot, setting it atop the stove until well heated, and then, sometimes, continuing the cooking in the oven. Little liquid is needed; the vegetables and other ingredients provide sufficient moisture, which eventually cooks down to a thick, tasty sauce. Sometimes a sour or tart liquid is added to balance the flavors. These include *koruk* (the Turkish version of verjuice), sumac water, tamarind, or pomegranate juice as well as such fruit flavorings as sour plums, dried lemons, or sour grape powder.

On a recent trip to Turkey, I visited the village of Sorkun, a small town of no more than fifty families, near Eskisehir in the central flatlands, where villagers specialize in making *guvec* pots used throughout the country. The people of Sorkun have been making these deep, straight-sided pots for centuries out of clay dug nearby. The children learn from their grandparents, and it was amazing to watch these young ones throw pots with an economy of movement that spoke of a lifetime of familiarity with clay.

I brought back several Sorkun *guvec* pots and used them to test this chicken recipe. You can also achieve excellent results substituting either a glazed or unglazed three-quart earthenware casserole. For more on Turkish *Guvec,* see page 133.

This recipe must be started a day or two in advance.

> **PREFERRED CLAY POT:**
>
> **A deep, 3-quart glazed or unglazed earthenware or flameware casserole, or a Turkish *guvec***
>
> **If using an electric or ceramic stovetop, be sure to use a heat diffuser with the clay pot.**

½ cup whole sumac berries

2 tablespoons juniper berries or 1 tablespoon dried menengic fruits

¾ teaspoon whole black peppercorns

5 garlic cloves, peeled

Sea salt and freshly ground black pepper

1½ teaspoons fresh thyme leaves or 1 teaspoon dried

¾ teaspoon ground coriander

½ teaspoon dried mint, preferably Egyptian

½ teaspoon grated lemon zest

Pinch of Turkish or Aleppo pepper

⅓ cup extra virgin olive oil

6 large chicken thighs (about 8 ounces each), preferably organic, trimmed of all excess fat

1 medium onion, finely chopped

2 cups peeled, seeded, and chopped Roma tomatoes or 1 can (14 ounces) diced tomatoes

1 pound Yukon Gold potatoes, peeled and thickly sliced

1 medium green bell pepper or Italian frying pepper, cut into ½-inch dice

2 tablespoons Turkish sweet red pepper paste or 4 canned or jarred piquillo peppers, drained and mashed to a puree

½ teaspoon whole cumin seeds, toasted

Pinch of sugar

1 A day in advance, bring ⅔ cup water to a boil in a small conventional saucepan. Add the sumac berries and press down to moisten. Remove from the heat and let them soak overnight.

2 Meanwhile, in a heavy mortar, pound the juniper berries with the pepper, garlic cloves, and 1 tablespoon salt until a smooth paste forms. Blend in the thyme, coriander, mint, lemon zest, red pepper, and olive oil. Pierce the chicken thighs all over with a skewer or the tip of a knife and coat with the marinade. Cover and refrigerate overnight.

3 About 2 hours before serving, bring the chicken to room temperature. Preheat the oven to 350°F. Press the sumac berries through a fine sieve set over the casserole to express all the flavorful liquid. Add the onion, tomatoes, potatoes, green pepper, sweet red pepper paste, cumin, 1 teaspoon salt, and ½ teaspoon pepper. Stir once. Place the pot over medium-low heat and warm up the contents for 15 minutes.

4 Cover the casserole with foil and transfer to the preheated oven. Immediately raise the oven temperature to 450°F and bake the vegetables for 45 minutes.

5 Transfer the casserole to a wooden surface or folded kitchen towel to prevent cracking. Discard the foil cover. Place the chicken thighs, skin side up, in a single layer on top of the vegetables. Carefully tilt the pan and spoon some of the juices up over the skin. Return the casserole to the oven and bake, uncovered, for 45 minutes.

6 Remove the casserole from the oven, setting it down on a wooden board or folded towel. Tilt the pan and pour all the juices into a saucepan. Add a pinch of sugar and boil down to about ¼ cup of thick syrup. Drizzle over the chicken and serve right from the casserole.

Chicken Guvec with Okra and Sour Grape Juice

SERVES 4

"All year long we have lemons, pomegranate molasses, sumac flakes and sumac berries to give an extra 'push' to our food," my food journalist friend, Ayfer Ünsal, tells me. "Then in summer," she adds, "we have sour grape juice, and that makes our dishes very tart and very special."

In this wonderful Turkish recipe, chicken and fresh young okra are cloaked in a delightful sweet-and-sour sauce, which slowly penetrates the chicken, melding to form a unique flavor. This dish is traditionally baked in a clay-lined oven environment that helps to produce a beautiful layer of oven-seared tomato slices on its surface. Serve with bulgur pilaf.

> **PREFERRED CLAY POT:**
>
> A deep 11-inch Spanish cazuela or flameware baking dish
>
> If using an electric or ceramic stovetop, be sure to use a heat diffuser with the clay pot.
>
> **SUGGESTED CLAY ENVIRONMENT:**
>
> Double slabs of pizza stones or food-safe quarry tiles set on the upper and lower oven racks

1 pound red ripe tomatoes, peeled, seeded, and chopped, plus 2 or 3 small tomatoes, thinly sliced

Coarse sea salt and freshly ground black pepper

½ cup verjuice (see Note)

2 pounds large chicken thighs, preferably organic, trimmed of all excess fat

12 ounces small, firm okra pods, rubbed with a towel to remove any fuzz

3 tablespoons cider vinegar

⅔ cup thinly sliced shallot

¼ cup extra virgin olive oil

1 medium green frying pepper or bell pepper, cut into 1-inch pieces

Pinch of Turkish or Aleppo pepper

Pinch of ground coriander

Pinch of ground cumin

Sugar

2 teaspoons finely chopped garlic

1 About 3 hours before you plan to serve the dish, sprinkle the chopped tomatoes with a little salt and let drain for up to 2 hours. Meanwhile, in a small nonreactive saucepan, boil the verjus until it is reduced to 3 tablespoons.

2 Season the chicken lightly with salt and black pepper and let stand at room temperature for 1 hour. At the same time, pare the cone tops of the okra pods and trim the tips if they are black, but do not cut into the pods. Place the okra on a flat tray; sprinkle with the cider vinegar and a few teaspoons of coarse salt. Let stand in a warm place for 1 hour.

3 Preheat the oven to 400°F. While the oven is heating, rinse the okra, drain well, and pat dry with paper towels. Pat the chicken thighs dry.

4 Set the cazuela over medium-low heat. Add the chicken, shallot, and 2 tablespoons of the olive oil. Cook for 5 minutes on one side without browning. Push the chicken thighs to one side of the pan. Add the chopped tomatoes, green pepper, verjus, red pepper, coriander, cumin, ½ teaspoon sugar, ½ teaspoon salt, and ¼ teaspoon pepper; mix gently and continue cooking for 5 minutes.

5 Meanwhile, heat the remaining 2 tablespoons oil in a large nonstick skillet. Add the okra and fry over medium-high heat for a minute to develop a bit of extra flavor and shine; add the okra to the cazuela. In the same oil, over low heat, cook the garlic until softened and fragrant but not brown, about 1 minute. Scoop out and add to the chicken and okra. Gently mix the ingredients in the cazuela, lifting the chicken thighs to the top of the tomatoes and peppers and arranging them side by side, skin side up. Garnish the top with the thinly sliced tomato. Drizzle the garlic oil from the skillet over the tomatoes and sprinkle with an additional pinch of sugar. Set the casserole in the oven and bake for 45 minutes.

6 Turn the oven off and leave the guvec inside without opening for 45 minutes longer. Remove the pot from the oven, place a cover on top to hold everything in place, and tilt to pour off the oil. Serve while the guvec is still warm.

NOTE TO THE COOK: If you can't find verjuice, substitute fresh lemon juice or 3 tablespoons dried sour grape powder, which is available at Persian grocers.

Moroccan Chicken Kdra With Almonds and Chickpeas

SERVES 4 TO 6

*H*ere's an updated version of one of the most famous *kdra* dishes, a style of cooking that features the preserved butter of Morocco called *smen* as well as pepper and saffron. The name also indicates the poultry or meat is cooked in a creamy sauce. In this recipe, the accompanying soft, fresh green almonds and peeled chickpeas are included to make a sensational velvety textured, aromatic chicken stew that is eaten with flat bread.

> **PREFERRED CLAY POTS:**
>
> A bean pot for cooking the chickpeas (optional)
>
> A 10- to 12-inch glazed earthenware or flameware shallow casserole with a tight-fitting lid
>
> If using an electric or ceramic stovetop, be sure to use a heat diffuser with the clay pots.

½ cup dried chickpeas

Kosher salt and freshly ground white pepper

6 large chicken thighs (2½ to 3 pounds), preferably organic

¼ teaspoon ground turmeric

¼ teaspoon ground ginger

Pinch of saffron threads

2 cups peeled green almonds (see Note) or 1 cup blanched whole almonds, boiled in water for about 2 hours until soft

2 tablespoons smen (see page 295) or unsalted butter

1 3-inch Ceylon cinnamon stick

2 large yellow onions, 1 grated and 1 quartered lengthwise and thinly sliced

¼ cup chopped fresh flat-leaf parsley

2 tablespoons fresh lemon juice

1 Place the chickpeas in a large bowl with enough water to cover by 3 inches. Measure the water as you add it; then add 1½ tablespoons kosher salt for each cup of water. Soak overnight.

2 The next day, drain the chickpeas, rinse well, and place in a bean pot or a use a conventional 3-quart saucepan. Add fresh water to cover and boil for 10 minutes. Drain and submerge the chickpeas in a bowl of cold water. Rub them between your palms or fingers to remove their skins. Return the chickpeas to the bean pot or saucepan, cover again with fresh water, and simmer until tender, about 1 hour.

3 Meanwhile, in the casserole, combine the chicken thighs, 1 teaspoon salt, 1 teaspoon white pepper, turmeric, ginger, saffron, almonds, and smen. Gently crush the cinnamon stick between two fingers to release its aroma and add to the casserole. Set over medium-low heat and warm the spices with the chicken, turning the thighs occasionally, for 10 to 15 minutes. Add the grated onion and ½ cup water. Cover and cook for 20 minutes.

4 Drain the chickpeas, reserving ½ cup of their cooking liquid. Add the chickpeas and reserved liquid to the casserole along with the sliced onion and parsley. Cover and cook until the chicken is very tender, 10 to 15 minutes.

5   Remove the chicken and set aside. Raise the heat to medium and bring the sauce to a boil; cook until thickened, about 15 minutes. Stir in the lemon juice, and season with additional salt and pepper to taste. Return the chicken to the casserole and reheat, basting with the sauce.

NOTE TO THE COOK: Fuzzy green almonds are available in June from some Middle Eastern grocers or from www.greenalmonds.com. To prepare green almonds, score each with a knife, break open the outer shell, and remove the sac. Soak the sacs in a mixture of salted water and milk to firm up for about 1 hour.

TAGINE

The very word *tagine* has reached folkloric status. People are charmed by both the promise of a complexly flavored dish and the visually seductive image of the cooking pot of the same name: a combination of low-rimmed, concave, and platelike bottom and conical top. This two-part vessel was devised to condense steam back into moisture, enhancing the slow-cooked stewing effect while maximizing cooking efficiency. At the same time, it provides a charming and attractive vessel in which to serve the dish when done.

Tagine pots are versatile, and I recommend that you acquire one, but you can still prepare all the following dishes by improvising with another clay pot to encourage slow, steady cooking and provide that coveted earthy taste. A Spanish cazuela with a crumbled sheet of wet parchment set atop will serve you well. The parchment will recirculate the steam, creating the almost mystical quality of succulent flesh and unctuous sauce that is the essence of the tagine cooking style.

Moroccan Chicken with Lemon and Eggs

SERVES 4 TO 8

*B*ack in the 1970s, when I was living in Tangier and working on my Moroccan cookbook, I was invited to Rabat to learn what was described to me as "a great dish that will be demonstrated for you by a virtuoso cook." The demonstrator turned out to be a short, squat, very dark-skinned Berber woman named Rakia, a specialist at making *djej mefenned,* one of the most difficult-to-execute dishes in Moroccan cuisine.

Rakia turned out to be quite a character. She cracked jokes as she worked and sang and belly danced around the kitchen, the whole while puffing on strong Koutoubia brand cigarettes. When she dropped something on the floor, which she did several times, she bent straight down from the waist like a jackknife blade to pick it up.

For all her amusing traits, her technique was truly dazzling, as she twirled a whole roasted chicken in sizzling fat while simultaneously basting it with seasoned beaten eggs. This procedure resulted in an herbed, silken cloak that bonded to the bird just before it was brought to the table.

"Yes, it's very hard to do," Rakia assured me with one of her signature laughs, implying that I would never be able to master the technique. "Of course there is an easier way, the one the sissy cooks down in Eassaouira use. But of course it's not the same at all," she added with another cackle.

A recipe for sissy cooks! For wimps! After that contemptuous description, I never even considered following up. Meanwhile I struggled to master Rakia's dish, finally publishing an adequate attempt. Although not an herbal omelet lying atop a chicken, which so many cooks have presented when stumped, it was still a far cry from the total encasement Rakia was able to achieve.

My mistake, as I discovered this year, though, as the Essaouira recipe for "wimps" is quite marvelous and totally different. It is its own dish. Basically, a cut-up, cooked chicken is served partially submerged in flavored eggs. My version, as given here, is easy, and the dish is delicious, the seasoned egg mixture becoming a kind of rich and smooth custard sauce that surrounds the chicken legs and thighs.

> **PREFERRED CLAY POT:**
>
> A 10- to 12-inch glazed or unglazed earthenware tagine or Spanish cazuela with a tight-fitting lid, or a 10- to 12-inch flameware tagine
>
> If using an electric or ceramic stovetop, be sure to use a heat diffuser with the clay pot.

4 large whole chicken legs, preferably organic,
   separated into drumsticks and thigh to make
   8 pieces

½ teaspoon saffron threads

3 large garlic cloves, peeled

Coarse salt and freshly ground black pepper

1 teaspoon ground ginger

Pinch of ground cinnamon

4 tablespoons (½ stick) unsalted butter,
   2 tablespoons softened to room temperature

1 tablespoon smen (page 295), or 1 more
   tablespoon unsalted butter

1 large onion, grated, rinsed, and squeezed dry

½ preserved lemon rind, trimmed and diced
   (page 317)

16 to 18 pitted picholine olives, washed, drained,
   and roughly chopped

2 tablespoons chopped fresh cilantro

2 tablespoons chopped fresh flat-leaf parsley

4 large eggs

2 tablespoons fresh lemon juice

1 About 2 hours before serving, rinse the chicken and pat dry; trim away any excess fat. Soak the saffron in ½ cup hot water. In a mortar, pound the garlic to a paste with 1 teaspoon salt. Blend in the ginger, ½ teaspoon black pepper, cinnamon, the softened butter, and the smen. Gradually stir in the hot saffron water, as if making a mayonnaise. Mix with half of the grated onion and pour into the tagine. Place the chicken pieces, skin side up, on top and let stand at room temperature for about 1 hour.

2 Cover the tagine, set over medium-low heat, and cook without disturbing for 45 minutes, or until the chicken is tender. Transfer the chicken pieces to a broiling pan, skin side up; pat dry.

3 Preheat the broiler. In a medium bowl, combine the preserved lemon, olives, cilantro, and parsley.

4 Skim off most of the fat from the liquid in the tagine, reserving about ¼ cup. Pour the degreased liquid into the bowl. Return the tagine to the heat and add the rest of the grated onion and half of the reserved fat. Cook over medium-low heat, stirring occasionally, until the onion is lightly caramelized, about 10 minutes. Scrape into the bowl and mix to combine. Set the sauce aside. Do not wash the tagine.

5 Brush the reserved fat over the chicken legs and thighs and run them under the broiler 6 inches from the heat for about 5 minutes to finish cooking the chicken and crisp the skin. Set aside in a warm place while you finish the sauce.

6 Melt the remaining 2 tablespoons butter in the tagine over medium-low heat. In a mixing bowl, whisk the eggs until well blended. Season with a pinch each of salt and pepper. When the butter is foaming, add the eggs and cook, stirring gently and continually scraping the bottom. As the eggs begin to thicken, gradually add the lemon juice 1 tablespoon at a time, stirring slowly to a creamy consistency. Immediately remove from the heat and fold in the warm sauce. Season with additional salt and pepper to taste. Nestle the broiled chicken, skin side up, in the custardy sauce, cover, and let stand for a few minutes. The sauce will continue to cook in the receding heat of the tagine. Serve while still warm.

Moroccan Chicken with Pumpkin, Sweet-and-Sour Plums, and Toasted Almonds

SERVES 3 OR 4

This has long been one of my favorite chicken tagines, one I was never able to share with readers before because I couldn't get the sweet-and-sour dried yellow or golden plums essential to the dish in the United States. Now that they're available at East Indian groceries, sold under the name *alu bokhara*, I'm delighted to be able to share this truly great dish, in which many of the essential parts of Moroccan cooking come together: slow and low cooking, delicate floral honey, crunchy almonds, sweet-and-sour fruit, and, if available, a mere teaspoon of the legendary *smen*.

PREFERRED CLAY POT:

A 10- to 12- inch glazed or unglazed earthenware or flameware tagine for the chicken

If using an electric or ceramic stovetop, be sure to use a heat diffuser with the clay pot.

24 sweet-and-sour dried yellow plums with pits

2 pinches of saffron threads

2 pounds organic chicken thighs (6 to 8)

Salt and freshly ground black pepper

1 onion, roughly cut up

1 garlic clove, chopped

1½ teaspoons Moroccan Spice Mixture: La Kama (page 316)

12 fresh cilantro sprigs, tied in a bunch

4 tablespoons (½ stick) unsalted butter

1 teaspoon smen (page 295; optional)

1 3-inch Ceylon cinnamon stick

¾ to 1 pound butternut squash, peeled and diced

2 tablespoons honey, preferably lavender, orange blossom, or acacia

1 tablespoon orange flower water

3 tablespoons whole blanched almonds, toasted

1 Put the dried plums in a saucepan, cover with water, and bring to a boil and cook for 10 minutes. Let soak for 30 minutes. At the same time, soak the saffron in ⅓ cup hot water.

2 Pierce the skin side of the chicken thighs with a thin needle or a toothpick. Season the exposed meat side with salt and pepper. Place the chicken skin side down in the tagine over medium-low heat and warm slowly until fat runs out of the skin. Use a bulb baster to remove the chicken fat and discard. Add the onion, garlic, La Kama spices, cilantro bundle, 1 tablespoon of the butter, the smen, and the saffron with its soaking water. Gently crush the cinnamon stick between two fingers to release its aroma and add to the tagine. Cover and cook for 20 minutes. Uncover, raise the heat to medium, and cook for 10 minutes longer. Remove and discard the cinnamon stick and cilantro.

3 In a 10-inch nonstick skillet, melt 2 tablespoons of the remaining butter over medium heat. Add the squash, cover, and cook until just tender, about 10 minutes. Drain the plums; pit and quarter using a small pair of scissors and add them to the skillet. Thin the honey with the orange flower water and add along with the remaining 1 tablespoon butter. Cook, uncovered, over medium heat until the butternut squash is glazed, about 5 minutes.

4 Working in batches, transfer the chicken to the skillet and turn it in the syrupy juices until lightly glazed, about 1 minute; return to the tagine. Repeat with the remaining chicken thighs. Spread the plums and butternut squash over the chicken, scrape the syrupy juices on top, and gently reheat the tagine until heated through. Scatter the almonds on top and serve.

Moroccan Chicken Tagine with Sweet Onions and Raisins

SERVES 4 TO 6

Unlike Western stews, just a few Moroccan tagines call for an initial intense sautéing. If browning is required, it is usually done in a hot oven, under a clay dish filled with hot coals, or under a broiler after the meat or chicken is simmered to perfection on top of the stove.

In my travels through southern Morocco I noticed that many of the tagine cooking pots were unglazed and made of a clay that shimmered due to high mica content. Such tagines, I was told, were particularly strong and could take direct flame heat. This corresponded to my observation that it is in southern Morocco that one finds tagine recipes, such as this one, that call for early browning. You can find an unglazed and mica rich tagine from the Moroccan Souss region at www.tagines.com. Here I brown the chicken legs and thighs in the tagine and at the same time slowly cook the sauce in a separate casserole to develop a rich intensity of flavor and color. After this stage, chicken and sauce are combined and then baked to glaze the onion topping.

PREFERRED CLAY POTS:

A 3-quart glazed or unglazed earthenware or flameware saucepan or casserole with a tight-fitting lid

A 10- to 12-inch flameware tagine or Spanish cazuela

If using an electric or ceramic stovetop, be sure to use a heat diffuser with the clay pots.

3 pounds large whole chicken legs, preferably organic

2 pounds large onions, quartered lengthwise and thinly sliced

3 tablespoons unsalted butter

Pinch of saffron threads

2 teaspoons ground cinnamon

1 teaspoon ground ginger

2 tablespoons sugar

Salt and freshly ground black pepper

½ cup raisins

2 tablespoons honey

(continued)

1 Separate the chicken legs at the joint into thighs and drumsticks. Trim off any excess fat. Let come to room temperature. Meanwhile, soak the saffron in ½ cup warm water for 15 minutes.

2 Place the onions, 1 tablespoon of the butter, the saffron and soaking water, cinnamon, ginger, sugar, and 1 teaspoon each salt and pepper in the 3-quart earthenware casserole. Cover and cook over medium-low heat, stirring occasionally, for 45 minutes. (If the onions begin to brown too quickly, reduce the heat to low.)

3 Remove the cover. Add the raisins, raise the heat to medium, and continue cooking, uncovered, until the onions are soft and glazed and the sauce is thickened and reduced to 2 cups, about 45 minutes longer.

4 Put 1 tablespoon of the butter in the tagine. Add the chicken and set over medium-low heat. Cook slowly until the butter sizzles and the chicken skin begins to release some fat. Raise the heat to medium and continue to brown the chicken, moving it around in the tagine to keep it from sticking, but always keeping it on the skin side, for 30 minutes. From time to time, tilt the tagine and spoon off excess fat. Note that you will have to adjust the heat to keep the chicken browning slowly and consistently. Use a wooden or silicone spatula to scrape up bits and pieces that attach to the bottom of the tagine.

5 Preheat the oven to 450°F. Reduce the heat under the tagine to medium-low, turn the chicken pieces over, and cook for 15 minutes longer. Turn over again and brush the skin side of the chicken with the honey.

6 Transfer the tagine to the oven and bake, uncovered, until the chicken is glazed, about 10 minutes.

7 Spread the onion sauce over the chicken, dot with the remaining butter, and bake until the onions turn golden brown, about 5 minutes.

Baked Moroccan Chicken with Charred Tomatoes

SERVES 4

In this super moist recipe from the city of Tangier, a quartered chicken bakes slowly in a spicy sauce of grated tomatoes and onions until the flesh is just tender and incredibly juicy. The thick, intensely flavored sauce is then sprinkled with cinnamon and raw sugar and broiled for the final few minutes until lightly charred on top with delectable crusty edges.

In the old days before home ovens, cooks placed a shallow earthenware plate over the filled tagine, then piled on glowing olivewood embers. This hot covering turned the top crusty and brown, sealed in the moisture, and infused the dish with a subtle smoky fragrance.

Serve with the Moroccan Country Bread on page 257.

1 chicken (3½ to 4 pounds), preferably organic, quartered and trimmed of excess fat

2 pounds red ripe tomatoes

1 medium red onion

1 3-inch Ceylon cinnamon stick

1 teaspoon Moroccan Spice Mixture: La Kama (page 316)

½ teaspoon cubeb berries, crushed to a powder (optional; see Note)

⅛ teaspoon saffron threads

Salt

2 tablespoons extra virgin olive oil

½ teaspoon ground cinnamon

3 tablespoons turbinado sugar

1   Preheat the oven to 275°F. Place the chicken quarters, skin side up and side by side, in the tagine. Halve the tomatoes and squeeze out and discard the seeds. Use the coarse side of a grater to grate the tomatoes; discard the skins. Strain the tomatoes to remove excess moisture. You should have about 2 cups thick grated tomato pulp. Grate, rinse, and squeeze dry the onion. Add the tomato, onion, cinnamon stick, La Kama spices, cubeb berries, saffron, 1 teaspoon salt, and oil to the tagine and mix well with the chicken. Gently crush the cinnamon stick between two fingers to release its aroma and add to the tagine. Set the tagine on the middle rack in the oven to bake without disturbing for 1 hour and 45 minutes. (You do not need the cover of the tagine.)

2   Transfer the tagine to a wooden surface or folded cloth. Turn on the broiler. Rearrange the chicken in the center of the dish and top with the thick, intensely flavored tomato. Pour any liquid in the baking dish into a small conventional skillet, add the ground cinnamon and sugar, and bring to a boil. Reduce to a thick sauce and drizzle over the chicken and tomato. Set the tagine on the oven center rack about 9 inches from heat source and quickly broil until the tomato coating is lightly charred. Discard the cinnamon stick and serve the chicken hot.

NOTE TO THE COOK: Cubeb berries are also known as *cubeb pepper* or *tailed pepper*. They have a peppery, aromatic, bitter flavor that binds well with La Kama spices. You can purchase the berries at www.Kalustyans.com.

Tunisian Chicken Tagine with Brik Pastry

SERVES 6

The Tunisian name for this dish is *tagine malsouka,* the latter being the Tunisian word for the crisp, paper-thin pastry Tunisians use to wrap up foods for deep frying, including their famous street dish: *brik.*

Brik pastry, which is as thin as phyllo dough, is also used in the capital city of Tunis as a wrapping for a Tunisian "tagine," which is not a stew cooked in a conical clay dish as in Morocco, but something akin to an Italian frittata with meat or chicken along with herbs, lots of egg, cheese, bread crumbs, or beans cooked in an earthenware dish. This particular version is quite quiche-like, with pastry surrounding the chicken, eggs, and cheese.

> **PREFERRED CLAY POT:**
>
> A 10- to 12-inch glazed or unglazed earthenware tagine or flameware tagine or skillet, or a Spanish cazuela
>
> If using an electric or ceramic stovetop, be sure to use a heat diffuser with the clay pot.

8 ounces skinless, boneless chicken breast, raw or cooked, cut into 1-inch cubes

Salt and freshly ground black pepper

Extra virgin olive oil

2 medium onions, chopped (about 1½ cups)

2 pinches of crushed hot red pepper

Pinch of ground turmeric

4 large eggs

2 hard-boiled eggs, peeled and crumbled with a fork

3 ounces Gruyère, Comté, or Monterey Jack cheese, grated

1½ cups soft bread crumbs

1 tablespoon small capers, drained and rinsed

2 tablespoons chopped fresh flat-leaf parsley

10 brik wrappers (about 6 ounces) or phyllo sheets

1 Season the chicken lightly with salt and pepper. Heat 1½ tablespoons of the olive oil in the tagine over medium-low heat. Add the onions and the chicken if it's raw and cook slowly, stirring, until the onions are golden, about 5 minutes. If using cooked chicken, add it now.

2 Add 1 cup hot water and bring to a boil. Cook, stirring, for 6 to 7 minutes if you used raw chicken and 2 minutes if cooked. Season with salt, black pepper, hot pepper, and turmeric. (The recipe can be made to this point up to 2 days in advance. Let the spiced chicken cool; then transfer it to another container, cover, and refrigerate.)

3 About 1 hour before serving, set a rack in the center of the oven and preheat the oven to 350°F. If it was prepared in advance, remove the spiced chicken from the refrigerator.

4 Whisk the raw eggs until well blended. Add the hard-boiled eggs, grated cheese, bread crumbs, capers, and parsley.

5 Generously oil the inside of the tagine. Unwrap the brik pastry, place 1 sheet on the bottom of the dish, and brush with olive oil. Arrange 5 more sheets, brushing each with oil, overlapping so that they cover the bottom of the dish and extend over the sides. Spread the filling evenly in the dish. Fold the overhanging pastry leaves over the top to cover the filling. Place the remaining pastry sheets, brushed with oil, on top and fold these neatly around the edges, as for tucking in sheets. Prick the top sheets of pastry in 2 or 3 places with a skewer.

6 Bake the tagine until the top is golden brown, about 25 minutes. Remove from the oven and let stand for 10 minutes to set before serving.

Inspired by a recipe in Klementine Konstantini's Traditions Culinaires de Tunisie.

Catalonian Chicken Sautéed with Red Peppers, Tomatoes, and Black Olives

SERVES 4

*H*ere's my version of the famous dish *poulet à la Catalane,* in which a rich Mediterranean-style sauce can make even a supermarket chicken taste good. Use a first-rate chicken and it will be superb! Serve with good crusty bread.

> **PREFERRED CLAY POT:**
>
> **An 11- or 12-inch Spanish cazuela or straight-sided flameware skillet**
>
> **If using an electric or ceramic stovetop, be sure to use a heat diffuser with the clay pot.**

1 chicken (about 3 pounds), preferably organic, quartered

Salt and freshly ground black pepper

3 tablespoons extra virgin olive oil

3 ounces thinly sliced pancetta, chopped

3 medium onions, sliced

8 large garlic cloves, unpeeled

Herb bouquet: 3 fresh flat-leaf parsley sprigs, 1 fresh thyme sprig, 1 small bay leaf, and 1 3-inch cinnamon stick, tied together

3 tablespoons dry white wine

2 red bell peppers, roasted, peeled, and seeded, cut into 1-inch pieces, or 1 jar (3 ounces) piquillo peppers, drained and cut up

1½ pounds red ripe tomatoes, peeled, seeded, halved, and cut into 1-inch chunks

12 dry-cured black olives, rinsed

Pinch of crushed hot red pepper

2 cups unsalted chicken stock, boiled until reduced to ⅔ cup

1½ tablespoons chopped fresh flat-leaf parsley

1 teaspoon grated lemon zest

(continued)

1 Generously season the chicken pieces with salt and pepper. Cut away any excess fat. Loosely wrap with plastic wrap and refrigerate for up to 2 days. About 1 hour before serving, remove the chicken from the refrigerator and pat dry.

2 In the cazuela, slowly heat 2 tablespoons of the olive oil over medium-low heat. When it is just sizzling, add the pancetta. Cover with a lid or foil and cook for 1 minute. Add the chicken pieces skin side down, half the onions, and the garlic cloves. Cook the chicken for 1 minute on each side, shaking the pan to prevent sticking. Reduce the heat to low, cover, and cook slowly for 10 minutes.

3 Uncover the cazuela and carefully tilt the pan so you can spoon off the fat. Turn the chicken over. Add the herb bouquet and the white wine. Cover and cook slowly for 10 minutes longer.

4 Meanwhile, in a 10-inch conventional skillet, cook the remaining onions, the red bell peppers, and the tomatoes in the remaining 1 tablespoon olive oil for 5 minutes, tossing often. Add the olives and hot pepper. Set the vegetables aside.

5 Transfer the cooked chicken breast quarters to a side dish; cover and keep warm. Add the reduced stock to the cazuela and continue cooking the legs and garlic, uncovered, for 5 minutes longer, or until the dark meat is tender. There should be about ¼ cup syrupy pan juices along with the garlic and pancetta. Remove and discard the herb bouquet.

6 Return the chicken breasts to the cazuela. Turn each piece of chicken and the garlic in the syrupy juices to glaze them with sauce. Add the vegetables from the skillet. Swirl over medium-high heat for 30 seconds. Season with salt and pepper. Top with parsley and lemon zest and serve right from the pot.

Chicken with Red Wine Vinegar, Tomato, and Shallots

SERVES 4 TO 6

I think of this popular French dish as "comfort" food. All the flavors are familiar yet greatly magnified by steady slow cooking of the sauce base. Something wondrous emerges as red wine vinegar, rich tomato sauce, sliced shallot, garlic, and a touch of honey slowly meld together in a clay pot. Long cooking of the vinegar softens acidity while deepening flavor, with the result that the sauce comes out perfectly balanced and never overwhelms the chicken.

> **PREFERRED CLAY POT:**
>
> A 10- or 11-inch straight-sided flameware skillet or a Spanish cazuela
>
> If using an electric or ceramic stovetop, be sure to use a heat diffuser with the clay pot.

8 large chicken thighs (about 3½ pounds), preferably organic

Salt and freshly ground black pepper

¾ cup plus 2 tablespoons red wine vinegar, preferably homemade (page 313)

1 tablespoon strong chicken stock or glace de poulet diluted in ½ cup water or ½ cup rich chicken stock

1 tablespoon honey

¼ cup thick tomato sauce or 1 tablespoon tomato paste

2 tablespoons unsalted butter

¾ cup thinly sliced shallot

2 tablespoons thinly sliced garlic

¾ cup dry white wine, such as Viognier, at room temperature

2 tablespoons crème fraîche

3 tablespoons chopped fresh tarragon

1 Rinse the chicken thighs; pat dry and trim away all excess fat. Season the chicken with salt and pepper. Let stand at room temperature while you prepare the sauce.

2 In a medium nonreactive saucepan, combine the vinegar, chicken stock, honey, and tomato sauce. Boil until reduced to ¾ cup. Remove from the heat and keep warm.

3 Set the flameware skillet over medium-low heat. Add the butter and, when foaming, slowly raise the heat to medium. Add half the pieces of chicken and brown well on all sides, 6 to 8 minutes. Transfer to a side dish and repeat with the remaining chicken.

4 Add the shallot and garlic to the pan and cook slowly until soft, about 5 minutes. Pour the warm sauce into the pan and slowly bring to a boil. Return the chicken thighs to the skillet, skin side up. Slowly pour in the wine. Season with 2 pinches of salt and 1 pinch of pepper. Cover, raise the heat to medium, and simmer until the chicken is tender, about 20 minutes. Remove the chicken, cover with foil, and let rest while you finish the sauce.

5 Stir the crème fraîche into the skillet and boil for a few minutes. Season with salt and pepper to taste. Return the chicken to the pot and top with the chopped tarragon.

Wine-Marinated Chicken Thighs with Almonds and Sweet Tomato Jam

SERVES 4

*D*ominique Bucaille, a highly talented chef working in the Grambois in the heart of the vineyards of the Luberon, France, sent me this recipe. (You'll find other recipes of Dominique's in the meat chapter, pages 122 and 150). His unusual dish is prepared in two steps. First, the thighs and legs are browned in a skillet without added fat while the wine is heated in a saucepan. Then the hot chicken is added to the hot wine and the whole is left to marinate for about an hour at room temperature. When ready to serve, the dish is finished with a rich flavorful sauce studded with almonds and a side of spicy sweet tomato jam.

In late spring Dominique uses soft, delicately flavored green almonds. If you're lucky enough to find fresh almonds, break open the shells; then soak the soft young nuts in salted water to firm them up. Otherwise, soak whole blanched almonds in warm water for several hours before adding to the dish.

> **PREFERRED CLAY POT:**
>
> A 10- or 11-inch straight-sided flameware skillet
>
> If using an electric or ceramic stovetop, be sure to use a heat diffuser with the clay pot.

Sweet Tomato Jam (recipe follows)

6 whole chicken legs (6 to 7 ounces each), preferably organic

Coarse sea salt and freshly ground black pepper

1 cup fruity white wine, preferably from Provence

4 garlic cloves, unpeeled but slightly crushed

½ cup diced onion

½ cup diced carrot

Aromatic bouquet: 1 small leek, quartered lengthwise and tied with 2 or 3 tender celery leaves, fresh thyme sprigs, fresh flat-leaf parsley sprigs and 1 bay leaf

Tiny pinch of saffron threads

24 fresh green almonds or 1 cup whole blanched almonds

1 cup chicken stock

1 Prepare the tomato jam in advance. Let it come to room temperature.

2 About 2 hours before serving, trim away and discard any excess fat from the chicken, but leave the skin on. Divide the legs at the joint into thighs and drumsticks. Season with salt and pepper.

3 In the dry flameware skillet, fry the chicken over medium-high heat until light brown on the bottom, 2 to 3 minutes. Turn over and brown on the other side.

4   Meanwhile, in a deep stainless-steel saucepan, bring the wine to a boil. Immediately ignite with a long match; stand back and avert your face as the flames appear. When the flames subside, remove the saucepan from the heat and slide the chicken into the hot wine.

5   Quickly return the skillet to medium-high heat. Add the garlic, onion, and carrot and sauté stirring, until lightly browned, 3 to 5 minutes. Use a slotted spoon to transfer the vegetables to the chicken and wine in the saucepan.

6   Discard any fat in the ceramic skillet. Add a few tablespoons of hot water to the skillet and bring to a boil, scraping up any browned bits from the bottom of the pan. Add to the chicken along with the aromatic bouquet and the saffron. Marinate for 45 minutes. Meanwhile, score each green almond with a knife, break open the outer shell, and remove the sac. Soak the sacs in a mixture of salted water and milk to firm them for about 1 hour.

7   Transfer the chicken, vegetables, and marinade from the saucepan to the skillet. Add the chicken stock and set over medium-heat; slowly bring to a boil. Cover with a crumpled sheet of parchment and a lid, and simmer until the chicken thighs are just cooked through and tender, about 20 minutes.

8   Transfer the chicken to a serving dish; cover with foil. Using a flat strainer, scoop out the solids from the sauce and discard. Boil down the remaining juices to a syrupy consistency, skimming often, 3 to 4 minutes. Season with salt and pepper to taste. Pour over the chicken. Drain the almonds and scatter them on top. Serve with the tomato jam as a condiment alongside.

Sweet Tomato Jam

MAKES ABOUT 1¾ CUPS

This easy condiment can be held in the refrigerator for up to four days.

> 2 pounds Roma or other flavorful ripe tomatoes
>
> 1 tablespoon extra olive oil
>
> 1½ tablespoons honey
>
> ¼ teaspoon ground cinnamon
>
> 1 teaspoon salt
>
> ½ teaspoon freshly ground black pepper
>
> 1 teaspoon orange flower water
>
> 2 teaspoons sesame seeds, lightly toasted

1   Preheat the oven to 450°F. Place the tomatoes on a rimmed baking sheet and roast until charred and soft, about 45 minutes, turning them after 20 to 25 minutes. Let cool completely, then peel, seed, and coarsely chop them.

2   In a flameware skillet, cook the tomatoes in the olive oil over medium-high heat, stirring occasionally to prevent scorching, until all the moisture is evaporated and the tomatoes are sizzling, about 10 minutes.

3   Stir in the honey, cinnamon, salt, and pepper. Reduce the heat slightly and simmer for 2 to 3 minutes longer. Remove from the heat and let cool. Stir in the orange flower water. Serve at room temperature in a shallow bowl, with the sesame seeds sprinkled on top.

Monastery Chicken with Linden Tea Sauce

SERVES 4

This fine chicken dish bears the unique flavor of tea made from the dried blossoms of a linden tree. It was this tea into which the narrator in Marcel Proust's *Remembrance of Things Past* dunked his madeleine in the famous passage of evoked nostalgia: "I raised to my lips a spoonful of the tea in which I had soaked a morsel of the cake. No sooner had the warm liquid mixed with the crumbs touched my palate than a shudder ran through me and I stopped, intent upon the extraordinary thing that was happening to me. An exquisite pleasure had invaded my senses."

In his captivating cookbook, *La Cuisine des Monastères* ("Monastery Cooking"), three-star chef Marc Meneau presents a delectable recipe using these blossoms to produce a sweet, aromatic sauce for chicken. The following recipe is inspired by his. When gently cooked in clay, it is exquisite.

> **PREFERRED CLAY POT:**
>
> A 10- or 11-inch straight-sided flameware skillet
>
> If using an electric or ceramic stovetop, be sure to use a heat diffuser with the clay pot.

4 large chicken thighs (about 2¼ pounds), preferably organic

Salt and freshly ground black pepper

1 garlic clove, crushed

⅓ ounce (10 grams) dried linden flowers and leaves (see Note)

¼ cup dry white wine

¼ cup heavy cream

¼ teaspoon fresh lemon juice

1   Prick the skin of the chicken with the tines of a fork or skewer. Season all over with salt and pepper. Rub the meat side with the garlic. Let stand at room temperature for up to 1 hour, until ready to cook.

2   Meanwhile, bring 2 cups of water to a boil in a small nonreactive saucepan. Add the linden blossoms and leaves and stir once. Remove from the heat and let infuse for 15 minutes. Strain the tea, return it to the pan, and boil until it is reduced to about ⅓ cup of reddish brown liquid. Add the white wine and set aside.

3   Place the chicken thighs, skin side down, in the flameware skillet, turn the heat to medium-low, and heat slowly, allowing the fat to run out and begin to fry the skin side of the chicken until just golden, about 10 minutes. Tilt the skillet and use a bulb baster to remove and discard most of the fat. Add the warm linden-wine mixture, cover with a sheet of parchment, and simmer for 10 to 15 minutes, or until cooked through and tender, turning the chicken once.

4   Transfer the chicken to a serving dish and skim off any fat from the surface of the cooking liquid. Raise the heat to medium-high and boil until the cooking liquid is reduced to about ⅓ cup. Add the cream, reduce the heat to medium, and boil until the sauce thickens slightly. Add the lemon juice and season with salt and pepper to taste. Spoon the sauce over the chicken and serve.

NOTE TO THE COOK: Linden blossom tea can be purchased from the following sources: www.mountain spiritherbals.com and www.mountainroseherbs.com.

Sautéed Chicken Livers with Vinegar and Onions

SERVES 4 TO 6

*I*n this special dish, chicken livers are served with sweet long-cooked onions combined with a subtle amount of anchovy. Begin this dish early in the day or prepare steps 1 through 3 a day in advance. Serve as a light lunch with thin rounds of French bread and a robust white wine.

PREFERRED CLAY POT:

A 3- or 4-quart glazed earthenware casserole

If using an electric or ceramic stovetop, be sure to use a heat diffuser with the clay pot.

---

12 ounces fresh or thawed chicken livers

¾ cup milk

Salt and freshly ground black pepper

3 pounds large Spanish onions, thinly sliced

3 tablespoons unsalted butter

3 tablespoons vegetable oil

2 ounces flat anchovy fillets, drained and crushed to a paste

2 teaspoons sugar

½ cup red wine vinegar

2 garlic cloves, finely chopped

All-purpose flour for dusting

1 cup unsalted chicken stock, boiled until reduced to ½ cup

1½ teaspoons chopped fresh flat-leaf parsley

1½ teaspoons minced fresh chives

6 thin round slices of a French baguette, toasted and rubbed with a cut garlic clove

1 Soak the chicken livers in a bowl of milk with 1 teaspoon salt for at least 3 hours or overnight in the refrigerator.

2 Meanwhile, place the onions, 2 tablespoons of the butter, 2 tablespoons of the oil, and ¼ cup water in the earthenware casserole over medium-low heat. Bring to a boil; cover tightly and reduce the heat to low. Cook slowly for 2 hours, or until the onions are soft and golden. Add the crushed anchovies and continue cooking for 30 minutes.

3 In a nonreactive conventional skillet, stir the sugar over medium heat for 30 seconds to warm it. Add ¼ cup of the vinegar and bring to a boil, stirring. When the sweetened vinegar begins to darken, stop the cooking with a spoonful of cold water, swirling the pan to combine it; then stir in another ¼ cup of water and cook, stirring, until the syrup is smooth, about 15 seconds.

4 Scrape the vinegar syrup into the casserole with the onions and add half the chopped garlic. Cover and cook over low heat for 30 minutes to blend the flavors. The onions should be a deep golden brown color. Season with salt and pepper to taste. (The onions can be prepared up to this point early in the day.) When cool, cover and refrigerate; reheat about 20 minutes before serving.

5 About 5 minutes before serving, drain and rinse the chicken livers. Pat them dry with paper towels, then dust lightly with flour seasoned with salt and pepper. In a large conventional skillet, melt the remaining 1 tablespoon butter in the remaining 1 tablespoon oil over medium-high heat. Add the remaining chopped

(continued)

garlic and the chicken livers and sauté, tossing, until the livers are lightly browned outside and still rosy pink in the center, about 1½ minutes per side. Transfer the livers to a side dish and toss with the reheated onions.

6 Quickly pour the remaining ¼ cup vinegar into the skillet and boil, scraping up any browned bits that cling to the bottom and sides of the pan. Add the stock and boil until reduced by half. Spoon the syrupy vinegar glaze over the livers and onions. Sprinkle the parsley and chives on top and divide among individual plates. Accompany with slices of toasted French bread rubbed with fresh garlic.

Duck Legs with Picholine Olives and Wild Mushrooms

SERVES 2

The nutty flavor of the picholine olives, the earthy taste of the cèpe mushrooms, and the thick meaty flavor of the duck legs give this dish, a specialty from the French Alps, a wonderful multi-dimensional quality in which the ensemble is strong yet each piece stands out. And it goes beautifully with another specialty of the region: Chestnut Potato Gnocchi (page 226).

PREFERRED CLAY POT:

A 10-or 11-inch straight-sided flameware skillet or Spanish cazuela

If using an electric or ceramic stovetop, be sure to use a heat diffuser with the clay pot.

⅓ cup dried cèpes or porcini mushrooms

Pinch of sugar

2 large duck legs, trimmed of excess fat

Salt and freshly ground black pepper

1 tablespoon extra virgin olive oil

2 medium tomatoes, peeled, seeded, and chopped

1 medium onion, finely chopped

3 large garlic cloves, finely chopped

1½ teaspoons tomato paste, canned or homemade (page 317)

½ cup dry red wine

Large herb bouquet: 1 bay leaf, 4 sprigs each fresh flat-leaf parsley and thyme, tied together

4 ounces picholine olives, rinsed and pitted

1 Soak the dried porcini with a pinch of sugar in 1 cup warm water to soften for 30 minutes. Drain the mushrooms, straining the liquid through a coffee filter or paper towels. Rinse the mushrooms briefly and sliver if large. Set the mushrooms and soaking liquid aside separately.

2 Meanwhile, rinse the duck legs and pat dry. Prick the skin with the tines of a fork or a skewer at 1-inch intervals. Season generously with salt and pepper.

3 Heat the olive oil in the ceramic skillet over medium heat. Add the duck legs, skin side down, and brown lightly on both sides, about 10 minutes. Transfer the duck to a side dish.

4 Pour off all but 2 tablespoons of the fat from the skillet. Add the tomatoes and a pinch of sugar. Raise the heat to medium-high and cook, mashing the tomatoes, until they are lightly scorched, 7 to 8 minutes. Reduce the heat to medium. Add the onion, garlic, tomato paste, and red wine. Cook, stirring, until a thick sauce forms, about 20 minutes.

5 Return the duck legs to the skillet. Add the herb bouquet and mushrooms, cover tightly, and cook over medium heat for 30 minutes. Meanwhile, preheat the oven to 300°F.

6 Discard the herb bouquet, tilt the skillet, and spoon off and discard all excess fat. Add the rinsed olives and reserved mushroom-soaking liquid and bring to a boil. Lift the duck legs so they are on top of the olives and mushrooms, skin side up. Place the skillet in the top third of the oven. Raise the temperature to 400°F and bake, uncovered, for 25 minutes, or until the duck legs are tender, the skin is browned and crisp, and the sauce is bubbling. Serve at once.

Slow-Cooked Duck Breast with Peppercorns and Golden Raisins

SERVES 2

For this great duck dish, a takeoff on steak *au poivre*, I've employed a low-temperature cooking method commonly used by professional chefs but rarely presented in recipes intended for home cooks. Large Peking duck breasts are seared quickly on both sides in a skillet and then transferred to a preheated earthenware serving dish and roasted in a low oven for about twenty minutes until perfectly cooked and incredibly tender. This is a perfect example of the superiority of clay over metal for slow cooking. If you transferred the breasts to a metal dish, it would quickly heat up and the breasts would overcook.

PREFERRED CLAY POT:
A 9- or 10-inch glazed earthenware or flameware skillet

2 large boneless Peking duck breast halves
  (5 ounces each)

1 teaspoon sea salt

2 tablespoons golden raisins

1 tablespoon cognac

1 tablespoon dry red wine

3 tablespoons unsalted butter

1½ teaspoons crushed black peppercorns

¾ cup poultry or meat stock

1 teaspoon Dijon mustard

2 tablespoons heavy cream

(continued)

1   About 1 hour before serving, use a thin-bladed knife to remove the skin and fat from the duck breasts. Season the duck breasts with the salt, cover loosely with paper towels, and let stand at room temperature for 30 minutes. In a small bowl, soak the raisins in the cognac mixed with the wine.

2   Place the earthenware skillet on the center rack of the oven. Set the temperature at 140°F or 150°F.

3   Pat the duck dry with paper towels. Spread half the crushed peppercorns on a sheet of wax paper and firmly press the duck into them. Turn, spread the remaining peppercorns on top of the duck, and use your palm to press them down firmly.

4   Set a dry stainless-steel or cast-iron skillet over medium heat. When it is hot, add 1 tablespoon of the butter and the duck and sear for 1 minute on each side. Immediately transfer the duck to the warm pan in the oven. Bake for 25 to 30 minutes.

5   While the duck roasts, begin the sauce: Pour off the fat and remove any loose peppercorns in the skillet. Set the skillet over low heat and add the raisins along with the cognac and wine. Warm for a minute or two, then carefully ignite with a match. When the flames subside, add the stock and bring to a boil. Scrape up any browned bits from the bottom of the skillet. Whisk in the mustard and cream, then remove from the heat and set aside.

6   Test the duck with your thumb and forefinger by pinching the flesh; it should just spring back. Transfer the cooked breasts to a carving board and let stand for a few minutes. Again, check the breast for doneness. If it is too rare for your taste, reheat the skillet and cook gently for another minute or two on each side. Immediately return to the wooden work surface. Meanwhile, quickly reheat the sauce and swirl in the remaining 2 tablespoons butter. Pour the sauce into a serving dish. Thinly slice the breasts crosswise on a diagonal and arrange overlapping on the raisin sauce. Serve at once.

Cazuela Duck Leg Confit

SERVES 4

I'm always looking for new ways to prepare duck confit. When I first started making it, I used an electric slow cooker and at least five pounds of duck fat. Such a large amount of fat ensured that the duck legs could be stored safely for months so that the wondrous alchemical maturing process that makes for great confit could take place. Later, I introduced the *sous vide* method, which requires very little fat. (Those methods are presented in detail in the revised edition of my book *The Cooking of Southwest France, 2007.*)

Here, now, is a third method—quicker and easier—in which fatted duck legs are baked slowly side by side in a clay pot. This method incorporates a small amount of purchased fat, and though it won't have quite the inimitable flavor of a traditional long-aged confit, it provides a fine, wonderfully flavorful meal within a week. As with the other methods, you will have plenty of lovely duck fat left over for cooking potatoes, stews, and soups or for making more duck confit.

Please note that the duck juices, fondly known as "duck Jell-O," should be saved to flavor the accompanying lentil ragout.

4 small Moulard duck legs (about 2 pounds total), with plenty of attached fat

4 teaspoons coarse salt, preferably Diamond Crystal (2 teaspoons per pound of duck legs)

1 tablespoon juniper berries, lightly cracked

1 tablespoon black peppercorns, lightly cracked

1 teaspoon coriander seeds, lightly cracked

1 clove, lightly cracked

⅛ teaspoon freshly grated nutmeg

3 garlic cloves, coarsely chopped

2 bay leaves, crumbled

1 tablespoon chopped fresh flat-leaf parsley

1 tablespoon chopped fresh thyme or 1 teaspoon dried

7 or 8 ounces rendered duck fat, homemade or store-bought

1 At least 5 days and up to a week in advance, rinse and dry the duck legs. In a mortar, coarsely pound the salt with the juniper berries, black peppercorns, coriander seeds, clove, nutmeg, garlic, and bay leaves. Mix with the parsley and thyme. Rub the duck with the mixture. Place in a zippered plastic bag or a covered glass or earthenware dish; cover and refrigerate for 24 hours.

2 The next day, preheat the oven to 225°F. Remove the duck from the refrigerator and wipe away all the flavoring and juices with a paper towel. Prick the fatty skin all over with the tines of a fork or a skewer.

3 Place the rendered fat in the cazuela and add the duck legs, skin side up, in a single layer. Cover with a round of parchment and a lid and set in the oven to cook without opening the oven door for 4 hours, or until the duck is very tender. Turn off the heat and leave the confit in the oven for 1 to 2 hours longer to cool in the fat.

4 Transfer the duck to a deep container. Ladle fat over the duck to cover. When cold, cover with plastic wrap and refrigerate. The confit will keep up to 6 days, submerged in its cooking fat in the refrigerator. Scrape off all fat before using.

Cazuela Duck Confit with a Ragout of Green Lentilles du Puy

SERVES 4

PREFERRED CLAY POT:

A 2½- or 3-quart earthenware or flameware casserole

If using an electric or ceramic stovetop, be sure to use a heat diffuser with the clay pot.

Cazuela Duck Leg Confit (preceding recipe)

½ ounce dried cèpes or porcini (⅓ cup)

1 tablespoon rendered duck fat

2 cups coarsely chopped scallions

Herb bouquet: 1 bay leaf, 3 fresh flat-leaf parsley sprigs, and a few tender sprigs of celery leaves tied together with string

1½ ounces thinly sliced lean pancetta, shredded

½ cup finely diced carrot

2 tablespoons homemade tomato paste (page 317)

1 cup green lentilles du Puy

2 cups chicken stock, simmering

1 tablespoon duck "Jell-O" (see preceding recipe)

1 teaspoon Dijon mustard

3 tablespoons crème fraîche or heavy cream

Salt and freshly ground black pepper

1 tablespoon chopped fresh flat-leaf parsley

1 tablespoon chopped celery leaves

1 Prepare the Cazuela Duck Leg Confit 5 to 7 days in advance. Remove from the refrigerator and let stand at room temperature for about 4 hours.

2 Crumble the dried cèpes into a bowl, add 5 tablespoons water, and soak for at least 20 minutes, until softened. Strain, pressing on the mushrooms to extract as much liquid as possible and saving the mushrooms and liquid separately.

3 In the earthenware casserole, slowly heat the duck fat along with the scallions and mushroom soaking liquid. Cover and cook over medium heat, stirring, until the scallions are soft, golden, and glazed, about 5 minutes. Add the herb bouquet, pancetta, soaked mushrooms, and carrot; fry lightly and stir over medium heat until golden, about 10 minutes. Add the tomato paste and fry gently until lightly caramelized.

4 Meanwhile, put the lentils in a saucepan, cover with 1 quart water, and bring slowly to a boil over medium-low heat. Drain and add to the casserole. Add the chicken stock and duck "Jell-O." Cover and cook over medium-low heat until the lentils are tender, about 30 minutes.

5 While the lentils are cooking, place a rimmed, nonstick baking sheet on the top rack in the oven and preheat the oven to 400°F.

6 Put the duck legs, skin side down, on the hot baking pan and bake until the skin is crisp, about 20 minutes.

7 Use a slotted spoon to transfer the lentils to a side dish. Pick out and discard the herbs from the liquid. Stir the mustard and cream into the liquid in the casserole; bring to a boil. Return about ¾ cup of the lentils to the casserole and cook, crushing and stirring, until the sauce thickens slightly. Return the remaining lentils to the casserole and season with salt and pepper to taste. Arrange the drained duck legs on top, garnish with a sprinkling of chopped parsley and celery, and serve hot, directly from the casserole.

Duck Agrodolce with Grape Syrup, Pine Nuts, and Almonds

SERVES 4

*H*ere's my adaptation of a recipe from Francesco Contrafatto's *Sicilia del Sole,* a cookbook I purchased in Palermo more than thirty years ago but didn't open until recently. I'm so glad I did! I love his notion of serving a dark syrupy sauce, made with the pulp and skin of Sicilian grapes, with poultry. I substitute northern Italian saba, which you can find online, or you can substitute similar Mediterranean syrups or grape molasses, such as Greek *petimezi,* Spanish *arrop,* or Turkish *pekmez,* thinned with a little water, to produce this exciting sweet-and-sour duck dish.

> **PREFERRED CLAY POT:**
>
> A 4- or 5-quart glazed or unglazed earthenware casserole with a tight-fitting lid
>
> If using an electric or ceramic stovetop, be sure to use a heat diffuser with the clay pot.

4 large Moulard duck legs (12 to 16 ounces each)

1 teaspoon black peppercorns

1 3-inch cinnamon stick

1 large onion, finely chopped, plus 1 slice of onion

4 celery ribs, sliced ½ inch thick

Sea salt and freshly ground black pepper

3 tablespoons extra virgin olive oil

1 carrot, finely diced

¼ cup plus 2 tablespoons grape molasses, diluted with ¼ cup water

½ cup pitted green olives, drained and rinsed

3 tablespoons currants or small black raisins, soaked in hot water to soften and drained

⅓ cup pine nuts

2 tablespoons capers, drained and rinsed

7 ounces sliced almonds, toasted

2 teaspoons red wine vinegar, or more to taste

2 teaspoons sugar, or more to taste

Celery leaf sprigs for garnish

1 Remove the excess fat from the duck legs; prick the skin all over with a fork or a skewer and place in the earthenware casserole. Add 2 cups water, the peppercorns, cinnamon stick, and onion slice. Slowly bring to a boil. Cover the duck with a sheet of parchment and a tight-fitting lid and poach gently over medium heat for 45 minutes.

2 Meanwhile, cook the celery in a medium conventional saucepan of salted water until tender, about 10 minutes; drain and set aside.

3 Lift each piece of duck out of the casserole, letting the fat and juices fall back into the pot, and set aside on a flat plate; salt lightly. Skim as much fat as possible from the cooking juices. Measure out and reserve ¾ cup of the juices. Save the remaining poaching liquid for some other purpose or discard.

(continued)

4 Wipe out the casserole and return it to medium heat. Add half the olive oil, the carrot, and the chopped onion and cook until tender, about 10 minutes. Stir in the ¾ cup reserved cooking juices and half the grape molasses. Add to the saucepan with the cooked celery and bring to a boil. Season with salt and pepper to taste. Set aside.

5 Put the remaining oil and grape molasses in the casserole, stir to mix, and add the duck. Cook over medium heat until the skin side is nicely coated with sauce, about 5 minutes. Add the olives, currants, pine nuts, capers, and almonds and mix gently to combine. Add the contents of the saucepan to the casserole. Bring to a boil; reduce the heat, cover, and cook slowly until the duck is completely tender, about 45 minutes. (On electric and ceramic ranges, the duck may need another 20 minutes.)

6 Use a slotted spoon to transfer the duck, vegetables, and other garnishes to a heated serving dish. Degrease the liquid in the pan. Add the vinegar and sugar to the cooking juices and bring quickly to a boil. Boil until reduced to a nice napping consistency (coats the back of a spoon), correct the seasoning with salt and pepper, and pour over the duck. Garnish with sprigs of fresh celery.

Cazuela Quail with Red Peppers and Pine Nut Picada

SERVES 6

Here's one of my favorite Catalan recipes from the vicinity of Tarragona: lean quail flesh wrapped in rich, silky sweet red peppers, cooked in a *picada*, a cinnamon-flavored tomato sauce thickened with toasted pine nuts.

> **PREFERRED CLAY POT:**
> An 10- to 12-inch straight-sided flameware skillet
> If using an electric or ceramic stovetop, be sure to use a heat diffuser with the clay pot.

6 bone-in quail (about 6 ounces each)

¼ cup plus 2 tablespoons extra virgin olive oil

1 tablespoon fresh thyme leaves

1 tablespoon chopped fresh flat-leaf parsley

¼ teaspoon freshly grated nutmeg

Coarse sea salt and freshly ground black pepper

1 large onion, grated (about 1 cup)

3 plum tomatoes, grated (1 cup)

Pinch of ground cinnamon

3 tablespoons pine nuts

1 large garlic clove

3 large red bell peppers

1 Cut off the wing tips at the second joint of each quail. With kitchen shears, remove the backbones. Flatten, skin side down, to loosen the breastbone. Cut or pull out the wishbone, tiny rib bones, and breastbone. Leave in place the thigh and leg bones. Place the quail in a medium bowl and toss gently with ¼ cup of the olive oil, the thyme, 2 teaspoons of the parsley, the nutmeg, and 1¼ teaspoons each salt and pepper. Cover and refrigerate for 1 to 3 hours.

2 About 1 hour before serving, preheat the oven to 450°F. Shake the marinade from the quail into the flameware skillet set over medium-heat. When hot, add the quail, skin side up, and sear for an instant; turn over and sear the skin side. Set aside on a plate. Add the grated onion to the skillet and cook, stirring, over medium heat until soft and golden, 7 or 8 minutes. Add the tomatoes, cinnamon, and 3 tablespoons water. Continue to cook, stirring occasionally, for 10 minutes.

3 Peel the red bell peppers with a swivel-bladed vegetable peeler, then cut each lengthwise in half; discard the membranes, seeds, and stems. Fold each quail into its natural shape and place breast side up in a pepper half.

4 In a small dry skillet, toast the pine nuts over medium heat until golden and fragrant, 3 to 4 minutes. Transfer to a mortar and let cool slightly. Add the garlic, 1 teaspoon coarse salt, and the remaining 1 teaspoon parsley. Crush to a paste. Stir into the tomato sauce in the skillet. Season with salt and pepper to taste.

5 Arrange the peppers stuffed with quail in a single layer in the tomato sauce. Brush the breasts with the remaining 2 tablespoons olive oil and sprinkle lightly with salt and pepper. Bake the quail-stuffed peppers in the top third of the oven for 20 minutes, or until they are just cooked through. Garnish with the remaining parsley and serve at once directly from the skillet.

Clay Pan–Roasted Guinea Fowl with Chanterelles, Walnut Oil, and Verjuice

SERVES 4

One of my favorite cookbooks of recent years is Chef Paul Bertolli's *Cooking By Hand*. In it, Paul is particularly eloquent on what he calls "bottom-up cooking" (from the Italian *fondo di cottura*)— the concept of developing flavor from the bottom of the pan by forcing caramelization and then working browned scrapings into the food. It's an earthy style of Italian home cooking particularly well suited to the preparation of a game bird such as guinea hen.

Pieces of the bird are browned in a large flameware or La Chamba skillet. Cooking with little or no fat encourages the juices to emerge and caramelize. All cooking is done on top of the stove. The result is fabulous, producing deep and intense flavor, and the technique isn't at all difficult, though it does require constant attention.

In autumn, I add chestnuts and chanterelles; in spring, cut-up artichoke bottoms. I serve the guinea fowl right from the ceramic flameware skillet, adding to the homey effect. And the method is economical: If you roast a three-pound guinea hen, it will feed two or three. But "bottom-up cooking" will yield four juicy portions.

> **PREFERRED CLAY POT:**
>
> An 11- or 12-inch straight-sided flameware or La Chamba skillet, or a Spanish cazuela
>
> If using an electric or ceramic stovetop, be sure to use a heat diffuser with the clay pot.

1 guinea fowl (2¾ to 3½ pounds), cut into
   8 pieces (see Note)

Coarse salt and freshly ground black pepper

2 tablespoons extra virgin olive oil

4 garlic cloves, sliced

8 ounces small fresh chanterelles

2 thin slices pancetta, diced

3 tablespoons chopped fresh flat-leaf parsley

¾ cup Guinea Hen Stock (recipe follows) or
   chicken stock

1 teaspoon walnut oil

3 to 4 teaspoons verjuice, white wine vinegar,
   or fresh lemon juice

1 Generously season the pieces of guinea fowl with salt and pepper.

2 Heat the olive oil in the flameware skillet over medium heat. Place the thigh and leg pieces, skin side down, in the hot oil and cook for 5 minutes. Surround with the breast pieces, skin side down, and continue browning, shifting the pieces from time to time for even coloring. If the breast pieces appear to be cooking too fast, lift and "park" them on top of the dark parts for a few minutes before returning them to the gently sizzling fat. Cook for 20 to 25 minutes, until nicely browned; turn the pieces over and repeat on the other side, cooking for 10 to 15 minutes longer. Transfer the pieces of guinea hen to a side dish.

3 Add the garlic slices, chanterelles, and a few tablespoons of water to the pan drippings in the skillet and cook for about 5 minutes, stirring, to scrape up any flavorful bits clinging to the bottom of the pan. Add the pancetta, parsley, and a few pinches of salt and pepper, and cook for 2 minutes longer. Pour in the stock and boil down until it's thick enough to coat a spoon.

4 Return the guinea hen to the skillet, skin side up, partially cover, and simmer in the reduced stock for 10 minutes. Add the walnut oil and verjuice and correct the seasoning with salt and pepper. Serve directly from the skillet.

NOTE TO THE COOK: To cut up the guinea fowl: First remove the backbone and wing tips. Then press down on the breastbone to weaken it. Divide the breast in half and cut each breast half into two parts. Separate each thigh-leg section at the joint. Save all the trimmings, giblets, and excess fat for the stock.

Guinea Hen Stock

MAKES ABOUT ¾ CUP

Backbone, neck, wing tips, liver, and excess fat from the guinea fowl

2 tablespoons olive oil

1 small onion, sliced

1 carrot, sliced

2 garlic cloves, bruised

1 bay leaf

4 to 5 fresh thyme sprigs

4 to 5 fresh flat-leaf parsley sprigs

1 cup dry white wine

1 Put the backbone, neck, wing tips, and excess fat from the guinea hen in a medium conventional saucepan over medium heat and slowly let the pieces brown, about 15 minutes.

2 Add the onion, carrot, garlic, bay leaf, thyme, parsley, and white wine and simmer until reduced to a glaze, about 30 minutes.

3 Use a strainer to scoop out and discard the vegetables. Add ½ cup hot water to the juices in the saucepan and bring to a boil. Remove from the heat and set aside until needed.

Roast Turkey with Sausage, Mushroom, and Walnut Stuffing

SERVES 10

Here's my adaptation of a terrific turkey dish from the beautiful, savagely rural area of France called the Aveyron near the French southwest. I learned it years ago from Chef Michel Bras, whose three-star restaurant is in Laguiole, a town famous for its knives. I've been making it on and off for Thanksgiving ever since. For best flavor, use a turkey that is tagged "Heritage." To find one in your area, check www.newfarm.org/features/1103/heritageturkey.shtml.

I offer two methods here so you can choose the one most appropriate for your kitchen: One calls for a large Romertopf baker, and the other uses a clay-lined oven. Both produce a turkey of great succulence and a wonderful parchmentlike skin.

> **PREFERRED CLAY POT:**
> Romertopf clay baker 14 pounds

1 young heritage turkey (10 to 12 pounds)

Salt and freshly ground black pepper

¼ cup dried cèpes or porcini (1½ ounces), crumbled

8 to 9 ounces fresh white-meat pork sausage, such as boudin blanc, weisswurst, or bratwurst

2 tablespoons unsalted butter

1½ ounces thinly sliced pancetta, slivered

8 ounces fresh white mushrooms, sliced

½ cup chopped scallion or shallot

2 garlic cloves, chopped

¼ cup chopped fresh flat-leaf parsley

2 tablespoons fresh thyme leaves

⅓ cup chopped walnuts

3 tablespoons cognac

1 cup cubed stale white bread without crusts

¼ cup milk

2 eggs, lightly beaten

1 Up to a day in advance, remove the giblets and the neck from the turkey cavity. Discard or save for another purpose. Rinse the turkey inside and out and pat dry with paper towels. Cut off the wing at the first joint and save for some other purpose. Season the turkey inside and out with salt and pepper.

2 Make the stuffing: Rinse the dried cèpes; soak in water to cover for 15 minutes. Then strain through a paper coffee filter or cheesecloth and reserve the cèpes and soaking water separately.

3 Meanwhile, prick the sausage. Cook in a small skillet over medium heat, turning, just until firm, about 5 minutes. Let cool slightly; then coarsely chop.

4 In a large skillet, heat the butter and pancetta, stirring, over medium heat without browning for about 5 minutes. Add the fresh mushrooms, raise the heat to medium-high, and sauté, stirring, until they are softened and well reduced, 5 minutes. Add the scallion, garlic, 3 tablespoons of the chopped parsley, and 1 tablespoon of the chopped thyme leaves and cook, stirring, for 5 minutes longer. Add the walnuts and stir until lightly browned, about 3 minutes. Add the cèpes, reserved soaking liquid, and chopped sausage to the skillet. Bring to a boil, stirring, and cook until the sausage is cooked through and the mixture is thick. Season with salt and pepper and let cool. (The recipe can be prepared to this point 1 day in advance. Cover the stuffing base and refrigerate.)

5 The following day, about 4½ hours before serving, remove the turkey and stuffing base from the refrigerator. Let stand at room temperature for about 1 hour.

6 Soak the Romertopf top and bottom in cold water to cover for 15 minutes. Meanwhile, soak the bread cubes in the milk for 5 minutes; then squeeze gently and toss to lighten. Add the bread and beaten eggs to the stuffing and mix thoroughly. Add 1 teaspoon salt and ¼ teaspoon pepper. Place a handful of the stuffing in the neck cavity and secure it closed with a small bamboo skewer. Fill the main cavity loosely with the remaining stuffing to allow room for expansion. Tie the legs close together.

7 Drain the Romertopf baker and shake off excess moisture. Grease the inside of the top and bottom with rendered fat or butter. Place the turkey in the Romertopf and brush all over with the remaining fat. Cover the pot and place in a cold oven. Turn the heat to 425°F and bake for 1½ hours.

8 Use heavy oven mitts to transfer the baker to a wooden surface. Carefully remove the cover, tilt the lower part of the baker, and use a bulb baster to transfer the juices into a shallow saucepan; skim the fat off the top and boil down to a glaze; set aside. Replace the cover on the Romertopf and return to the oven; bake for 30 minutes. Remove the top and cook for 30 minutes longer, or until the turkey thigh meat registers 165°F to 170°F and the skin is brown and crisp.

9 Let the baker stand, uncovered, on a wooden surface for about 20 minutes. Transfer the turkey to a carving board. Pour the juices from the baker into the saucepan with the reserved glaze. Skim off the fat and boil over high heat until reduced to 2 cups, about 5 minutes, skimming often. Season with salt and pepper to taste. Carve the turkey and arrange on a serving dish. Surround with the stuffing. Pour the reduced pan juices into a sauceboat and serve alongside.

Roast Turkey without a Romertopf

> **SUGGESTED CLAY ENVIRONMENT:**
> **Double slabs of pizza stones or food-safe quarry tiles set on the upper and lower oven racks.**

¼ cup rendered duck fat, lard, or softened unsalted butter

About 4 hours before serving, preheat the oven to 325°F. Generously rub the bird with the softened fat. Place the turkey, breast side up, on a low cake rack in a shallow roasting pan. Set in the oven, feet toward the back, and roast for about 2½ hours. Midway, remove the turkey from the oven, pour the pan juices into a saucepan, skim the fat off the top, and boil until reduced by half. Return the turkey to the oven without basting. If the turkey begins to brown too quickly, cover it loosely with foil. Remove the foil during the last 30 minutes of roasting.

Meats

Slow-Roasted Glazed Lamb Shoulder with Spring Vegetables

SERVES 6 TO 8

*T*his terrific method for slow-roasted lamb shoulder was taught to me by Michelin-rated chef Dominique Bucaille of Haute-Provence, who was adamant that a clay cooking environment is crucial to its success.

Dominique slow roasts the shoulder in a shallow earthenware saucepan called a *poêlon* in a wood-burning beehive oven. Lacking this oven, he suggests using a Provençal tian, a wide-at-the-top and narrow-at-the-bottom earthenware bowl, so that the meat is surrounded by clay on three sides. (I recommend roasting in a cazuela in a clay environment.)

When the lamb is partially cooked, Dominique removes it and adds carrots, peas, fava beans, and spring onions, all subtly flavored with thyme twigs, to the pan. Then he sets the meat on top of the vegetables and continues roasting. In this way, the vegetables aromatize the meat, and the meat drippings impart their flavor to the vegetables. At completion, the lamb is so soft it can be cut with a spoon, while the vegetables retain their shapes.

After cooking, the pan juices are degreased, reduced, and poured back over the lamb and vegetables. The completed dish is presented at the table farmhouse style, in its cooking pot.

PREFERRED CLAY POT:

A large *poêlon de terre*, or an 11- or 12-inch Spanish cazuela, or a straight-sided flameware skillet

SUGGESTED CLAY ENVIRONMENT:

Double slabs of pizza stones or food-safe quarry tiles set on the upper and lower oven racks

1 boneless lamb shoulder roast (4 pounds) at room temperature

Salt and freshly ground black pepper

5 or 6 fresh thyme sprigs

Herb bouquet: 2 imported bay leaves, 1 leek, 10 fresh flat-leaf parsley sprigs, and 3 fresh lemon thyme sprigs, if available, tied with kitchen string

10 large garlic cloves, unpeeled

¼ cup extra virgin olive oil

1 bunch of spring onions or scallions

12 ounces small carrots

6 ounces fresh fava beans, shucked and peeled

8 ounces grape or cherry tomatoes

6 ounces frozen baby peas, thawed

3 tablespoons unsalted butter

1 tablespoon chopped fresh flat-leaf parsley

1 About 5 hours before serving, trim any excess fat from the lamb and season the meat generously with salt and pepper. Scatter the thyme, herb bouquet, and garlic cloves in the bottom of the cazuela. Place the lamb, fat side up, on top and pour the olive oil over the meat. Cover with a lid or foil and place in a cold oven. Set the temperature at 450°F and bake for 1 hour.

2 Reduce the oven temperature to 350°F and bake for another hour. Turn the meat over, reduce the heat to 300°F, and continue cooking, covered, for a third hour. Remove the lamb from the baking dish; leave the oven on. Discard the thyme and herb bouquet. Pour the juices into a small saucepan and set aside.

3 Scatter the spring onions, carrots, fava beans, tomatoes, and peas over the bottom of the cazuela. Dot with the butter and season with salt and pepper to taste. Set the lamb on top, fatty side up, and return it to the oven. Bake, uncovered, for 1 hour. Turn the oven off and leave the casserole in the oven without opening the door for 30 minutes longer.

4 Meanwhile, skim all the fat off the reserved cooking juices. Bring to a boil and cook until reduced to about ⅔ cup. Season with salt and pepper to taste.

5 Carefully transfer the cazuela to a wooden surface or folded kitchen towel to prevent cracking. Spoon the reduced juices over the lamb and vegetables. Garnish with the chopped parsley and serve directly from the dish.

COOKING MEAT IN A CLAY POT

Every Mediterranean country boasts its own particular clay pots for cooking meat. These come in remarkably similar shapes and sizes, which make it easy to substitute one for another. Whether it's a round French marmite or pot-bellied *daubière,* deep Turkish *guvec* or Greek *yiouvetsi,* brown-glazed Italian *pignata, tegame,* or *tiella,* tall Spanish olla or wide cazuela, or cone-topped Moroccan tagine, they all share a common quality: The clay makes the meat taste better.

Most home cooks around the Mediterranean region that I interviewed still prefer these traditional cooking vessels to the new, flashier metal alternatives. Whenever I asked why, I got pretty much the same set of answers: Clay pots produce tender, juicier, tastier meat without basting and often with less fat; they heat evenly; they retain moisture so the food remains succulent; they impart an earthy aroma; and they look great on the table.

One Turkish cook insisted that her *guvec* pot had a kind of "memory" of the dishes she always cooked in it. "Each time I use it, the *guvec* is a little better," she told me. When I recounted this tale to a Turkish friend, she told me there was a saying that amounted to the same thing: "If a clay pot recognizes an old tenant, it will produce a delicious dish when you bring the pot back to life."

Bell-Cooked Lamb Shanks with Lemon Potatoes

SERVES 4

The Ionian island of Cephalonia is known for its beautiful beaches, underground waterways, and also for its two famous lamb dishes: a mixed meat pie and this juicy lamb shank preparation.

Normally I braise lamb shanks, but here they are roasted over a bed of lemon-flavored potatoes beneath a clay dome, or "bell," cover. The moist heat results in crusty brown lamb that is packed with flavor and extremely juicy, with a unique buttery texture. Lemon-scented potatoes pair beautifully with the velvety meat, providing a wonderful one-pot meal.

The original recipe calls for a special two-part pot made of clay and hay called a *tserepa,* which is heated in a fireplace until extremely hot. Then the pot is filled with the lamb, potatoes, and carrots, the cover is put back in place, and the food cooks in the residual heat as the pot slowly cools down.

> **PREFERRED CLAY POT:**
>
> A Cephalonian *tserepa,* La Cloche stoneware domed baker, or a 4-quart round, covered stoneware casserole suitable for use in an oven heated to 475°F

1¼ pounds waxy medium potatoes, preferably Yukon Gold, peeled and quartered lengthwise

½ cup fresh lemon juice

3 garlic cloves, chopped

1½ teaspoons dried Greek oregano

1½ teaspoons coarse salt

½ teaspoon freshly ground black pepper

5 tablespoons extra virgin olive oil

4 lamb shanks (about 1 pound each), cracked

3 tablespoons chopped fresh flat-leaf parsley

1 About 5 hours before serving, soak the cut potatoes in water to cover for 30 minutes. Drain the potatoes and shake them dry. In a stainless-steel saucepan, combine ¼ cup of the lemon juice, one of the chopped garlic cloves, ½ teaspoon of the dried oregano, ½ teaspoon of the salt, ¼ teaspoon of the pepper, 3 tablespoons of the olive oil, and ½ cup cold water. Add the potatoes, stir to coat with the liquid, cover, and let stand in a cool place for up to 2 hours. Do not refrigerate.

2 Meanwhile, rinse the lamb shanks and wipe dry; trim away any excess fat. Massage with the remaining ¼ cup lemon juice. Combine 1 tablespoon of the parsley with the remaining oregano, garlic, salt, and pepper. Roll the lamb shanks in the seasonings to coat; let stand at room temperature for up to 2 hours.

3 Preheat the oven to 400°F. Place the lamb shanks in the bottom of the tserepa. Cover and place in the oven. Immediately raise the oven temperature to 475°F and bake for 30 minutes. Reduce the temperature to 350°F and bake for 1 hour longer.

4 Set the saucepan with the potatoes and marinating liquid over medium heat and bring to a boil. Meanwhile, carefully transfer the hot casserole to a wooden work surface or folded kitchen towel to prevent cracking. Do the same when you remove the top. Spoon the hot potatoes around the lamb and pour the cooking liquid into the casserole. Replace the cover, return the casserole to the oven, and bake for 1 hour.

5 Remove the lid and place on a wooden work surface or folded kitchen towel to prevent cracking. Reduce the oven temperature to 250°F and bake, uncovered, without opening the oven door for 30 minutes longer.

6 Remove the lamb shanks and arrange them on a warmed serving platter; surround with the potatoes. Skim the fat off the cooking juices in the casserole and pour over the lamb. Serve at once, with the remaining parsley sprinkled on top.

HAOUARI'S TUNISIAN LAMB BAKED IN A CLAY JAR

My friendship with Tunisian chef Haouari Abderrazak goes back fifteen years. Over that time I've stayed in his house, come to know his wife and children, and accompanied him as he picked herbs and vegetables from his garden. My books are filled with the numerous dishes he's taught me, including a method of baking lamb in a disposable clay jar.

On Haouari's native island of Djerba, an inexpensive amphora-shaped unglazed terra-cotta pot called a *gargoulette* is stuffed with lamb along with vegetables, spices, and olive oil and then baked slowly immersed in hot embers. Just before service, Haouari brings the pot out to the table, breaks it open with a mallet, and pours the contents into terra-cotta bowls. I offer a recipe for this dish in *The Slow Mediterranean Kitchen.*

Tile-Roasted Lamb Shepherd's Style

SERVES 2

On my last trip to Turkey I spent a day at a lovely outdoor restaurant, Ayso, in the town of Silivri near the Marmara Sea. The owner, Kemal Sofuoğlo invited me into the kitchen to observe the preparation of his popular clay pot dishes, including this one, *Çomlekte Çoban Kavurma,* which he translated as "shepherd's roast lamb cooked on an earthen plate."

It's an easy recipe, but it must be cooked as directed: hot meat on a hot dry concave clay tile or a thick, unglazed ceramic skillet, such as La Chamba. To accomplish this, the meat is first sautéed in a skillet and then transferred to a slowly preheated clay tile to finish along with finely chopped shallots and diced tomatoes. You'll hear the lamb cubes sizzle when they hit the hot tile, and that's part of the fun. You'll also get a wonderful herbal aroma conveyed by the released steam.

This method is fairly common around the Mediterranean and much appreciated for the special earthy flavor it conveys. I've even seen pairs of hot concave roof tiles with meat, fish, or poultry sandwiched between them.

PREFERRED CLAY POT:

An unglazed and untreated concave roof tile or a La Chamba skillet, or a *comal*, well scrubbed and completely dried

1 large tomato

½ teaspoon coarse salt

12 ounces boneless lamb loin

Salt and freshly ground black pepper

2 pinches of Greek oregano

1 tablespoon unsalted butter

3 medium shallots, finely chopped

1 About 45 minutes before serving, temper the tile or ceramic dish by placing it in a cold oven on the lowest rack, close to the door. Set the oven temperature at 250°F and heat for 15 minutes. Raise the oven temperature to 400°F and heat the tile for 30 minutes.

2 Meanwhile, peel and chop the tomato. Sprinkle with the salt and drain on a paper towel–lined plate.

3 Trim as much fat as possible from the lamb and cut the meat into 12 cubes. Season the lamb with salt, pepper, and a pinch of oregano. Set aside at room temperature.

4 About 10 minutes before serving, lightly oil a heavy 10-inch conventional skillet and set it over high heat. Add the lamb to the skillet and sauté, tossing, for 2 minutes. Remove from the heat. Sprinkle the shallots and salted tomatoes over the meat.

5 Open the oven door, quickly scrape the contents of the skillet onto the heated tile, and immediately close the oven door. Cook the meat on the tile for 3 to 4 minutes. Transfer the hot tile to a wooden surface or folded kitchen towel to prevent cracking. Serve at once, sprinkled with an additional pinch of oregano and salt.

Moroccan Mechoui

SERVES 6 TO 8

My husband, Bill, is a midwestern carnivore, so I usually defer to him on roasting big pieces of meat. In his opinion, the gold standard for slow-roasted lamb is Moroccan *mechoui*, with its delicious crusty exterior and awesomely juicy flesh. I agree.

Moroccans prepare *mechoui* in a number of different ways. The most common is slow, steady spit roasting, done outdoors (often at festivals) over embers. This method is excellent, but it requires constant basting.

Another method, which Bill and I first observed in the Saharan south of the country, reminded us of a clambake. The men set a wood fire at the bottom of a brick-lined pit, and when it was extremely hot, they buried a whole dressed lamb in it and then closed off the top of the pit with a mixture of mud and grass. As the lamb steamed, it basted itself and emerged after a few hours meltingly tender, with a juiciness that spit-roasted lamb cannot acquire.

Here you'll find my way of simulating this Saharan method, cooking a lamb shoulder inside a Romertopf clay baker, which produces a slow release of steam that tenderizes tough lamb shoulder. When all the moisture has evaporated, the outside starts to crisp and turn golden brown while the meat continues to soften. I learned the seasoned butter formula years ago from a retired cook from the palace kitchen of King Mohammed V. It's still the best *mechoui* seasoning I know.

PREFERRED CLAY POT:
Romertopf clay baker, 5 to 7 pounds

1 bone-in lamb shoulder (6 to 7 pounds)

1 garlic clove, coarsely chopped

1 teaspoon coarse sea salt

5 tablespoons unsalted butter, at room temperature

1½ tablespoons ground coriander

1½ teaspoons ground cumin

1 teaspoon sweet paprika

Small bowls of coarse sea salt and ground cumin
for serving

1 About 4 hours before serving, remove the lamb from the refrigerator. Trim away as much fat as possible and most of the thick outer skin, or fell.

2 In a small bowl or mortar, use a pestle to crush the garlic and salt to a smooth paste. Add the butter, coriander, cumin, and paprika and mix well. Rub the spiced butter all over the lamb, and let stand at room temperature for 15 minutes.

3 Meanwhile, soak the top and bottom of the Romertopf baker in water to cover for 15 minutes. Drain the baker and shake off excess moisture. Place the lamb, fat side up, in the pot, cover with the lid, and place in a cold oven. Set the oven temperature at 475°F and bake for 3 hours.

4 Carefully transfer the entire hot Romertopf baker to a wooden work surface or folded kitchen towel to prevent cracking. Uncover and let the lamb rest for 10 minutes before removing it from the baker. Carve and serve with small dishes of salt and cumin to dip or sprinkle over the meat.

Stuffed Breast of Lamb in the Style of Diyarkabir

SERVES 5 TO 6

This Turkish stuffed lamb breast, called *kaburga dolmasi*, is the most popular item at the Kurdish-style restaurants of famous restaurateur Selim Amca'nin's in Ankara and Diyarkabir. It's a dish for spring, when young lamb is available. The rice stuffing is scented with allspice, cinnamon, and dark opal basil, spiked with pine nuts, almonds, and raisins.

While the closed compartment of the clay baker may make you think of steaming, in fact the cooking is a two-step process. First the stuffed meat does steam in moist heat, which tenderizes it, but once the water evaporates from the clay, the meat dry roasts until crisp and brown.

> **PREFERRED CLAY POT:**
> **Romertopf clay baker, 5 to 7 pounds**

2¾ to 3 pounds breast of lamb

½ cup whole-milk yogurt

1 tablespoon tomato paste

Salt and freshly ground black pepper

1¼ cups Arborio, Baldo, or Spanish paella rice

4 tablespoons (½ stick) unsalted butter

¼ cup blanched almonds

¼ cup pine nuts

¼ cup dried currants

1 tablespoon dried opal basil (optional)

¼ teaspoon Turkish Spice Mixture (recipe follows)

1 One day in advance, rinse the lamb breast and pat it dry. Trim off as much fat as possible and the thick outer skin, or fell. Create a pocket for stuffing by sliding a thin-bladed knife along the top of the rib bones to separate the meat from the bones. Mix together the yogurt, tomato paste, ½ teaspoon salt, and ¼ teaspoon pepper, and rub all over the lamb breast inside and out. Wrap in plastic or butcher's paper and refrigerate overnight.

2 The following day, about 4 hours before serving, remove the lamb from the refrigerator. Soak the rice in 2 cups of very hot water for 15 minutes; drain into a sieve.

3 Melt 2 tablespoons of the butter in a medium conventional skillet. Add the almonds and sauté over medium-low heat until golden, about 3 minutes. Stir in the pine nuts and cook for 2 to 3 minutes longer, until fragrant. Add the currants, stir once, and remove from the heat. Spread the drained rice over the nuts and currants. Add 1½ cups water, 2 teaspoons salt, ½ teaspoon pepper, the basil, and the spice mixture. Cover and cook over medium heat until the water is absorbed, about 10 minutes. Remove from the heat and let cool completely.

4 Soak the Romertopf baker in water to cover for 15 minutes. Stuff the lamb with the rice filling, and sew the end shut with white kitchen string. Place the roast, skin side up, in the bottom part of the baker and dot with the remaining 2 tablespoons butter. Cover and place in the oven. Set the temperature at 400°F and bake for 2 hours without opening the oven door.

5 Turn off the heat and leave the baker in the hot oven for 30 minutes longer.

6 Carefully transfer the hot baker to a wooden surface or folded kitchen towel to prevent cracking. Transfer the meat to a carving board and let rest for 10 minutes. Pour out and discard the fat that has accumulated in the pot. Cut away all the string from the lamb breast and pull out any protruding rib bones. Carve into ½-inch-thick slices. Arrange on a heated platter and serve at once.

NOTES TO THE COOK:

❋ Because there isn't much demand for lamb breasts, which can be fatty, butchers tend to cut them up and sell the meat for stewing. To make sure a breast is available, order ahead.

❋ If you don't have a Romertopf baker, you can roast the lamb breast by rigging a clay environment using double slabs of pizza stones or food-safe quarry tiles set on the upper and lower oven racks, or you can use a La Cloche stoneware domed baker. Preheat the stones or tiles in the oven at 250°F. Place the stuffed breast of lamb, skin side up, in a shallow roasting pan, cover with foil, and set in the oven to roast for 3 hours. Raise the oven heat to 450°F and roast until the lamb is well browned, about 1 hour. If using a La Cloche stoneware domed baker, preheat the oven to 400°F. Line the shallow pan with foil. Place the lamb in the pan, cover with the dome, and bake in a preheated oven for 2½ hours.

Turkish Spice Mixture

MAKES ABOUT 2 TABLESPOONS

This is one of several blends popular in the eastern Mediterranean region for meat dishes, and vegetable stuffings.

1 teaspoon mixed pickling spice

2 teaspoons allspice berries or 1 teaspoon ground

1½ teaspoons ground cinnamon

1 teaspoon whole black peppercorns

½ teaspoon freshly grated nutmeg

4 cloves

Combine all the ingredients in an electric spice grinder or blender, and process until finely ground. Strain through a sieve. Store in a tightly covered jar at room temperature. Keeps fresh up to 3 months.

Stuffed Breast of Lamb Aegean Style

SERVES 4 TO 6

I've adapted this recipe from one in Dora Parisi's fine cookbook *Tastes of the Aegean*. Dora, who lives on the Island of Lesbos, kindly invited me over for a meal and then pointed me toward dishes that are cooked in the *gastra*, a dome-shaped ceramic vessel that works like a miniature beehive oven.

This stuffing for the lamb is quite amazing: sautéed potatoes, onions, and cubes of bread are tossed with lots of black currants and then mixed with a generous amount of ricotta and myzithra cheese, which brings it into perfect balance.

> **PREFERRED CLAY POT:**
> **Romertopf clay baker, 5 to 7 pounds**

2¾ to 3 pounds breast of lamb

½ lemon

Salt and freshly ground black pepper

⅓ cup extra virgin olive oil

1 medium Yukon Gold potato, peeled and finely diced

¾ cup cubed stale firm white bread with crust

Pinch of sugar

½ cup dried currants

1 medium onion, chopped

2 eggs

⅓ cup ricotta cheese

8 ounces myzithra, kefalotyri, or pecorino Romano cheese, grated (about 2 cups)

2 tablespoons chopped fresh flat-leaf parsley

1 tablespoon yogurt

1 tablespoon Dijon mustard

1 garlic clove, minced

1 Rinse the lamb breast and pat it dry. Trim off as much fat as possible as well as the thick outer skin, or fell. Create a pocket for stuffing by sliding a thin-bladed knife along the top of the rib bones to separate the meat from the bones. Rub all over with the juice of the lemon half. Sprinkle with salt and pepper. Let the lamb stand at room temperature while you prepare the stuffing.

2 Heat ¼ cup of the olive oil in a large conventional skillet. Add the potatoes, bread, and sugar and sauté over medium-high heat, stirring often, until golden, about 5 minutes. Scrape into a side dish. Heat the remaining olive oil in the skillet, add the onion, and sauté until golden, about 5 minutes. Return the potatoes and bread to the skillet, add the currants and toss once to mix. Remove from the heat and let cool.

3 Soak the Romertopf baker in water to cover for 15 minutes. Meanwhile, in a large bowl, lightly beat the eggs. Stir in the ricotta and grated cheese. Add the potato-bread mixture and the parsley; mix well. Stuff the lamb with this filling, and sew the end shut with white kitchen string. Fold the thinner part of the breast underneath and shape into a flat oblong roast.

4   In a small bowl, mix together the yogurt, mustard, and garlic. Spread all over the lamb. Drain the Romertopf, shaking off any excess moisture. Place the stuffed breast of lamb in the baker, cover with the lid, and place in a cold oven. Set the oven temperature at 400°F and bake for 2 hours without disturbing.

5   Turn off the oven. Leave the baker in the hot oven without opening the door for 30 minutes longer. Transfer the hot pot to a wooden surface or folded kitchen towel to prevent cracking. Pour out and discard the fat that has accumulated around the meat. Let the meat rest for 10 minutes. Cut away all the string and pull out any protruding ribs. Carve into 1½-inch-thick slices. Arrange on a heated platter and serve at once.

NOTE TO THE COOK: If you don't have a Romertopf, you can roast the lamb breast in a La Cloche stoneware domed baker. Preheat the oven to 400°F. Place the stuffed breast of lamb, skin side up, in a shallow roasting pan, cover, and set in the oven to roast for 2½ hours.

Pignata of Lamb Stewed with Sheep's Milk Cheese

SERVES 4

Pignatas are cooking vessels shaped like bean pots, and they play many roles in the Italian kitchen. For this Easter dish from the town of Bari in Puglia, you can substitute any flameproof ceramic pot to cook cubes of lamb shoulder slowly along with onions, tomatoes, and parsley. At a certain point, a huge amount of greens is added along with additional flavorings; then cooking continues slowly until the stew reaches luscious, succulent perfection.

Up to this point the dish can be prepared in advance and left to mellow in the refrigerator. In the final step, the stew is spread out in a shallow clay baking dish, covered with two types of cheese—one soft and creamy, the other hard and pungent—and baked until the cheeses have melted and the top is golden.

> **PREFERRED CLAY POTS:**
>
> A 3- to 4-quart *pignata*, a glazed earthenware or flameware casserole, a bean pot, or a Spanish olla
>
> A 10- to 12-inch shallow round earthenware, stoneware, or flameware baking dish
>
> If using an electric or ceramic stovetop, be sure to use a heat diffuser with the clay pots.

(continued)

1½ pounds boneless lamb shoulder

1 medium onion, chopped

2 large garlic cloves, sliced

½ cup packed coarsely chopped fresh flat-leaf parsley

¼ cup chopped celery rib

¼ cup chopped celery leaves

1 cup halved cherry tomatoes

Coarse salt

½ teaspoon freshly ground black pepper

5 tablespoons extra virgin olive oil

1¾ to 2 pounds broccoli rabe

1 ounce sliced pancetta or salami, shredded

½ teaspoon crushed hot red pepper

2 ounces soft pecorino Toscana fresco or ricotta salata, crumbled

2 ounces grated hard pecorino cheese

1 Trim off any excess fat and cut the lamb into 1-inch cubes. Place in the pignata and add the onion, garlic, parsley, celery ribs and leaves, cherry tomatoes, ½ teaspoon salt, ¼ teaspoon of the pepper, and 3 tablespoons of the olive oil; stir to mix well. Cover with a sheet of parchment and a lid, set over medium-low heat, and cook for 1 hour.

2 Meanwhile, trim off and discard the thick stalks from the broccoli rabe. Cut the florets and leaves into 1-inch chunks. Place in a colander; sprinkle with 3 to 4 tablespoons coarse salt and toss to coat. Let stand for 45 minutes. Rinse the greens in plenty of water to remove the salt; drain and squeeze out as much moisture as possible. Add to the casserole along with the pancetta, hot pepper, ½ teaspoon salt, and the remaining ¼ teaspoon black pepper. Cover and cook for 45 minutes.

3 Transfer the meat and greens to the baking dish. If there is a lot of liquid in the casserole, pour it into a small conventional saucepan and boil until reduced to a syrupy glaze. Mix the glaze with the remaining 2 tablespoons olive oil and the two cheeses and spread evenly over the meat and greens.

4 Set in a cold oven, turn the heat to 450°F, and bake until the cheese is melted, about 30 minutes. Serve at once.

TURKISH GUVEC

Just as *tagine* may refer to both a specific Moroccan cooking vessel and the type of food prepared in it, so the Turkish word *guvec* describes a pot and also a dish. The famous *guvec* pot of Turkey has dozens of different names in Balkan countries, but whatever they call it, they are talking about the same basic cooking vessel: a wide medium-tall, glazed or unglazed earthenware pot in which food is cooked slowly with little or no additional liquid.

My friend, Turkish food writer Ayfer Ünsal, brought me to Beypazari, a town about half an hour out of Ankara, which is famous for its *guvec* preparation. The mayor himself greeted us. He proudly told me that his recipe was so good he'd patented it! Later I heard that the townspeople joked that those who followed their own recipes felt they had to close their kitchen curtains lest the mayor find out.

One of the most popular *guvecs* is a thick summer dish of lamb cooked slowly with a variety of late summer vegetables: eggplant, tomatoes, beans, okra, and peppers. An important rule of the dish is that no water or stock be added; the meat and vegetables are sufficient to contribute just the right amount of moisture.

Traditionally, a *guvec* was prepared at home and then sent out to a commercial bakery for cooking in a wood-burning oven. The finished dish was returned to the household on the cushioned head of a delivery boy. Today most *guvecs* are both assembled and cooked at specialty bakeries with wood-fired ovens and then delivered in panel trucks.

The top such establishment in Beypazari is run by third-generation *guvec* baker Adil Değirmencioğlu. He told me that his customers order their *guvec* a day in advance. Unless an order includes rice, no water is added to the pot. If a customer does not return the empty pot promptly, further orders from that house are ignored.

See page 90 for another *guvec* recipe using chicken and okra and page 248 for one with white beans and *basturma* (a spicy, air-dried meat).

Summer Lamb and Vegetable Guvec

SERVES 6

This is Ayfer Ünsal's unabridged version of a famous Turkish casserole containing lamb, green beans, okra, eggplant, and tomatoes—the *guvec* equivalent of a "pizza with the works." After Ayfer puts her *guvec* together, she drops the pot off at her local bakery, goes for a two-hour swim, and then picks it up on her way home. She usually serves it at room temperature with bulgur or rice pilaf later in the day.

> **PREFERRED CLAY POT:**
>
> A 3½- or 4-quart wide earthenware or stoneware casserole or a Turkish *guvec*
>
> **SUGGESTED CLAY ENVIRONMENT:**
>
> Double slabs of pizza stones or food-safe quarry tiles set on the upper and lower oven racks

1 pound boneless lean lamb shoulder

2 teaspoons Turkish sweet red pepper paste

Coarse salt and freshly ground black pepper

½ teaspoon ground allspice

12 large garlic cloves, 6 thinly sliced and 6 whole

2 lemons, thinly sliced

5 tablespoons extra virgin olive oil

1 pound long, thin eggplants

8 ounces small, firm okra pods, rubbed with a towel to remove any fuzz

1 pound fresh green beans, trimmed

8 ounces small red potatoes, scrubbed and halved

1 medium green bell pepper, diced

1 medium red bell pepper, diced

4 ounces small shallots, thinly sliced

12 ounces zucchini, trimmed and cut into 1-inch chunks

2 medium tomatoes, grated, plus 3 large tomatoes, thinly sliced

½ teaspoon sugar

1 One day in advance, trim any excess fat from the lamb. Cut the meat into 1½-inch cubes. In a large plastic bag, combine the Turkish pepper paste, 1 teaspoon black pepper, the allspice, sliced garlic, one of the sliced lemons, and 2 tablespoons of the olive oil. Add the lamb, seal the bag, and massage the marinade gently into the lamb. Refrigerate overnight.

2 The following day, bring the meat and marinade to room temperature. Using a swivel-bladed vegetable peeler, remove the eggplant skin lengthwise in 1-inch-wide strips. Wrap the skins in plastic so they don't dry out and set aside. Cut the eggplant into 1-inch cubes, toss with 1 tablespoon coarse salt, and drain in a colander for 30 minutes.

3 Grease the earthenware casserole and spread the meat and its marinade evenly over the bottom of the dish. Pick out the lemon slices and toss them with the okra in a bowl. Season the okra with ½ teaspoon salt and a pinch of black pepper.

4 Scatter the green beans over the meat. Arrange the potatoes on top. In a bowl, mix the diced peppers, shallots, whole garlic cloves, zucchini, and grated tomatoes and spread on top of the potatoes. Season lightly with salt and pepper.

5 Rinse the eggplant under cold running water and drain well. Wrap in paper towels and press to squeeze out as much moisture as possible. Spread the eggplant cubes over the mixed vegetables. Scatter the okra and lemon slices on top. Arrange the reserved eggplant skin, black side up, in a spoke pattern on top. Layer the slices of fresh tomato over the eggplant and sprinkle with the sugar and a little salt and pepper. Drizzle the remaining 3 tablespoons olive oil over all.

6 Place in a cold oven, set the temperature at 400°F, and bake for 1½ hours. Turn off the heat and continue to bake for another 30 minutes in the receding heat. Cover the dish if the tomatoes are browning too fast. Serve at room temperature.

MAKE IT AND BREAK IT: DRAMA IN THE DINING ROOM

The Story of Testi of Lamb from Cappadocia

The Turkish area of Cappadocia is famous for many things, including rock outcroppings that resemble a lunar landscape and, in the culinary sphere, *testi kebap*, a savory lamb stew. An amphora-shaped clay vessel is stuffed with lamb, vegetables, and spices, sealed with dough, and baked in a wood-fired oven for four to five hours. For serving, the pot is broken open at the table, and the stew is poured out onto the dinner plates.

Aydin Ayhan Guney, owner of the Somine Restaurant in Ürgüp, Turkey, told me how a group of visiting Japanese restaurateurs, who fell in love with the dish, worked out a deal with him to bring it to Japan. He now ships tens of thousands of clay pots a year filled with this lamb stew. His Turkish restaurant prepares the dish, cooks it, cools the pots down, and flash-freezes them for shipping to Japan. When one is ordered in Japan, the vase is defrosted, resealed with a fresh piece of dough, reheated, and served with the neck whacked off at table.

Greek Lamb Yiouvetsi with Pasta, Tomatoes, and Cheese

SERVES 8

This is one of the most famous of all Greek Island lamb dishes. Like *guvec*, the word *yiouvetsi* applies to both the dish and also the pot in which it's cooked. The *yiouvetsi* pot closely resembles a Turkish *guvec*, but what's put into it is quite different. Leg of lamb or lamb shoulder is cooked slowly with tomatoes, herbs, spices, and pasta and then served sprinkled with grated Greek cheese. Like so many eastern Mediterranean casseroles, its best served warm rather than hot.

> **PREFERRED CLAY POT:**
>
> **A 12-inch-wide earthenware casserole or Spanish cazuela or straight-sided flameware skillet**
>
> **If using an electric or ceramic stovetop, be sure to use a heat diffuser with the clay pots.**
>
> **SUGGESTED CLAY ENVIRONMENT:**
>
> **Double slabs of pizza stone slabs or food-safe quarry tiles set on the upper and lower oven racks**

2 pounds lean boneless lamb shoulder

1 teaspoon dried Greek oregano

Coarse salt and freshly ground black pepper

¼ cup extra virgin olive oil

2 medium onions, chopped

Pinch of sugar

6 garlic cloves, peeled

1 can (14 ounces) diced tomatoes

1½ tablespoons tomato paste, preferably homemade (page 317)

2 imported bay leaves

¼ teaspoon Aleppo pepper

1 3-inch Ceylon cinnamon stick

1 pound kritharaki or orzo

1 cup grated Greek myzithra, kefalotyri, or pecorino Romano cheese

2 teaspoons chopped fresh flat-leaf parsley

1 Trim any excess fat from the lamb. Cut the meat into 1½-inch cubes and pat dry. Season with ½ teaspoon of the oregano and ¼ teaspoon black pepper.

2 Heat 2 tablespoons of the olive oil in the earthenware casserole set over medium-low heat. Add the lamb and cook slowly, tossing once or twice, for 3 minutes. Add the onions, ½ teaspoon salt, and the sugar and cook, stirring occasionally, for 10 minutes.

3 Add the garlic, diced tomatoes, tomato paste, bay leaves, Aleppo pepper, and 2 cups hot water. Gently crush the cinnamon stick between two fingers to release its aroma and add to the casserole. Cover and simmer for 1½ hours, or until the meat is tender and the tomato sauce is thick. Remove and discard the cinnamon stick and bay leaves. Let the dish cool; then remove all surface fat. (The recipe can be prepared to this point up to 2 days in advance.)

4 About 2 hours before serving, preheat the oven to 300°F. Reheat the lamb and sauce over low heat on top of the stove. Meanwhile, in a large saucepan of salted water, cook the pasta for 3 minutes; drain and add to the lamb. Raise the heat to medium and bring to a boil. Season with the remaining ½ teaspoon oregano and with salt, black pepper, and Aleppo pepper to taste. Stir in 1 cup hot water. Cover the casserole and transfer to the oven. Immediately raise the temperature to 450°F and bake for 30 minutes.

5 Remove the cover and drizzle the remaining 2 tablespoons olive oil on top and sprinkle with 2 tablespoons of the cheese. Continue to bake, uncovered, for 15 minutes longer, or until the top is crusty and brown. Turn off the heat and leave the casserole in the oven to cook in the receding heat for 30 minutes. Serve with the parsley sprinkled on top. Pass the remaining grated cheese on the side.

CONFIT OF LAMB IN A SPANISH CAZUELA

Writing in *Spain Gourmetour* magazine, food journalist Vicky Hayward describes a Spanish method of preparing confit of baby lamb in a clay pot. The recipe comes from the restaurant Meson Loba Parda in the village of Urueña situated in the center of the Iberian Peninsula.

Hayward describes how the restaurant cooks chunks of baby lamb in olive oil infused with garlic and bay leaf and rendered pork fat until tender and just barely browned. After several days of maturing, the lamb chunks are browned in the oven and then served along with potatoes cooked in some of the cooking fat. Sounds delicious!

Turkish Stuffed Dried Eggplant and Peppers

SERVES 8

My friend Ayfer Ünsal is a self-assured cook whose recipes often tread the culinary edge. She has an uncanny knack for discovering some of the most interesting and delectable Turkish dishes. Here she uses dried eggplants and peppers, which probably don't sound very appealing, but which, after rehydration and cooking, render one of the best stuffed vegetable dishes you'll ever eat.

Serve warm with a bowl of yogurt and garlic sauce.

> **PREFERRED CLAY POT:**
>
> A 3½- or 4-quart glazed or unglazed earthenware casserole
>
> If using an electric or ceramic stovetop, be sure to use a heat diffuser with the clay pot.

24 dried eggplants (see Sources)

1 dozen dried sweet red peppers (see Sources)

8 ounces lean ground lamb

6 garlic cloves, finely chopped

3 medium onions, finely chopped

2 tablespoons sweet Turkish red pepper paste

2 tablespoons tomato paste, canned or homemade (page 317)

1 tablespoon Turkish or Aleppo pepper flakes

2 tablespoons dried mint

½ teaspoon ground coriander

½ teaspoon ground cumin

½ teaspoon freshly ground black pepper

2 tablespoons crème fraîche or slivered fresh Teleme cheese

1⅓ cups coarse bulgur (8 ounces)

3 tablespoons extra virgin olive oil

4 teaspoons salt

12 dried sour prunes or dried sour yellow plums (see Sources)

2½ tablespoons fresh lemon juice

Yogurt and Garlic Sauce (recipe follows)

1 Place the dried eggplants in a conventional saucepan, cover with water, and bring to a boil. Lower the heat and simmer for 15 minutes. Drain the eggplants and soak again in fresh cold water for 1 hour. At the same time, place the dried peppers in a bowl, cover with boiling water, and let stand for 1 hour.

2 In a medium bowl, combine the lamb, garlic, onions, pepper and tomato pastes, Turkish pepper flakes, dried mint, coriander, cumin, black pepper, and crème fraîche. Knead with your hands until well blended. Gently tilt the bowl with the soaking eggplants and scoop out ½ cup water and put in a mixing bowl. Add the bulgur, 2 tablespoons of the olive oil, and the salt and knead until well blended. Then add the meat mixture and knead until smooth.

3 Soak the sour plums in hot water to cover for 10 minutes; drain. Flatten with the palm of your hand, remove the pits, and pat dry.

4 Drain the eggplants and peppers; blot them dry with paper towels. Loosely stuff each vegetable with 2 to 3 tablespoons of the lamb and bulgur mixture. Place the vegetables, open side up, in the casserole. Arrange the plums in between the vegetables and on top and cover with a heavy, inverted plate; gently press down so that the vegetables will remain in place during cooking. Pour 2 cups hot water, the remaining olive oil and the lemon juice around the plate. Cover the pot with a tight-fitting lid, set it over medium heat, and bring to a boil. Reduce the heat to low and simmer gently for 1 hour.

5 Transfer the hot casserole to a wooden surface or folded kitchen towel to prevent cracking. Let stand without removing the cover for 30 minutes. Carefully remove the lid and the plate and transfer the stuffed vegetables one by one to a serving platter. Scatter the prunes or plums on top and serve warm, with the Yogurt and Garlic Sauce on the side.

Yogurt and Garlic Sauce

MAKES 2 CUPS

3 cups unflavored yogurt

1 tablespoon crushed garlic

Salt

1 Line a sieve with a coffee filter or several layers of cheesecloth. Set over a bowl and dump in the yogurt. Let drain for 1 to 2 hours at room temperature, until the yogurt is reduced to 2 cups.

2 Transfer the thickened yogurt to a bowl. Beat in the garlic. Add salt to taste and let stand for a few hours to mellow before serving.

Clay Pot Tianu with Lamb, Potatoes, and Onions

SERVES 4

Like every other culinary writer who's been to Puglia in southern Italy, I've fallen in love with its cuisine. On a recent visit to the town of Salento, I purchased a massive, heavily illustrated volume filled with stories and tempting regional recipes. My favorite, presented here, marinates lamb shoulder chops with rosemary, garlic, and capers and then has you cook the meat with potato slices, onions, and pecorino Sardo cheese in a shallow clay rectangular baker called a *tianu* or *teglia di terra-cotta*. It's a perfect example of simple southern Italian cooking at its foolproof best.

> **PREFERRED CLAY POT:**
>
> **A 10- × 11-inch stoneware baking dish or lasagne pan (oven safe to 400°F)**
>
> **If using an electric or ceramic stovetop, be sure to use a heat diffuser with the clay pot.**

1 pound bone-in shoulder lamb chops

3 tablespoons finely chopped fresh flat-leaf parsley

5 tablespoons extra virgin olive oil

1 fresh rosemary sprig

3 garlic cloves, chopped

1 tablespoon small capers, drained and rinsed

Sea salt and freshly ground black pepper

1 large onion, sliced

1¾ pounds Yukon Gold potatoes

1½ ounces pecorino Sardo cheese or other dry sheep's milk cheese, grated (about ⅓ cup)

½ cup dry bread crumbs

1 One day in advance, trim any excess fat from the lamb and divide the chops into 12 chunks, leaving the bones in. In a medium bowl, combine the parsley, 2½ tablespoons of the olive oil, the rosemary, garlic, capers, ½ teaspoon sea salt, ¼ teaspoon pepper, and ⅓ cup cold water. Add the lamb, toss to coat with the marinade, cover, and refrigerate overnight.

2 About 3 hours before serving, use a slotted spoon to lift out the lamb and set aside. Discard the rosemary sprig. Pour the rest of the marinade into a conventional skillet. Add the onion and a pinch of salt. Cook over medium heat, stirring occasionally, until the liquid evaporates and the onion turns pale golden, about 15 minutes. Add the reserved lamb to the skillet, cover with a sheet of crumpled parchment and a lid, and cook for 30 minutes. With a slotted spoon, transfer the lamb and onion to a plate. Bring the liquid in the skillet to a boil and cook until reduced to a thickened juice, about 10 minutes.

3 While the liquid is reducing, preheat the oven to 400°F. Lightly oil the baking dish. Peel the potatoes and slice them into thin rounds. Cover the bottom of the baking dish with half the potato slices. Top with the lamb, onions, and oily juices from the skillet. Cover with half the cheese and half the bread crumbs. Make another layer of potatoes; season with salt and pepper. Sprinkle the remaining cheese and bread crumbs on top. Drizzle the remaining 2½ tablespoons olive oil over all. Cover with a sheet of foil, transfer to the oven, and bake for 30 minutes.

4 Remove the foil cover and continue baking for another 30 minutes. The potatoes should form a beautiful golden brown crust on top. Turn off the heat and leave the pan in the oven without opening the door for another 30 minutes before serving.

Adapted from a recipe in Lucia Lazari's Odori, Sapori, Colori della Cucina Salentina in 629 ricette de Ieri e di Oggi.

Tunisian Lamb and Cheese Tagine

SERVES 4

This popular lamb tagine from the city of Tunis bears no resemblance to a Moroccan tagine. It is, in fact, similar to an Italian frittata, with delectable crusty edges and a glazed brown-speckled top. City cooks obtain this lovely brown sheen simply by baking the tagine first and then broiling it for the final five minutes of cooking.

> **PREFERRED CLAY POT:**
> A 10-inch Spanish cazuela, or an earthenware or flameware tagine
> If using an electric or ceramic stovetop, be sure to use a heat diffuser with the clay pot.

1 pound boneless lean lamb shoulder

2 tablespoons extra virgin olive oil

Coarse salt and freshly ground black pepper

½ cup chopped onion

1 teaspoon Tunisian Mixed Spices (recipe follows)

1 cup boiling water

⅛ teaspoon saffron threads

6 eggs

3 tablespoons fresh bread crumbs

1 scant cup (3 ounces) Gruyère cheese, shredded

1 scant cup (3 ounces) Gouda cheese, shredded

1 tablespoon butter, melted

1 Trim any excess fat from the lamb, and cut the meat into 12 cubes. Heat the olive oil in a medium conventional skillet. Add the lamb and sauté over medium-high heat until lightly browned, 3 to 4 minutes. Season with ½ teaspoon salt and ¼ teaspoon pepper.

2 Add the onion, cover, and reduce the heat to medium. Cook for 10 minutes. Add the Tunisian mixed spices and the boiling water. Reduce the heat to low and simmer, covered, until the lamb is very tender, about 1 hour.

3 With a slotted spoon, transfer the lamb to the cazuela and cover with foil to keep it moist. Boil the cooking juices in the skillet until reduced to ½ cup. Let cool; then skim off as much fat as possible.

4 Set an oven rack on the middle shelf of the oven. Preheat the oven to 350°F. In a small bowl, soak the saffron in ⅓ cup warm water.

(continued)

5 In a mixing bowl, beat the eggs until frothy. Whisk in the cooled cooking juices, bread crumbs, Gruyere, and ¼ teaspoon black pepper. Pour the egg mixture over the lamb and scatter the Gouda cheese on top. Loosely cover the dish with foil and bake for 15 minutes.

6 Raise the oven temperature to 450°F. In a small bowl, combine the melted butter and the saffron with its soaking water. Remove the foil from the cazuela and drizzle half the buttered saffron water over the eggs. Bake, uncovered, for 5 minutes.

7 Drizzle on the rest of the saffron water and bake for 5 minutes longer, or until the eggs are just set and the cheese is lightly browned. Transfer the hot pan to a wooden surface or folded kitchen towel to prevent cracking. Let stand for 20 to 30 minutes to set. Serve warm, cut into wedges.

Tunisian Mixed Spices

MAKES 2 TABLESPOONS

This spice mixture, called *tabil* in Tunisia, is available on line from www.seasonedpioneers.com.uk, or you can make it yourself.

1½ teaspoons ground caraway seeds

1½ teaspoons ground cumin

1½ teaspoons ground coriander

1½ teaspoon cayenne

Mix together the caraway, cumin, coriander, and cayenne. Store in a covered jar at room temperature for up 2 months.

Moroccan Lamb Tagine with Melting Tomatoes and Onions

SERVES 4 TO 6

The Moroccan word for this type of cooking is *bennaraïn*, which means "between two fires." In rural areas, home cooks place a tagine filled with meat and vegetables over glowing olivewood embers and cook the dish three-quarters of the way. Then the conical top is removed, a flat earthenware pan is placed over the food, and hot coals are piled on top. The resulting dish is crusty on both top and bottom and infused with a smoky fragrance. My kitchen adaptation produces a light charring under a broiler.

You'll want to serve torn pieces of flat bread with this tagine. Consider them implements for grasping hold of the lamb and sauce and then transporting them to the mouth.

> **PREFERRED CLAY POT:**
>
> A glazed or unglazed earthenware or flameware tagine, or a 10- or 11-inch Spanish cazuela with a cover
>
> A heat diffuser is suggested for slow, steady cooking on all stovetops.

2½ pounds thick, bone-in lamb shoulder arm chops

3 tablespoons golden raisins

3 large red onions, 1 grated and 2 thinly sliced

2 teaspoons Moroccan Spice Mixture: La Kama
(page 316)

¼ teaspoon ground cubeb berries (see Sources)
or cayenne

⅛ teaspoon saffron threads

1 3-inch Ceylon cinnamon stick, lightly crushed

Salt

1 tablespoon smen (optional, page 295)
or unsalted butter

3 tablespoons mild olive oil

6 plum tomatoes, preferably Roma, peeled,
quartered lengthwise, and seeded

Freshly ground black pepper

2 tablespoons turbinado sugar mixed with
1 teaspoon ground cinnamon

6 loaves Moroccan Country Bread (page 257)
or soft flour tortillas

1 tablespoon chopped fresh flat-leaf parsley

1 Trim any excess fat from the lamb. Cut the chops into 1½-inch chunks with the bones.

2 Soak the raisins in warm water for 15 minutes.

3 Place the lamb, grated onion, La Kama spices, cubeb berries or cayenne, saffron, cinnamon stick, 1 teaspoon salt, smen or butter, and half the oil in the tagine. Place on a heat diffuser over low heat until the aroma of the spices is released, about 10 minutes. Do not brown the meat. Add ½ cup hot water and slowly bring to a boil.

4 Drain the raisins. Cover the meat with the onion slices and raisins and spread the tomatoes, cut side down, on top. Cover the tagine, reduce the heat to low, and cook for 2 hours.

5 Set an oven rack on the middle shelf of the oven. Preheat the oven to 350°F.

6 Remove the top of the tagine and tilt the pot to pour all the liquid into a medium conventional skillet. Skim the fat off the top of the liquid; then boil it down to ¾ cup. Season with salt and pepper to taste. Spread the reduced juices over the tomatoes in the tagine. Remove and discard the cinnamon stick. Scatter the sugar and ground cinnamon on top. Place in the oven and bake, uncovered, for 45 minutes. Switch the oven heat to broil, dribble over the remaining oil, and cook until crusty and lightly charred, about 5 minutes. Serve at once or reheat gently over medium heat.

7 Just before serving, reheat the bread, tear it into large pieces, and spread about one-third over a large serving platter. Spoon about half of the contents of the tagine on top. Repeat with another third of the bread and the remaining contents of the tagine. Top with the last of the bread and a sprinkling of parsley and serve at once.

NOTE TO THE COOK: Ceylon cinnamon is light tan and delicate and is used frequently in Moroccan cooking. It is often sold as Mexican cinnamon. The sticks are soft, making them very easy to bruise.

Moroccan Lamb Tagine with Winter Squash and Toasted Pine Nuts

SERVES 4

This tantalizing recipe utilizes two kitchen tricks employed by Moroccan home cooks. Onions are treated in two ways for different effect: grated onions added early in the cooking melt into the sauce, and sliced onions added later provide heft.

A second trick concerns the handling of pumpkin, butternut, or kabocha squash. The vegetable is grated and the pulp macerated in sugar until it "weeps," giving up its excess water. A small portion of the expressed liquid is then used to aid caramelization of the vegetable as it's sautéed down to the consistency of jam. This develops a lovely aroma, and, most important, concentrates the flavor.

> **PREFERRED CLAY POT:**
>
> A glazed or unglazed earthenware or flameware tagine, or a 10- or 11-inch Spanish cazuela with a cover
>
> A heat diffuser is suggested for slow, steady cooking on a stovetop.

2 pounds thick bone-in lamb shoulder arm chops

2½ to 3 pounds butternut squash

Coarse salt

⅛ teaspoon saffron threads

1 large onion, grated, plus 2 medium onions, sliced

Salt and freshly ground black pepper

2 teaspoons Moroccan Spice Mixture: La Kama (page 316)

2 teaspoons smen (optional; page 295)

Pinch of ground cinnamon

Pinch of ground ginger

1 tablespoon lavender or orange flower honey

3 tablespoons unsalted butter

2 tablespoons pine nuts, toasted

1 Trim any excess fat from the lamb. Cut the chops into 1½-inch chunks with the bones.

2 Peel the squash and scrape out the seeds and membrane. Using the shredding disk on a food processor or the large holes on a box grater, shred the squash. Sprinkle liberally with coarse salt and drain in a colander for about 1 hour. At the same time, soak the saffron in ⅓ cup warm water.

3 Place the lamb, grated onion, saffron and its water, 1 teaspoon salt, 1½ teaspoons of the spice mixture, and the smen in the tagine. Stir to mix well. Cover and cook over low heat for 1½ hours.

4 Stir in the sliced onions and continue to cook, covered, for 1 hour longer. Pick out the pieces of lamb and let stand until cool enough to handle. Cut out and discard the bones. Skim the fat off the cooking liquid in the tagine. Season the meat with salt and pepper and return to the tagine.

5 Rinse the grated squash under cold running water and squeeze in your hands over a bowl to catch the juices. Measure out and reserve 2 tablespoons of the juice; discard the remainder. Place the grated squash in a 10-inch nonstick skillet. Add the cinnamon, ginger, honey, remaining La Kama spices, 2 tablespoons of the butter, and the reserved 2 tablespoons squash liquid. Slowly fry until the squash is thickened to a jamlike consistency and colored a golden caramel, about 15 minutes.

6 Preheat the oven to 300°F. Ladle half the sauce from the tagine over the squash and stir to combine. Spread the squash evenly over the lamb. Dot with the remaining 1 tablespoon butter and place the tagine in the top third of the oven. Raise the heat to 425°F and bake, uncovered, until the squash is lightly glazed, about 30 minutes. Remove from the oven, be sure to set the tagine down on a wooden surface. Serve the tagine hot or warm, with the toasted pine nuts scattered on top.

Lamb Kofte Kebabs with Shallots

SERVES 4

Back in the 1990s, when I first began to explore Turkish cuisine, I received a fax from a woman who had heard that I was interested in the cooking of her native Gaziantep, a city located on an ancient caravan route, near the Syrian border. It is Turkey's gastronomic capital, known for its red pepper–based cooking, cooling yogurt soups, bright green pistachio baklava, grilled lamb kebabs, and hand-chopped lamb kebabs *(koftes)*, which come in numerous shapes and sizes.

"Everyone knows that Turkey is the home of shish kebab and baklava," she wrote. "Everyone in Turkey knows that the best examples of each are found here in Gaziantep. And everyone in Gaziantep knows that you will find the best of both at Burhan Cagdas's simple restaurant near the market in the center of town."

The fax was signed by a Ms. Ayfer Ünsal, a political journalist on staff at the local newspaper. In the years since, Ayfer has become a very close friend and has emerged as one of the top food writers in Turkey. But back then I took her fax as simply local chauvinism. Still, when I arrived in Gaziantep, I hastened to meet her, and she immediately led me to Burhan Cagdas's restaurant so I could see for myself that what she'd written was true. It was! Both the kebabs and the baklava were out of this world.

The dining room on the first floor is presided over by Burhan himself, a burly, mustachioed middle-aged man, with a sweet nature and an unexpected openness about how and why his kebabs are superior. "My great-grandfather founded this restaurant," he told me. "I still do things the way he did. I'm a traditional guy, and this is a traditional kebab house."

(continued)

His lamb is hand-chopped by master meat cutters using long, two-handled, half-moon-shaped knives. Working like surgeons, they rapidly cut the meat and some lamb tail fat into tiny dice. The chopped meat is then kneaded until it reaches the correct consistency for sticking to the skewers. Since lamb tail fat is nearly impossible to find here, I've worked up a method to reproduce its effect by kneading a bit of crème fraîche into the meat. This works exceptionally well, keeping the kofte meat rich tasting and meltingly tender.

Once the *koftes* are prepared, they are interspersed on skewers with a seasonal fruit or vegetable and then grilled. Among Burhan's seasonal additions are chunks of eastern Mediterranean truffles, halves of summer loquats, tiny sour apples, whole garlic heads, slices of seedless eggplant, chunks of tomato, and whole shallots. Some of these preparations are served with a sauce, others dry.

"Ground meat kebabs skewered along with shallots have to be on the fire longer so they will cook properly," Burhan explained. "But this produces dryness, so we remove the skewers along with the shallots when the meat is only half-done. Then we slowly finish the cooking in a covered clay *tava* with a little water or pomegranate molasses—in effect brewing and then sweating the meat to maintain juiciness."

In Turkey, I found numerous cooks using a lovely shallow clay dish, called a *tava* in the southeastern part of the country and a *tepsi* along the Mediterranean Sea. Both are oval or round, glazed or unglazed, and used extensively for ground lamb dishes. As with many clay pots, the cooking vessels double as serving dishes. Cazuelas are excellent substitutes.

1 pound lean ground lamb

3 tablespoons crème fraîche or slivered soft Teleme cheese

1 garlic clove, crushed

Fine salt and finely ground black pepper

12 large shallots (1 pound)

1 tablespoon extra virgin olive oil

1 teaspoon pomegranate molasses

1 teaspoon fresh lemon juice

1 tablespoon chopped fresh flat-leaf parsley

2 tablespoons chopped scallion

Warm pita bread

1 About 1¼ hours before serving, prepare a hot fire using lump charcoal in an outdoor grill. Or preheat a gas grill. Meanwhile, place the ground lamb, crème fraîche, garlic, 1 teaspoon salt, and ½ teaspoon pepper in a large bowl or on a wooden surface. Knead by dipping your knuckles in cold water and using them to press down and work the mixture until it is well blended and smooth. Form into 16 sausage shapes.

2 Peel the shallots and cut them lengthwise in half. Trim the root ends, leaving enough intact to hold the shallots together. Alternately, skewer the lamb kebabs and shallot halves onto 4 long metal skewers, pressing meat and shallot firmly.

3 Brush the meat and shallots with olive oil and grill, turning once, until the lamb and shallots are nicely browned on the outside, about 3 minutes; they will still be fairly raw inside. Remove from the grill and slip the meat and shallots off the skewers into the clay pot, being careful not to break the kebabs. Stir together ¾ teaspoon of the pomegranate molasses, the lemon juice, and ⅓ cup water and add to the pot. Cover and cook the meat and shallots over medium-low embers on the grill or over low heat on top of the stove until almost all the liquid has been absorbed, 25 to 30 minutes.

4 Gently turn the kebabs to glaze the meat and shallots all over with the sauce. Dilute the remaining ¼ teaspoon pomegranate molasses with 3 tablespoons water, add to the pot, and continue to turn and baste over medium heat for about 1 minute. Scatter the parsley and scallion on top and serve directly from the cazuela, with warm pita on the side.

GRILLING OVER A FLOWER POT

Since this book is about cooking in clay, I'd feel remiss if I didn't share a method of grilling over an unglazed terra-cotta flowerpot, especially if you bought one to do some upside-down roasting:

Set your flowerpot on a flowerpot saucer, fill it halfway up with sand, set hot coals (from the fireplace) on the sand, and, when the pot has reached the proper temperature, arrange an oiled heavy metal grill across the top. Then place the ground meat kebab skewers between the grates so the meat won't stick to the grill.

Turkish Lamb Pancake with Tomato and Pepper

SERVES 6

*H*ere's a wonderful recipe for a smooth, rich pancake of ground lamb, which explodes with flavor thanks to the popular seasoning mix of mint, cumin, and mild Turkish Marash red pepper. It is baked in a clay dish deep enough to keep the meat from drying out as the interior cooks and the surface browns to a crisp shell.

When I first tasted this dish in Kilis in southeastern Turkey, it had a particularly luscious, buttery texture due to the addition of lamb tail fat. No lamb tail fat available? Don't substitute ordinary lamb fat, which has too strong a taste; instead follow my method for adding richness and tenderness by kneading a little crème fraîche into the ground lamb. Serve with lightly buttered, warm flat bread.

> **PREFERRED CLAY POT:**
> An 11- or 12-inch Spanish cazuela or La Chamba skillet or enchilada pan

2 pounds lean ground lamb

3 ounces crème fraîche.

1 packed cup fresh flat-leaf parsley leaves, chopped

2 teaspoons freshly ground black pepper

2 tablespoons Turkish or Aleppo pepper

1 teaspoon dried Mediterranean oregano

1 teaspoon dried mint, preferably Egyptian

1 teaspoon ground cumin

1 teaspoon salt

1 red ripe tomato, thinly sliced

1 Anaheim pepper, cut into 2-inch strips

1 tablespoon tomato paste, canned or homemade (page 317)

1 In a mixing bowl, combine the ground lamb, crème fraîche, parsley, black pepper, Turkish pepper, oregano, mint, cumin, and salt. Blend thoroughly. Place the seasoned meat in the clay pan and press to cover the bottom, forming a flat pancake. Arrange the tomato slices in a circle on top. Decorate with the pepper strips. Thoroughly blend the tomato paste with ⅓ cup of water and pour over the meat.

2 Place the dish in the top third of a cold oven. Set the temperature at 350°F and bake for 1¼ hours. Turn off the oven and let cook in the receding heat for 30 minutes longer.

3 Remove from the oven and pour off excess fat. Be sure to set the hot dish down on a wooden surface or folded kitchen towel to prevent cracking. Let cool slightly; then cut the lamb into wedges. Serve warm or at room temperature.

With thanks to Fethiye Akbulut Miller, who lives nearby in northern California and writes a wonderful culinary blog (www.yogurtland.com), for sending me this recipe for the book. Fethiye credits her version called tray kebab *to a Turkish book,* Proceedings of the Second Hatay Cuisine Symposium.

THE DAUBIÈRE

Bulbous pots are ideal for cooking all sorts of meats, for turning tough cuts buttery soft. The French *daubière*, instantly recognizable by its tall, potbellied shape and distinctive lid, is designed so that the ingredients can be packed inside with only a small amount of liquid and then set over low heat to braise. The ingenuity of the type of pot lies in the way they slowly convey heat up from the bottom, causing the tough connective tissues in meat, called collagen, to transform into gelatin rather than simply dissolve and melt away, as occurs when more direct high heat is applied during roasting in a hot oven.

In a *daubière* you use as little liquid as possible; the clay pot prevents the meat from drying out by controlling the temperature and recycling the moisture. Traditionally the cover has a trough to hold water, which heats up rather quickly and evaporates and must be replenished from time to time. As the water boils off as steam, heat is pulled off the lid, keeping the top relatively cool, the same way evaporation of sweat cools our skin.

Because the shape of the pot ensures the top is cooler than the bottom, this continuous action recycles the aromatic vapors produced by the cooking meat and vegetables, which condense at the top and fall back onto the food. Juices left in the pot at the end of cooking are intensely flavored, concentrated, and syrupy.

Another benefit of the design is the way it minimizes shrinkage of tough cuts of meat, including beef shanks, cross ribs (the cut between the shoulder and the rib), and beef cheeks. Slow low-temperature cooking allows firm root vegetables such as turnips and carrots, not only to retain their shape but to provide flavor while absorbing some of the meat juices. Stable temperature and stable moistness are what endow a daube with its unique succulence.

In the old days, when the *daubière* sat in the fireplace embers, cooking over many hours, sometimes through the night, the final product was butter-tender meat. Since most of us will not be cooking our daubes in the fireplace, I've found the following method works well in the modern kitchen. I place a wet piece of crumpled parchment directly on the meat and vegetables and then set a tight-fitting lid over the pot, thus ensuring recycling of moisture.

Those who prefer to cook their daubes in an oven should warm the pot very slowly on top of the stove for an hour before moving it to a preheated 275°F oven. Since oven heat will surround the pot, the meat may shrink and cook too quickly. To prevent this, it's a good idea, after an hour, to remove the cover, leaving the crumpled parchment in place and continue cooking until the meat is tender.

In his beautiful book *From the French Country Table: Pottery & Faience of Provence*, Bernard Duplessy advises readers on how to choose an earthenware *daubière*:

"The daube must always 'breathe' and so it's best for a daubière to be only partially glazed, leaving the lower half of the belly and the inside of the lid untreated. Resistant clay has to be used, as a daubière must withstand the heat of an oven. However, Madame Daubière is still not ready. Once home, it must be filled with water or milk. Placed upon a diffuser over a gas burner, it is then brought to a boil. Then, with each use, it is wise to rub the daubière inside and out with a clove of garlic. A magical and tasty hint."

The two most beautiful *daubières* I own were made by master potter Philippe Beltrando, whose studio is located in the Provençal town of Aubagne, France (see Sources). Philippe and I have been corresponding for some years about why daubes taste better when cooked in clay *daubières*. To learn about his views on this fascinating topic, see page xi.

There is a reason I have two *daubières*: I use one for cooking meats (beef, lamb, pork, and wild boar) and the other for octopus.

If you're interested in acquiring a Philippe Beltrando *daubière*, go to Barbara Wilde's website (www.frenchgardening.com) where she sells and ships Philippe's *daubieres*, *poêlons*, mortars, and other clay pots.

Provençal Daube of Beef Short Ribs with White Wine, Oven-Roasted Tomatoes, and Green Olives

SERVES 6

This wonderful beef daube was inspired by a dish from Dominique Bucaille, who taught me a revolutionary method for marinating meat in wine that not only improves flavor but also saves a day of preparation. I call it *hot-to-hot marination.* Here's how it works:

A bottle or a few cups of wine are brought to a boil in a braising pot and then flamed or boiled and reduced. At the same time, chunks of meat or poultry are browned quickly in hot oil, butter, or duck fat and then flamed with cognac. After the flames subside, the hot meat is transferred to the hot wine and left to marinate at room temperature for one to two hours. What happens is that when the hot surface of the meat meets the hot wine, the marinade penetrates the meat deeply.

During this quick hot-to-hot marination, all the vegetables and herbs are sautéed in the meat browning skillet, which is then deglazed. The vegetables and the deglazing liquid are added to the daube pot as soon as the marination is complete and the meat has cooled down.

You start cooking cold with cool meat in the bottom of the pot, vegetables and other ingredients packed over, and the marinade poured on top. Bring the pot slowly to a simmer on top of the stove, reduce the heat, place a piece of crumpled parchment on the food, put the lid on the stew pot, and cook the daube slowly to perfection.

Note: For best flavor, prepare the dish through step 8 at least a day in advance. Serve the daube with rice, pasta, Chestnut Flour Gnocchi (page 217 or Oven Polenta in a Clay Pot (page 206).

PREFERRED CLAY POTS:

A 4-quart *daubière*, deep earthenware casserole, bean pot, Chinese clay pot, or Spanish olla

A 10- or 12-inch shallow stoneware or earthenware baking dish

If using an electric or ceramic stovetop, be sure to use a heat diffuser with the clay pots.

---

3 pounds bone-in beef short ribs (12 pieces), trimmed of excess fat

1 bottle (750 ml) dry white wine

Herb bouquet: 2 leafy celery tops stuck with 4 whole cloves, 3 fresh thyme sprigs, 2 imported bay leaves, 1 small cinnamon stick, and 3 strips orange zest tied together

¼ cup dried cèpes or porcini mushrooms

1½ teaspoons coarse salt

¾ teaspoon freshly ground black pepper

2 tablespoons unsalted butter

1 tablespoon extra virgin olive oil

4 ounces pancetta, cut into slices ½ inch thick

2 medium onions, sliced

6 large carrots, cut into 2-inch pieces

2 pinches of sugar

1 tablespoon all-purpose flour

¼ cup red or white wine vinegar

2½ tablespoons tomato paste, canned or homemade (page 317)

3 garlic cloves, peeled and bruised

1 cup picholine olives, pitted, rinsed

5 Oven-Roasted Tomatoes (recipe follows)

3 tablespoons chopped fresh flat-leaf parsley

⅛ teaspoon freshly grated nutmeg

1 One to two days in advance, bring the meat to room temperature. Pour the wine into the daubière and bring to a boil. Boil until reduced by half, about 20 minutes. Add the herb bouquet and set aside, covered, to keep the liquid hot.

2 While the wine is reducing, soak the dried cèpes in ¾ cup hot water until softened, about 15 minutes. Lift out the mushrooms and squeeze any excess liquid back into the bowl. Strain the mushroom-soaking liquid through a coffee filter or double layer of cheesecloth, and set aside the liquid and mushrooms separately.

3 Season the meat with ½ teaspoon of the salt and ¼ teaspoon of the pepper. Melt the butter in the olive oil in a large conventional skillet over medium-high heat until sizzling. Add the meat and sauté, turning, until lightly browned on all sides, about 5 minutes. Immediately transfer the ribs to the hot wine, leaving the fat in the skillet. Gently swirl the daubière to coat the short ribs with the hot wine and marinate at room temperature for 1 hour.

4 Meanwhile, add the pancetta and the onions to the fat remaining in the skillet. Cover and cook over medium-low heat until the onions are soft, about 10 minutes. Add the carrots and a pinch of sugar. Raise the heat to medium and cook, uncovered, stirring occasionally, until the carrots are glazed, about 5 minutes longer. Using a slotted spoon, transfer the contents of the skillet to a side dish.

5 Pour off all but 2 tablespoons fat from the skillet. Add the flour and cook over medium-low heat, stirring often, until it turns golden brown, about 5 minutes. Whisk in the vinegar, tomato paste, and reserved mushroom-soaking liquid. Bring to a boil, stirring to dissolve the tomato paste. Cook over medium heat, stirring, until the liquid is smooth, about 2 minutes. Add the garlic and mushrooms and cook, stirring, for 1 minute longer. Add to the onions and carrots. Season the vegetables with the remaining 1 teaspoon salt and ½ teaspoon pepper.

6 Slip the pancetta beneath the meat; tuck in the herb bouquet and spread the vegetables on top. Pour the reduced wine marinade into the skillet and, without heating it, scrape up any bits and pieces of meat clinging to the bottom; pour the marinade back into the daubière and press down gently to compact the ingredients. (The wine does not need to cover the contents of the pot.) Place a sheet of crumpled parchment directly on top. Cover the clay pot with its lid and set over medium-low heat to cook for 1 hour. Reduce the heat to low and continue to cook for 3 hours longer.

(continued)

7 Transfer the hot daubière to a wooden surface or folded kitchen towel to prevent cracking. Be sure to put the lid down on a similar surface. Let the daube stand until cool; then transfer to a deep container. Cover and refrigerate for up to 2 days.

8 About 2 hours before serving, remove the daube from the refrigerator. Pick out and discard the herb bouquet. Lift out the short ribs and carrots; trim away all the congealed fat, bones, and gristle from the ribs. Arrange the meat and carrots in the stoneware baking dish, cover with a piece of foil, and place in the oven. Set the temperature at 300°F and bake for 1½ hours.

9 Meanwhile, press the cooking liquid and remaining vegetables through a strainer into a conventional saucepan; discard any solids that remain. Bring to a boil over high heat, skimming to remove the fat and the scum that rises to the surface. Then push the saucepan half off the heat and let the sauce boil slowly, skimming, for another 10 minutes, or until the sauce has reduced by one-third.

10 While the sauce is reducing, soak the olives in a bowl of water for about 20 minutes to remove excess saltiness. Drain them and add to the sauce. Add the whole oven-roasted tomatoes and half the parsley and bring to a boil. Adjust the seasoning of the sauce with a pinch of sugar, grated nutmeg, and salt and pepper to taste. Remove the baking dish from the oven and spread the hot sauce over the meat and carrots. Return to the oven, raise the temperature to 400°F, and continue to bake, uncovered, until the topping is thick and brown and the sauce is bubbling around the edges, about 20 minutes. Serve with the remaining chopped parsley sprinkled on top.

NOTES TO THE COOK:

❊ To finish the daube in the oven after the first hour, preheat the oven to 275°F. Transfer the clay pot to the oven and bake for 1¼ hours. Set the cover of the clay pot ajar and continue to bake for 1¼ hours.

❊ If you don't want to discard the pancetta, remove it from the sauce and pat dry. Slowly fry it on a griddle or stovetop grill until lightly browned on both sides. Cut into chunks and serve alongside the daube.

Oven-Roasted Tomatoes

These are fleshier and softer than sun-dried tomatoes and are easy to make.

5 large plum tomatoes, preferably Roma
½ teaspoon sugar
Salt and freshly ground black pepper
1½ tablespoons extra virgin olive oil

1 Preheat the oven to 275°F.

2 Halve the tomatoes horizontally. Arrange them in an oiled shallow rimmed baking dish just large enough to hold them all in a single layer. Dust with the sugar and sprinkle lightly with salt and pepper. Drizzle ¼ to ½ teaspoon extra virgin olive oil over each tomato half.

3 Bake for 1¾ hours. Turn the tomatoes over and continue baking for 1¾ hours longer. Let cool; then store in a covered container in the refrigerator.

Charentaise Daube of Beef with Red Wine and Cognac

SERVES 4 TO 6

Few beef stews have as rich a flavor, as buttery a texture, and as heady an aroma as this famous daube from the beautifully and gastronomically fascinating Charentes region on the Atlantic coast of France.

Traditionally, chunks of beef, a pig's or calf's foot, pork rind, carrots, and shallots are cooked together slowly with red wine in an earthenware pot, shaped much like a bean pot, called a *câline* locally. After several hours the food and rind are removed, cut into small pieces, and returned to the pot to break down further as cooking proceeds. Thus the liquid portion of this stew becomes wonderfully thick and rich.

To bring this daube off, I always use a fairly big red wine, one with plenty of tannin. I suggest a full-bodied Rhône or a young California Cabernet Sauvignon. To achieve smoothness, the wine and cognac are flamed together and their flames extinguished before they die out. This may seem like an unnecessary step, but Charentaise cooks swear that it's important since, if the flames are allowed to go out on their own, the wine may "burn" and develop bitterness.

Note: It's important to prepare steps 1 through 5 a day ahead. That way the fat will have time to congeal and can all be scraped off the top.

The dish is traditionally served with butter-glazed carrots and grilled French bread rubbed with garlic.

> **PREFERRED CLAY POT:**
>
> A 4½- to 5-quart glazed or unglazed earthenware or flameware casserole
>
> If using an electric or ceramic stovetop, be sure to use a heat diffuser with the clay pot.

2 pounds beef top blade roast

Salt and freshly ground black pepper

1½ tablespoons vegetable oil

5 ounces pancetta, sliced

2 tablespoons unsalted butter

1 pig's foot, split lengthwise

1 onion, thinly sliced

8 ounces carrots, peeled and cut into ½-inch-thick rounds

12 large shallots, peeled

½ pound fresh or salted pork rind, blanched 5 minutes, cut into wide strips (see Note, page 154)

1 bottle (750 ml) dry red wine, such as Cabernet Sauvignon

¼ cup cognac

½ head of garlic (about 5 cloves), cloves separated and peeled

Herb bouquet: 3 fresh Italian flat-leaf parsley sprigs, 3 fresh thyme sprigs, and 1 bay leaf tied together

(continued)

1 One day in advance, trim the beef of all surrounding fat; then cut into 12 pieces of approximately equal size. Thoroughly dry the meat and season with salt and pepper. Heat the oil in a large, heavy conventional skillet. Add the meat and sauté in batches over medium-high heat, turning, until browned, about 5 minutes per batch. Drain in a colander set over a bowl to catch the drippings. Pour ½ cup water into the skillet and bring to a boil, scraping up any brown bits from the bottom of the pan. Add to the drippings in the bowl.

2 Cut the pancetta into 1 by ¼-inch lardons. Melt the butter in the same skillet used to sauté the beef. Add the lardons and the pig's foot. Sauté over medium heat, turning, until lightly browned all over, about 10 minutes. Using a slotted spoon, transfer the lardons and pig's foot to the colander with the meat.

3 Add the onion, carrots, and shallots to the skillet and cook over medium heat until golden, about 20 minutes. Transfer the vegetables to a side dish, leaving the juices in the skillet. Slip the pork rind, fat side down, into the casserole. Top with the pig's foot, beef, vegetables, and lardons in that order. Skim the fat off the drippings in the skillet and add them to the earthenware pot.

4 Rinse and dry the skillet and return to medium heat. Add the wine and cognac and warm until hot but not boiling. Remove from the heat and carefully ignite, averting your face. Let the alcohol burn for 2 minutes; then cover the skillet to extinguish the flames. Pour into the casserole. Add the degreased drippings from step 1, garlic, and herb bouquet. Slowly bring to a simmer over medium-low heat. Reduce the heat to low, cover with a sheet of parchment and the lid, and cook for 2½ hours.

5 Transfer the beef to a deep bowl and cover to keep it moist. Remove the bones and gristle from the pig's foot while it is still warm. With a large sharp knife, chop the skin and meat together with the lardons until spongy and light. Spread this chopped mixture over the beef. Top with the vegetables. When cool, cover and refrigerate overnight. Refrigerate the juices separately.

6 The next day, about 3½ hours before serving, remove the bowl from the refrigerator and scrape the congealed fat off the juices. Let the meat stand at room temperature for 1 hour. Meanwhile, preheat the oven to 300°F.

7 Put the meat, vegetables, and sauce back into the earthenware pot. Set over low heat and bring to a simmer. Cover with parchment and partially cover with the lid. Transfer to the oven and bake for 2 hours.

8 Remove the meat from the casserole. Strain the sauce and vegetables through a sieve set over a large saucepan. Press down on the solids to extract as much flavor as possible. Bring to a boil, slide the skillet half off the heat, and continue to cook, skimming off the impurities that rise to the top, until the sauce reaches napping consistency (coats the back of a spoon), about 10 minutes. Season with salt and pepper to taste and pour over the meat.

NOTE TO THE COOK: Pork rind can be cut off either fatback or lean salt pork, or it can be purchased separately from a pork butcher. Do not substitute bacon rind, which is smoked.

Marrakech-Style Veal Tangia with Smen and Preserved Lemons

SERVES 4

J tasted my first *tangia* in Marrakech, where it was baked over burning acorns behind a bathhouse, the fire having been set to warm the bath water inside. As so often when Moroccans build a fire for warmth, they figure out a way to use it for cooking too.

In this case, tall amphora-shaped clay jars called *tangias* were nestled in the embers. Some of these *tangias* contained bony parts of veal or lamb such as shoulder, feet, and tails; others were filled with lamb and beef short ribs; and some with gazelle and camel meat.

I've had great success making this dish in a bean pot with veal, achieving a fine balance between the flavor of the meat, garlic, preserved lemons, spices, and preserved butter, or *smen*. Basically everything is packed into the pot at the same time, the top is covered with paper, and then the dish is cooked very slowly. In a good *tangia* the meat juices become *très savoureux* due to the mixing of salt, steam, aromatics, and the special flavor imparted by the clay cooking vessel. Serve with warm bread.

> **PREFERRED CLAY POT:**
> A 2½- or 3-quart bean pot, Spanish olla, or any earthenware casserole that is taller than it is wide

1¾ pounds boneless veal shoulder or 3 pounds bone-in veal shanks or beef short ribs

⅛ teaspoon saffron threads

½ teaspoon salt

1 tablespoon ground cumin

½ teaspoon ras el hanout or La Kama spices (page 316)

¼ teaspoon freshly ground black pepper

¼ teaspoon ground ginger

¼ teaspoon ground cinnamon

¼ teaspoon freshly grated nutmeg

4 large garlic cloves, lightly crushed

2 tablespoons homemade smen (page 295) or unsalted butter

1 preserved lemon (page 317), rinsed and quartered

1 Preheat the oven to 250°F. Cut the veal into 4 roughly equal pieces. Soak the saffron in ¼ cup warm water for 10 minutes.

2 Place all the ingredients in the bean pot; use a wooden spoon to mix them gently; then press them down to a compact mass. Cover with a small sheet of crumpled wet parchment and a lid. Set in the oven and bake for 4 hours.

3 Let cool down; then pour the stew into a bowl. Skim off the fat and reheat in a conventional pan just before serving. Serve in a warm serving bowl.

Catalan Estofat with Roast Vegetables

SERVES 6

Stewing is a great way to tenderize a tough piece of meat, in this case beef shin, which, being highly gelatinous, develops an especially luscious texture when cooked slowly. Traditionally, an *estofat* is made in a wide clay-covered casserole, smothered in hot coals.

My recipe, adapted and updated from a version served at the famous Hostal de Sant Jordi restaurant in Barcelona, Spain, bakes the casserole in an oven for 4 hours, which produces excellent results. Such long cooking requires a strong, sharp red wine, such as a Priorato from Tarragona, a Torres Gran Sangre de Toro, an Italian Barbera, or a good, strong domestic red, such as a Central Coast Syrah. I use the hot-to-hot marination method (see page 150) to flavor the meat right from the start.

Unlike a French daube, which is cooked on top of the stove, a Spanish *estofat* is slow-cooked in the oven with a tight-fitting lid to seal in the aromatic flavorings. A sealed pot will attain a higher internal temperature, all to the good when cooking a tough cut of beef. For best results, prepare steps 1 through 6 a day in advance.

PREFERRED CLAY POTS:

A 4½- to 5-quart glazed or unglazed earthenware or flameware casserole, or Chinese clay pot

A 12-inch shallow stoneware or earthenware baking dish for oven roasting the vegetables and serving the assembled dish

If using an electric or ceramic stovetop, be sure to use a heat diffuser with the clay pots.

3½ pounds boneless beef shin

1 bottle (750 ml) dry red wine

1 tablespoon herbes de Provence

3 cloves

1 3-inch cinnamon stick

1 tablespoon black peppercorns, lightly crushed

1 slab (4 ounces) pancetta or blanched salt pork, cut into 1- by ¼-inch lardons

½ cup extra virgin olive oil

2 large yellow onions, cut into 1-inch chunks

2 large carrots, sliced, plus 12 small carrots, peeled

1 celery rib, into 1-inch pieces

Coarse sea salt and freshly ground black pepper

3 tablespoons red wine vinegar

Pinch of sugar

2 heads of garlic, separated into cloves but unpeeled, plus 8 garlic cloves, peeled

¼ cup anise-flavored liqueur such as anisette, ouzo, pastis, raki, or sambuca

¼ cup sweet wine such as Black Muscat, muscatel, or a fortified wine like Madeira

18 small white onions, peeled

18 small whole new potatoes, scrubbed

¼ teaspoon fennel seeds

2 fresh thyme sprigs

3 tablespoons chopped fresh flat-leaf parsley

1 Trim any excess fat from the beef. Using a boning knife, follow the natural lines to separate the beef muscles into large pieces; then cut each piece against the grain into 2-inch chunks.

2 In a large nonreactive saucepan, combine the wine, herbes de Provence, cloves, cinnamon stick, and peppercorns. Bring to a simmer over medium heat.

3 Meanwhile, in the earthenware casserole, cook the lardons in 2 tablespoons of the olive oil over medium heat, stirring, until the fat is rendered and the lardons are browned lightly, about 5 minutes. With a slotted spoon, transfer the lardons to a large bowl. In batches, without crowding, add the pieces of beef to the fat in the casserole and brown lightly on all sides, about 10 minutes per batch. As it is browned, transfer the beef to the simmering wine. Immediately remove the saucepan from the heat and let stand for 1 hour.

4 While the meat is marinating, cook the yellow onions, sliced carrots, and celery in the same earthenware casserole over medium heat until golden, about 10 minutes. Scrape into the bowl with the lardons and season lightly with salt and pepper. Pour the vinegar into the casserole and stir in the sugar. Return the browned vegetables, lardons, and 8 peeled garlic cloves to the casserole.

5 Preheat the oven to 250°F. Reheat the contents of the casserole on top of the stove. Lift the meat out of the marinade and place on top of the vegetables. Bring the wine to a boil and pour it over the meat and vegetables; cover with wet crumpled parchment and a tight-fitting lid. Transfer to the oven and bake until the meat is fork-tender, 4 to 4½ hours.

6 Using a slotted spoon, transfer the beef to a plate and cover loosely with foil to keep it moist. Strain the cooking liquid into a large conventional saucepan, pressing down on the vegetables to extract the juices. Skim the fat off the top of the liquid. Bring to a boil and cook, skimming frequently, until the liquid reduces to about 2 cups, about 15 minutes. Stir in the liqueur and the sweet wine and return it to a boil. Remove from the heat and let cool; then pour the sauce over the meat, cover, and refrigerate overnight.

7 The following day, about 2 hours before serving, remove the meat and sauce from the refrigerator and bring to room temperature. Scrape the congealed fat from the surface of the sauce and the chunks of beef.

8 Meanwhile, pour the remaining 6 tablespoons olive oil into the baking dish. Add the unpeeled garlic cloves, whole small carrots, white onions, and potatoes, 1 teaspoon salt, ½ teaspoon pepper, and the fennel seeds. Toss to coat with the oil. Tuck in the thyme sprigs. Place in the cold oven and set the temperature at 350°F. Roast, uncovered, for 1½ hours.

9 Arrange the chunks of meat over the roasted vegetables and pour the sauce on top. Return to the oven and bake for 30 minutes. Serve hot, with the chopped parsley and coarse sea salt sprinkled on top.

Beef Stew with Mloukia Leaves

SERVES 12

"You'll either love this or hate it!" a cook in the Tunisian city of Gabès told me, referring to a very dark, blackish-green-sauced beef stew that had simmered for seven hours over hot coals. In fact, I liked it a lot and am including the recipe here along with her caveat. This dish won't be to everyone's taste, but here it is for the delectation of all you culinary adventurers out there.

The principal flavoring is powdered dried *mloukia* leaves, which are green but turn very dark when fried in olive oil. The taste of *mloukia* leaf powder is highly exotic, fascinating in that it tastes like nothing else. Dried *mloukia* or *molokhiya* leaves can be purchased at any Middle Eastern grocery. Because like okra or filé powder *mloukia* is mucilaginous, it endows this beef dish with a particularly rich and much prized viscous sauce.

This dish is best if made one or two days in advance. The marinade is strong and will penetrate the meat in about a day. Long, slow cooking does the rest of the work. This is one of a number of Tunisian dishes traditionally served on the buffet table on the first day of the year. It is supposed to bring luck and good health to all who those who partake of it.

> **PREFERRED CLAY POT:**
>
> A 4-quart wide, glazed earthenware or flameware casserole
>
> If using an electric or ceramic stovetop, be sure to use a heat diffuser with the clay pot.

3 pounds boneless beef chuck, cut into 1¼-inch chunks

2 tablespoons ground coriander

12 garlic cloves, minced

1 tablespoon dried mint, crumbled

1¾ teaspoons harissa

Salt and freshly ground black pepper

7 ounces dried mloukia leaves, pressed through the finest sieve to a powder (2 cups)

1⅓ cups extra virgin olive oil

2½ quarts boiling water

2 imported bay leaves

Pinch of salt

1 At least 1 day before cooking, toss the meat with the coriander, garlic, dried mint, harissa, and 1½ teaspoons black pepper. Cover and refrigerate overnight.

2 In the earthenware casserole, mix the mloukia powder and the olive oil to a smooth paste. Set over medium heat and bring to a boil, stirring constantly. Reduce the heat to medium-low, and use a wooden spatula to stir the mixture constantly for 10 minutes so it does not burn. (During this time, the mloukia will "toast" and develop a darker color and deeper flavor.) Reduce the heat to low and gradually stir in 2 quarts of the boiling water; be careful, because the mixture will splatter. (At this point, the mloukia will be lumpy.) Cover and cook over the lowest possible heat for 3 hours, stirring occasionally and adding simmering water if the mixture becomes dry.

3 When the mloukia sauce loses its gluey appearance and turns smooth, add the meat, bay leaf, and a pinch of salt. Add the remaining 2 cups boiling water. Simmer, uncovered, over medium heat for 2 hours.

4 Reduce the heat to very low and simmer for 1 hour longer. The dish is ready when the oil separates and mounts to the surface of the sauce in one continuous sheet. Correct the seasoning and serve very hot.

Stifado with Beef and Caramelized Onions

SERVES 6

This, I hasten to say, is my personal version of *stifado,* to which several of my Greek friends gently object. For one thing, I brown the beef first to deepen the flavor, something most Greek cooks don't do. For another, I make my stew a day ahead to allow the flavors to mellow completely. This also gives me time to remove the bones, cut the meat into smaller pieces, and remove all the fat from the sauce.

Serve the stew hot along with chunks of feta cheese and plenty of crusty bread.

> **PREFERRED CLAY POT:**
>
> A 5-quart glazed or unglazed earthenware or flameware casserole
>
> A 10- or 12-inch earthenware baking dish or Spanish cazuela
>
> If using an electric or ceramic stovetop, be sure to use a heat diffuser with the clay pots.

1 large yellow onion, chopped

⅓ cup extra virgin olive oil

3 garlic cloves, bruised

1 can (28 ounces) tomatoes, packed in tomato juice, crushed by hand

4 pounds meaty beef short ribs, well trimmed and cut into 10 to 12 individual pieces

Salt and freshly ground black pepper

1 cup dry red wine

3 pounds small white boiling onions, about 1 inch in diameter, peeled

1 teaspoon sugar

¼ cup red wine vinegar

Spice bag: 2 imported bay leaves, 1 tablespoon allspice berries, and 2 3-inch Ceylon cinnamon sticks wrapped in cheesecloth

1 tablespoon chopped fresh flat-leaf parsley

8 ounces feta cheese

(continued)

1 Set the casserole over medium-low heat. Add the chopped onion, half the olive oil, and ¼ cup water. Cook until the water has evaporated and the onion is soft and translucent, about 10 minutes. Add the garlic and tomatoes and cook, stirring, until the tomato sauce is thick, about 20 minutes.

2 Meanwhile, quickly rinse the beef, drain, and pat dry. Season lightly with salt and pepper. Heat the remaining olive oil in a large, heavy conventional skillet until hot. Working in batches, brown the beef chunks on all sides over high heat, 2 to 3 minutes. Transfer to the earthenware casserole. Pour off all the fat in the skillet. Add the red wine and bring to a boil, scraping up any brown bits from the bottom of the pan. Add the peeled onions and sugar and cook over medium-high heat, stirring, until the wine is reduced to a glaze and the onions are lightly browned all over, 5 minutes. Add 3 tablespoons of the vinegar and bring to a boil, stirring. Add the cheesecloth packet of spices to the beef and tomato sauce in the casserole along with the small white onions and the skillet juices. Cover with a sheet of parchment and a lid and cook over low heat for 2 to 2½ hours without disturbing.

3 Transfer the hot casserole to a wooden surface or folded kitchen towel to prevent cracking. Uncover and let stand until cooled. Skim the fat off the surface. Discard the packet of spices. When the meat is cool enough to handle, remove all bones and gristle. Cut the meat into 1-inch pieces and place in a large bowl. Use a slotted spoon to remove the onions from the sauce and add them to the meat. Cover and refrigerate overnight. Strain the tomato and cooking liquid into a second bowl. Let cool; then cover and refrigerate separately.

4 The following day, about 2 hours before serving, scrape any fat off the meat and onions and the sauce. Combine them in the baking dish and reheat in a 300°F oven or over low heat on top of the stove. Season with salt and pepper to taste. If you think the sauce needs it, stir in the last tablespoon of vinegar. Sprinkle with parsley and serve hot along with bite-sized portions of feta cheese and plenty of crusty bread.

NOTE TO THE COOK: To make small onions easier to peel, drop them into simmering water, soak for 1 minute, and drain. Use a small knife to remove the root end; peel off the outer skin.

Gratin of Veal Shanks with Spiced Tomato Sauce and Pasta

SERVES 4

Here's my updated recipe for *pastitsatha*, a particularly popular dish on the Ionian Island of Corfu, where the food is spicy rather than herbal as in most of Greece. It's nearly impossible to pass by a kitchen door in Corfu without catching the aroma of sweet paprika cooking in oil, but you'd be hard-pressed to find paprika used elsewhere in Greece.

Pastitsatha is truly an outstanding meal-in-one-pot dish. Chunks of farm-raised chicken or rosy veal shanks are cooked slowly with spices, garlic, wine, and vinegar, simmered with an onion and tomato sauce enriched with a little honey, and finally tossed with pasta. The combination of different peppers—cayenne, black, and paprika—is essential to obtain the deep spicy flavor that makes this dish so good.

> **PREFERRED CLAY POTS:**
>
> A 3-quart earthenware casserole, such as a Greek *yiouvetsi* or a Turkish *guvec*, or a wide glazed or unglazed earthenware or flameware casserole
>
> A 3½- to 4-quart (13- × 9- by 2-inch) stoneware or earthenware baking dish
>
> If using an electric or ceramic stovetop, be sure to use a heat diffuser with the clay pots.

2½ pounds veal shanks, cut into large chunks (ask your butcher to do this)

Salt and freshly ground black pepper

3 large garlic cloves, thinly sliced

¼ cup extra virgin olive oil

1 cup dry white or red wine

2 to 3 tablespoons red wine vinegar

1 small Ceylon cinnamon stick

2 cloves

1 bay leaf

2 medium red onions, finely chopped

1 can (28 ounces) whole San Marzano–style tomatoes, seeded and drained in a colander

1½ tablespoons honey, preferably thyme honey

¾ teaspoon sweet paprika

⅛ teaspoon crushed hot red pepper

12 ounces tubular pasta, such as bucatini, perciatelli, or ziti

5 tablespoons unsalted butter

3 ounces freshly grated kefalotyri or pecorino Romano cheese (about ¾ cup)

1 About 3½ hours before serving, preheat the oven to 300°F. Wipe the surface of the veal; rub it with 1 teaspoon salt and ½ teaspoon pepper. Slip half of the garlic slices between the bones and the meat.

2 Heat 2 tablespoons of the olive oil in the earthenware casserole over medium-low heat. Add the veal and cook, turning, until golden brown all over, about 10 minutes. Meanwhile, warm the wine and 2 tablespoons of the vinegar in a small saucepan; add the remaining garlic, the cinnamon, cloves, and bay leaf and boil over medium-high heat until reduced by half, about 5 minutes. Pour over the browned meat. Cover with a sheet of parchment and a lid and transfer to the oven. Bake for 1 hour.

(continued)

3 While the veal shanks are cooking, in a large conventional skillet cook the onions in the remaining 2 tablespoons olive oil, stirring, until softened, about 10 minutes. Add the tomatoes to the skillet along with the honey, paprika, and hot pepper. Season with salt and black pepper to taste. Cook, stirring occasionally, for 10 minutes longer. Raise the heat to medium-high and sauté until the onions and tomatoes begin to thicken, about 10 minutes.

4 Pour the tomato and onion sauce over the meat in the casserole. Replace the parchment and the lid and continue to bake for 2 hours, or until the veal is fork tender.

5 Transfer the hot casserole to a wooden surface or folded kitchen towel to prevent cracking. Pick out and discard the bay leaf and cinnamon stick from the sauce. Let the casserole rest for 10 minutes; then carefully tilt the pot and skim off the oil that rises to the surface; discard all but 2 tablespoons. Use the reserved oil to grease the baking dish. Transfer the veal shanks to a cutting board. Remove the bones and cut the meat into bite-sized pieces; wrap in foil and set aside. Reserve the tomato sauce in the casserole. Raise the oven temperature to 375°F.

6 In a large pot of boiling salted water, cook the pasta until it is just tender, about 10 minutes; drain well and return to the saucepan. Stir in the butter, and half the cheese; toss to mix. Season lightly with salt and pepper. Add the pasta to the tomato sauce in the casserole and stir gently to mix. Fold in the reserved chunks of veal. Cover with a sheet of aluminum foil and bake for 10 minutes. Uncover and bake for 10 minutes longer. Sprinkle the remaining cheese on top and serve at once.

Aegean-Style Koftes

SERVES 4

I learned this recipe for light, juicy, butter-tender beef or lamb meatballs from a motel chef in the town of Assos on the North Aegean coast of Turkey. Motel chef? Yes, indeed. My friend Ayfer Ünsal took me to the Terrace Motel, assuring me that the chef, Ilker Kaya, was immensely talented and that his *koftes* were divine. How right she was.

In Ilker's recipe, the *koftes* are very slowly poached in an onion sauce scented with cumin, red pepper, and *kekik* (Turkish oregano) and then served smothered in a soft sheet of grated sheep's milk cheese. The poaching is done in a clay pot made especially for this dish; I substitute a Spanish cazuela. *Kofte*, or meatballs, are typically cooked for about ten minutes, but simmering them longer over low heat creates a very tender texture, which allows them to absorb more flavor, at the same time imbuing the sauce with more "meatiness."

1 pound ground beef or lamb

1 teaspoon Marash or Aleppo pepper

½ teaspoon ground cumin

½ cup crumbled crustless day-old bread

1 garlic clove, crushed

Salt and freshly ground black pepper

2 tablespoons extra virgin olive oil

½ cup chopped onion

½ cup chopped scallion, white part only

1 small mildly hot green pepper, such as Anaheim, chopped

2 medium tomatoes, peeled, seeded, and chopped

2 tablespoons chopped fresh flat-leaf parsley

½ teaspoon dried Turkish kekik or Mediterranean oregano

3 tablespoons sweet Turkish pepper paste

1½ tablespoons unsalted butter, melted

½ cup grated sheep's milk cheese, such as kasseri or kashar

1 About 45 minutes before serving, knead the ground beef with the Marash pepper, cumin, crumbled bread, garlic, 1 teaspoon salt, and ⅛ teaspoon black pepper until the mixture is smooth. Divide into 8 ovals about 2½ inches long and 1 inch thick. Working on an unglazed clay saucer or a wooden work surface, gently roll—do not knead—the first oval around on itself until you can feel the thinnest veil of a skin develop over the surface of the meat, 1 to 2 minutes. Set aside and repeat with the remaining ovals.

2 Heat the olive oil in the cazuela over medium-low heat. Add the onion, scallion, and green pepper and cook until softened but not browned, about 5 minutes. Place the kofte ovals in a single layer on top of the onion. Add ¼ cup water, cover the pot with foil, and cook without disturbing for 20 minutes.

3 Carefully turn over each kofte. Scatter the chopped tomatoes between them, partially cover, and cook for 10 minutes.

4 Meanwhile, combine the parsley, oregano, Turkish pepper paste, and a pinch each of salt and pepper. Mash with a fork to blend well, adding 1½ tablespoons water. Sprinkle evenly over the koftes in the cazuela. Turn off the heat and immediately drizzle on the melted butter. Sprinkle the grated cheese and more black pepper on top and serve at once.

Beef Paupiettes with Tomatoes and Wild Capers

SERVES 4

In France this rich, wonderful dish is called *alouettes sans têtes*, meaning "doves without heads." The beef slices are stuffed with pancetta, garlic, and herbs and sautéed until brown on the outside. Then they are simmered in a delicious tomato sauce until meltingly tender. The addition of citrusy orange zest, piquant wild capers, and sweet fragrant thyme to a finished dish is particular to some parts of Provence. When you serve this rich, radiant dish directly from the clay pot, accompany it with a platter of buttered noodles or mashed potatoes.

> ### PREFERRED CLAY POT:
>
> A 12-inch Spanish cazuela, a straight-sided flameware skillet, or a French *poêlon de terre*
>
> If using an electric or ceramic stovetop, be sure to use a heat diffuser with the clay pot.

8 slices boneless lean beef, cut ¼ inch thick from a cross rib roast, each roughly 7 by 4 inches (about 1¾ pounds total)

Salt and freshly ground black pepper

8 ounces pancetta, diced

1 tablespoon mashed garlic plus 4 garlic cloves, halved

⅓ cup chopped fresh flat-leaf parsley

1½ tablespoons chopped celery leaves

¼ teaspoon freshly grated nutmeg

½ ounce dried cèpes or porcini, broken into small pieces

2 tablespoons extra virgin olive oil

1 medium onion, chopped

1 carrot, minced

1 cup dry white wine

Herb bouquet: 3 fresh flat-leaf parsley sprigs, 2 fresh thyme sprigs, 1 bay leaf, 1 celery rib stuck with 2 cloves, and 1 strip orange zest wrapped in cheesecloth

3 tablespoons tomato paste, canned or homemade (page 317)

3 cups meat or poultry stock, heated

1 teaspoon red wine vinegar

2 tablespoons capers, drained and rinsed

1 tablespoon each chopped fresh flat-leaf parsley and thyme, minced garlic, and grated orange zest for garnish

1 Lay the slices of beef out on a work surface and pound gently to flatten slightly. Season with salt and pepper. In a mixing bowl, combine the pancetta, mashed garlic, parsley, celery, nutmeg, 1 teaspoon salt, and ½ teaspoon pepper. Mix with your hands to blend well. Divide the stuffing evenly among the beef slices. Roll each slice up over the filling at the wider end, fold in the sides, roll up, and secure with white kitchen string or toothpicks.

2 Place the dried cèpes in a small bowl and cover with 1 cup hot water; let stand for 30 minutes to soften. Remove the cèpes from the soaking liquid, squeezing the mushrooms to release the liquid into the bowl. Reserve the liquid. Chop the cèpes.

3   Heat the olive oil in the cazuela set over medium-low heat. Add the onion and carrot and cook until soft and golden, about 10 minutes. Add the meat rolls and sauté slowly, turning, until browned all over, 20 minutes. Add the white wine, herb bouquet, garlic halves, tomato paste, cèpes, reserved mushroom-soaking liquid, and stock. Raise the heat to medium and bring to a simmer. Cover with a sheet of parchment and a lid. Reduce the heat to low and simmer for about 2 hours, turning the beef rolls once after an hour. Transfer the beef rolls to a side dish and cover with foil. Strain the cooking juices, pressing down on all the vegetables and any bits of pancetta that may have fallen out. Let the beef rolls and sauce cool separately; then cover and refrigerate. (The recipe can be made to this point up to a day in advance.)

4   About 1½ hours before serving, completely degrease the sauce. Cut away the strings from the beef rolls. Return the beef rolls and the sauce to the cazuela. Cook, uncovered, over medium-low heat for 1 hour, turning the beef rolls in the sauce from time to time. Stir in the vinegar and capers and simmer for a few minutes longer. Correct the seasoning with salt and pepper. Garnish with the chopped parsley and thyme, garlic, and orange zest and serve at once.

NOTE TO THE COOK: There is an art to pounding beef for paupiettes. Use a kitchen mallet and a combination swoop and tap, working from the center to the outer edge to achieve even thickness. Be sure not to pound too forcefully, or the beef slice will tear.

Loretta Keller's Beef Tripe Florentine

SERVES 12

In 2008, I was discussing tripe and *tripières* with San Francisco star chef Loretta Keller of restaurant Coco500. Loretta is a true soul mate, and, as it turns out, she adores tripe, owns a half dozen *tripières,* and uses them as often as she can. Learning of my interest, she offered to come up to Sonoma on a Sunday so we could cook together.

Loretta brought cleaned and blanched tripe with her. As soon as she arrived, she started a classic mirepoix of finely diced onion, carrot, and celery and then began to add flavorings—garlic, tomato, prosciutto, and dried Parmigiano-Reggiano rind. This enhanced mirepoix became the base for the braising liquid, the tripe was added, and the casserole was set in a low oven to braise for several hours. The tripe cooked so slowly that when she uncovered the dish, the shape had hardly changed, but it fell apart at the touch of a fork.

> **PREFERRED CLAY POT:**
> A 5-quart earthenware or flameware casserole or a *tripière*
> If using an electric or ceramic stovetop, be sure to use a heat diffuser with the clay pot.

3 pounds cleaned or "ready to cook" beef honeycomb tripe (ask for the reticulum)

3 tablespoons cider vinegar

3 tablespoons extra virgin olive oil

3 medium onions, cut into ½-inch dice

1 large carrot, cut into ½-inch dice

2 celery ribs, cut into ½-inch dice

6 garlic cloves, coarsely chopped

3 tablespoons brandy or cognac

1 cup dry white wine

3 ounces prosciutto in 1 piece (ask for the end)

1 square (3 inches) Parmigiano-Reggiano rind

1 can (28 ounces) imported San Marzano or other good canned tomatoes

2 to 3 tablespoons tomato paste, preferably homemade (page 317)

Pinch of crushed hot red pepper

Herb bouquet: 1 bunch of fresh basil, 1 bunch of fresh flat-leaf parsley, 1 bunch of fresh thyme, 1 bunch of fresh marjoram, and 2 imported bay leaves tied with white kitchen string

3 cups chicken stock, heated

Salt and freshly ground black pepper

2 tablespoons fresh lemon juice

1½ pounds fresh pappardelle pasta

1 cup grated pecorino cheese, preferably Sardo or Toscana

Chopped fresh flat-leaf parsley for garnish

1 Rinse the tripe under cold running water. Soak in a bowl with 3 cups water mixed with the vinegar for 1 hour; rinse again and drain well. Place the tripe in a deep kettle and cover with fresh cold water. Bring slowly to a boil over medium heat. Reduce the heat and simmer for 15 minutes; drain. As soon as the tripe is cool enough to handle, cut it into ½-inch-thick strips about 2½ inches long.

2 Meanwhile, in the casserole, heat the oil. Add the onions, carrot, and celery and cook over medium-low heat, stirring occasionally, until the vegetables are soft and golden, about 10 minutes. Add the garlic and cook until it turns golden, about 10 minutes longer. Pour in the brandy and ignite, averting your face. When the flames subside, add the white wine and boil until reduced by half, about 5 minutes. Add the tripe, prosciutto, Parmigiano-Reggiano rind, tomatoes, tomato paste, hot pepper, herb bouquet, and stock. Bring to a boil, add 1 teaspoon salt and ½ teaspoon pepper, lay a crumpled piece of wet parchment directly over the contents of the casserole, cover with a lid, and simmer over low heat until the tripe is "al dente" but tender and the cooking juices are very aromatic, 3 to 3½ hours.

3 Transfer the hot casserole to a wooden surface or folded kitchen towel to prevent cracking. Be careful where you set the lid as well. Remove and discard the herb bouquet, prosciutto, and Parmigiano-Reggiano rind. The dish can be prepared to this point up to 5 days in advance. Transfer it to a storage container and let cool; then cover and refrigerate.

4 About 1½ hours before serving, slowly reheat the tripe and sauce in a conventional saucepan over medium-low heat until it is meltingly tender, about 10 minutes. Season with the lemon juice and salt and pepper to taste.

5 About 20 minutes before serving, in a large pot of boiling salted water, cook the fresh pasta until it is just tender; drain and arrange in a warm serving dish. Pour the tripe and sauce over the pasta and toss to mix. Dust lightly with grated cheese and parsley and serve at once.

Roast Pork Shoulder with Glazed Turnips

SERVES 6 TO 8

My late friend Mario Ruspoli, whose French-language book on Tuscan cooking, *Petit Bréviaire de la Cuisine Étrusque et Romaine* is filled with terrific clay pot recipes, cooked this dish for me at his mother's home in Tangier, with a slow-roasted boned leg of suckling pig he'd purchased from the only Spanish butcher in town. It was meltingly tender with a crackling crisp skin, and he served it with glazed baby turnips.

Mario advised me it would have tasted even better if he had sent it to a baker's oven, but because of the Muslim prohibition against pork, that was not possible in Morocco. However, if you create a clay baker's style environment in your home oven (see page xvii), you will be able to prepare this dish at its very best.

Years later I learned another garnish that works fabulously with it: grilled Tuscan pecorino cheese with a drizzle of honey.

So long as you start with meat from a quality heritage pig, you won't go wrong, even if you don't roast it in a clay-lined oven. In this recipe I substitute a pork shoulder blade. Ask your butcher to butterfly the blade so it can be stuffed and rolled into a cylinder with the grain of the meat running lengthwise.

> **PREFERRED CLAY POT:**
>
> **A 10- to 12-inch Spanish cazuela**
>
> **If using an electric or ceramic stovetop, be sure to use a heat diffuser with the clay pot.**
>
> **RECOMMENDED CLAY ENVIRONMENT:**
>
> **Double slabs of pizza stones or food-safe quarry tiles set on the upper and lower oven racks**

3 pounds boneless pork shoulder blade, preferably heritage quality

4 garlic cloves

Sea salt

3 tablespoons chopped fresh rosemary

½ teaspoon freshly grated nutmeg

½ teaspoon freshly ground black pepper

3 tablespoons extra virgin olive oil

¾ cup dry red wine at room temperature

Glazed Turnips (recipe follows)

1 tablespoon red wine vinegar, preferably aged

1 About 5 hours before serving, bring the pork to room temperature. Place the pork, fatty side down, on a work surface. Pound the garlic in a mortar with 1 teaspoon sea salt until smooth. Blend in the rosemary, nutmeg, and pepper to make a smooth paste. Spread the seasonings over the meat, roll it up, and tie with string.

2 Preheat the oven to 275°F. Put the olive oil in the cazuela. Add the pork and roll to coat it all over. Place in the oven and roast for 2 hours, or until the internal temperature of the thickest part of the meat registers 140°F on an instant-read thermometer.

3 Baste the pork with the wine and continue to roast for 2 hours, or until an instant-read thermometer registers 175°F to 180°F. While the pork is roasting, prepare the turnips.

4 Transfer the pork roast to a carving board and cover loosely with foil; let rest for 20 to 30 minutes. Skim the fat off the pan drippings. Add the vinegar, ⅔ cup water, and the glazed turnips. Warm over medium-low heat. Serve with the sliced pork.

NOTE TO THE COOK: To serve the pork cold: Let the roast cool; then wrap and refrigerate overnight. The following day, slice 2 medium red onions paper thin and soak in 3 tablespoons red wine vinegar for 30 minutes. Slice the pork and serve with the drained red onions.

Glazed Turnips

> **PREFERRED CLAY POT:**
>
> A 2½- to 3-quart unglazed or glazed earthenware casserole, such as a large Chinese sandpot, a Colombian La Chamba casserole, or a medium Italian Vulcania casserole

2 pounds small turnips, peeled

3 tablespoons unsalted butter

2 teaspoons sugar

¾ teaspoon salt

¼ teaspoon freshly ground black pepper

Place the turnips, butter, sugar, salt, and pepper in a 2½- to 3-quart earthenware casserole. Add ½ cup water, cover with a sheet of crumpled parchment and a lid, and cook over low heat, shaking the pot occasionally without lifting the lid, for 45 minutes.

Roast Pork Shoulder with
Grilled Tuscan Pecorino Cheese

Prepare the recipe as directed, but serve the following grilled cheese alongside the pork slices.

Grilled Tuscan Pecorino

8 ounces fresh pecorino Toscana, chilled for easier slicing

⅓ cup orange flower honey or chestnut honey

Cut the cheese into 6 to 8 even slices. Heat a lightly oiled nonstick grill pan until hot. Add the slices and grill for less than a minute on the first side, or until just browned on the surface. Carefully turn over with a wide spatula and repeat on the second side. Place on the platter alongside the slices of pork, drizzle the honey over the cheese, and serve at once.

Roast Loin of Pork with Golden Raisins

SERVES 6

This excellent French recipe calls for an exotic ingredient: walnut wine (*vin de noix*). I like to make my own and offer a recipe for it in *The Cooking of Southwest France* revised edition (2007). But it does require access to a walnut tree and a year and a half of aging. If you wish to make this recipe in a timelier fashion, I suggest substituting the Italian green walnut liqueur *nocino* or a mix of good red wine with a little port wine or cognac.

> **PREFERRED CLAY POT:**
>
> An earthenware skillet, such as a French *poêlon de terre*, or an 11- or 12-inch Spanish cazuela or straight-sided flameware skillet
>
> If using an electric or ceramic stovetop, be sure to use a heat diffuser with the clay pot.

¾ cup golden raisins

¼ cup vin de noix or nocino or 3 tablespoons red wine mixed with 1 tablespoon port wine or cognac

4 garlic cloves

1 tablespoon coarse salt

1 tablespoon herbes de Provence

1 teaspoon fennel seeds

6 to 8 fresh sage leaves

1½ teaspoons whole black peppercorns

3 tablespoons extra virgin olive oil

1 boneless pork loin roast (2 to 2½ pounds), preferably from the blade end

3 medium onions, thinly sliced

½ teaspoon red wine vinegar

Salt and freshly ground black pepper

1 Soak the golden raisins in 1 cup hot water with 1 tablespoon of the vin de noix for 1 to 2 hours.

2 In a mortar, pound 3 of the garlic cloves with the salt to a paste. Add the herbes de Provence, fennel seeds, sage leaves, and peppercorns and pound until smooth. Alternatively, grind garlic, herbs, and spices in an electric spice mill. Stir in 2 tablespoons of the olive oil. Rub this seasoning paste all over the pork roast and let stand at room temperature for 1 hour.

3 Preheat the oven to 300°F. Cut the last garlic clove in half and rub it over the bottom and sides of the earthenware skillet. Grease with the remaining 1 tablespoon olive oil. Add the onions, vinegar, 2 tablespoons water, and pinches of salt and pepper; toss and set in the oven. Bake the onions, uncovered, for 1 hour, or until soft and golden.

4 Raise the oven heat to 400°F. Stir the onions, flatten slightly into a bed, and place the pork roast on top, fat side up. Return the skillet to the oven and roast for about 1 hour, until the internal temperature of the pork registers 140°F.

5 Transfer the pork roast to a carving board and let rest for 10 minutes before slicing. Meanwhile, use a slotted spoon to transfer the onions to a side dish. Pour out any fat from the skillet, set it over low heat, and add the remaining vin de noix. When warm, ignite, averting your face. When the flames subside, add the golden raisins with their soaking liquid and the cooked onions. Bring to a boil, stirring. Correct the seasoning and turn off the heat. Slice the pork, place over the onion-raisin sauce, and serve directly from the cazuela.

Slow-Cooked Pork in Milk with Pumpkin

SERVES 8

This recipe comes from Siglinda Scarpa, a sculptor, potter, and filmmaker who was born in Italy but now lives in North Carolina, where she makes beautiful flameproof terra-cotta pots. "When I was a very little girl, I used to wake up to the smell of food that my great-grandmother was cooking on the woodstove in terra-cotta pots. She had many of them in various shapes and sizes, and each one was used for a specific food and that food only," she told me.

Siglinda also teaches Italian clay pot cooking, and she kindly shared her recipe for *arrosto di maiale al latte* (pork braised in milk) with me. It's a dish known for its great taste but plain appearance. White-wine-and-vinegar-marinated pork poaches in milk along with slices of butternut squash in a heavy clay pot in the oven. The vinegar encourages the milk to curdle; then the sauce is cooked down to a creamy caramelized brown. All the while the steady slow heat in the unglazed clay helps to intensify the flavor and the sweetness of the dish.

> **PREFERRED CLAY POT:**
>
> A 4-quart unglazed earthenware casserole with a tight-fitting lid
>
> If using an electric or ceramic stovetop, be sure to use a heat diffuser with the clay pot.

1 boneless pork loin (about 4 pounds)

¾ cup dry white wine

¼ cup white wine vinegar

2 tablespoons unsalted butter

Salt and freshly ground black pepper

1 quart milk, heated

3 pounds pumpkin or butternut squash, peeled and thickly sliced

Herb and spice packet: 1 fresh sage sprig, 5 imported bay leaves, 4 cloves, and 12 whole black peppercorns tied in cheesecloth

½ teaspoon freshly grated nutmeg

1 One day in advance, place the pork in a deep mixing bowl. Add the wine, vinegar, and ½ cup water. Cover and refrigerate overnight.

2 The following morning, remove the pork from the marinade and pat completely dry with paper towels. Reserve 1 tablespoon of the marinade; discard the remainder.

3 Preheat the oven to 400°F. Place the earthenware casserole over medium-low heat. Add the butter and cook until it turns light brown, about 5 minutes. Add the pork, fat side down, and cook, turning, until browned all over, about 10 minutes. Raise the heat to medium and season the roast with a sprinkling of salt and pepper. Add 1⅓ cups of the hot milk and cook until it reduces to a thick, light brown glaze, about 30 minutes.

(continued)

4   Stir in the remaining warm milk, scraping up any golden brown bits from the bottom and sides of the casserole. Arrange the slices of butternut squash around the pork, and add the packet of herbs and spices and the reserved tablespoon marinade. Cover with a tight-fitting lid and cook over low heat for 45 minutes.

5   Uncover the pot, turn the pork over, pile the squash on top, and scrape up the curds along the sides and bottom of the casserole. Replace the squash around the pork and continue cooking, uncovered, stirring from time to time, until the pork is tender when pierced with a fork, about 45 minutes. Transfer the pork to a carving board. With a slotted spoon, transfer the squash to a bowl and cover with foil to keep warm.

6   Remove and discard the packet of herbs and spices from the casserole. Raise the heat to medium and boil the milk until it is reduced to a thick caramel-brown cream, about 20 minutes. Pour into a bowl and let stand until the fat rises to the top, about 5 minutes; then skim it off. Season the sauce with salt and pepper to taste. Slice the pork and arrange on a heated serving dish. Surround with the squash, spoon the curds over the pork, ladle the sauce on top, and serve at once.

Pork Tiella with Wild Mushrooms and Potatoes

SERVES 4

This recipe is from the Silana Mountains area of Calabria, Italy, where the wonderful cow's milk cheese called *caciocavallo* is made. You may have seen pairs of the pear-shaped cheese connected by a rope hanging over a beam in Italian groceries, a shape resembling the legs of an equestrian, which explains its name (*cavallo* means "horseman" in Italian).

A *tiella* is a wide, medium-high glazed earthenware cooking vessel popular in Calabria and Puglia; the word also refers to the dish cooked in the pot. Success depends on proper evaporation of moisture, the quality of the mushrooms, the meat, and the potatoes, as well as on the cooking time, which must be calculated perfectly so that everything becomes meltingly tender at the same moment. Happily, a Spanish cazuela will work perfectly well in this savory recipe.

> **PREFERRED CLAY POT:**
>
> A 12-inch Spanish cazuela or a *tiella* from southern Italy
>
> If using an electric or ceramic stovetop, be sure to use a heat diffuser with the clay pot.

¾ cup dried porcini or cèpes mushrooms (¾ ounce)

3 tablespoons extra virgin olive oil

3 garlic cloves, crushed

3 ounces thinly sliced pancetta, shredded

1 pound boneless pork shoulder, cut into 1½-inch chunks

1 pound red potatoes, peeled and thickly sliced

1 pound Italian brown mushrooms, quartered

1 long fresh rosemary sprig

¼ teaspoon crushed hot red pepper

Salt and freshly ground black pepper

4 ounces caciocavallo or aged provolone cheese, shredded

1 tablespoon chopped fresh flat-leaf parsley

1 Soak the porcini in 1 cup hot water for 20 to 30 minutes. Rub the mushrooms together to loosen any dirt and grit; then remove them from the water and coarsely chop. Strain the soaking liquid through a coffee filter or double layer of cheesecloth and set aside.

2 Heat 2 tablespoons of the olive oil in the cazuela. Add the garlic and pancetta and cook over medium-low heat, stirring, until golden, about 5 minutes. When the cazuela is warm, raise the heat to medium, add the pork, and cook, stirring, until lightly browned, about 10 minutes. Add the potatoes, chopped porcini, quartered fresh mushrooms, rosemary, hot red pepper, 1 teaspoon salt, ½ teaspoon pepper, and the reserved mushroom-soaking liquid. Cover and simmer over low heat for 45 minutes. (The recipe can be prepared to this point up to 1 day in advance. Bring back to room temperature before continuing.)

3 About 1½ hours before serving, scrape any surface fat from the pork dish. Carefully pick out as many potatoes as possible and set aside. Arrange the meat and mushrooms in one layer and top with a layer of the potatoes. Gently press down to make the dish compact. Scatter the remaining tablespoon olive oil and the cheese on top and set in a cold oven. Set the temperature at 400°F and bake for 30 minutes. Turn off the heat, and let the dish continue to cook in the receding heat for 45 minutes. Serve hot or warm, with the chopped parsley sprinkled on top.

Pork Daube with Wild Mushrooms

SERVES 6

I've been corresponding for years with expat Barbara Wilde, who shared this recipe with me. Barbara is passionate and highly knowledgeable about the food of Haute-Provence, France, where the fine local ingredients include lamb, honey, truffles, wild mushrooms, olives, olive oil, chestnuts, lavender, and, of course, the legendary herbal mix herbes de Provence. We share a love of the tender daubes of the region.

"Daubes often appear in the novels of the great regional writer Jean Giono," Barbara told me. "Giono describes them as dishes that 'nurture your body and your soul.'"

The best cooks reheat a daube at least three times. Why? Because at each reheating the sauce reduces further, becoming particularly intense and voluptuous. That is why the best daubes are sometimes called "caramels" of beef, lamb, or, in this case, pork or wild boar. You can serve this daube with pasta or rice garnished with sautéed chestnuts.

It's best to make this dish with meat from hogs raised the old-fashioned way. Brands such as Flying Pigs Farm, Certified Berkshire Pork from Eden Farms, and Vann Rose Duroc hogs are all highly recommended. The truly adventurous cook can order wild boar directly from D'Artagnan or Broken Arrow Ranch—in which case ½ cup of red wine vinegar should be added to the marinade.

Pork shoulder works beautifully. Being one of the tougher cuts, it's perfectly suited to the long, slow simmering that is the basis of daube cookery.

> **PREFERRED CLAY POT:**
>
> A 4- to 5-quart *daubière,* deep earthenware casserole, bean pot, Chinese clay pot, or Spanish olla
>
> If using an electric or ceramic stovetop, be sure to use a heat diffuser with the clay pot.

2½ to 3 pounds boneless pork shoulder or wild boar, cut into 2-inch chunks

1 bottle (750 ml) Viognier or Gewürztraminer

2 medium onions, thinly sliced

2 medium carrots, thickly sliced

Herb bouquet: 6 each fresh flat-leaf parsley, thyme, and winter savory sprigs plus 2 bay leaves and 1 leaf celery top tied with string

Spice bundle: ½ teaspoon lavender flowers, 12 crushed peppercorns, and ten crushed juniper berries tied in cheesecloth

5½ tablespoons extra virgin olive oil

1 ounce dried cèpes or porcini, plus 1 cup hot water

1 tablespoon all-purpose flour

2½ tablespoons brandy

4 teaspoons plus 1 pinch of coarse sea salt

1½ teaspoons coarsely ground black pepper

4 ounces fresh pork skin with a thin layer of fat, cut into 2- by ½-inch strips

9 juniper berries, bruised

1 head of garlic, separated into cloves but not peeled, plus 4 garlic cloves, chopped

1½ pounds fresh oyster and/or crimini mushrooms, halved if large

⅓ cup finely chopped fresh flat-leaf parsley

1 teaspoon red wine vinegar

1 Put the pork in a large bowl. Add the wine, half the sliced onions and carrots, the herb bouquet, spice packet, and 1½ tablespoons of the olive oil. Cover and refrigerate for at least 12 and up to 48 hours.

2 Drain the pork into a colander set over a bowl to catch the marinade. Discard the onions and carrots. Squeeze the spice bundle over the meat; then discard the bundle.

3 Soak the dried porcini in 1 cup hot water until softened, about 20 minutes. Drain the soaked mushrooms through a coffee filter or cheesecloth in a sieve set over a bowl. Squeeze them lightly to extract as much liquid as possible. Coarsely chop the mushrooms. Reserve the soaking water separately.

4 Pat the meat dry with paper towels. Heat 1½ tablespoons of the remaining olive oil in a large conventional skillet. In 2 batches, add the pork and sauté over medium-high heat until browned, about 5 minutes per batch.

5 Return all the meat to the skillet and sprinkle on the flour. Continue to cook, tossing, until all traces of flour disappear, about 1 minute. Remove from the heat. Immediately add the brandy and carefully ignite it with a long match; shake the skillet until the flames die down. Transfer the meat to a plate, tip the skillet, and sponge off the fat with a couple of paper towels (thus conserving all the browned bits clinging to the pan).

6 Add 1 tablespoon of the remaining olive oil to the skillet along with the remaining onions and carrots. Season with 1 teaspoon of the coarse sea salt and cook over medium-low heat, stirring occasionally, until the vegetables are lightly browned and just beginning to caramelize around the edges, about 15 minutes.

7 Preheat the oven to 250°F. Line the bottom of the earthenware casserole with the strips of pork skin, fat side down. Place one-third of the browned pork over the skin. Top with one-third of the sautéed onions and carrots. Sprinkle on 1 teaspoon of the remaining sea salt, ½ teaspoon of the pepper, 3 of the juniper berries, and one-third of the whole garlic cloves.

8 Repeat this layering two more times. Bury the reserved herb bouquet in the middle of the layers. Press gently to compress everything in the casserole tightly together.

9 Return the skillet to medium heat. Add the mushroom-soaking water and reserved marinade and bring to a boil, scraping up the browned bits from the bottom of the pan. Shift the skillet half off the heat. Simmer, skimming off the thick foam that forms on the cooler side of the skillet, until the juices are almost clear and have turned caramel brown, about 5 minutes.

10 Pour this liquid over the casserole. Top with a sheet of parchment directly on the surface of the meat and cover with the lid. Place in the oven and bake for 2½ hours.

11 Transfer the hot casserole to a wooden surface or folded kitchen towel to prevent cracking. Uncover and let cool completely. Then refrigerate the daube in the pot overnight.

(continued)

12 Remove as much fat as possible from the top of the daube. Let stand at room temperature for at least 2 hours so it's not cold when it goes into the oven. Preheat the oven to 250°F.

13 Heat the remaining 1½ tablespoons olive oil in a large conventional skillet. Add the fresh mushrooms and sauté over medium-high heat until shiny and light brown, about 3 minutes. Mix in the chopped garlic, parsley, and a pinch of salt. Remove from the heat and add the vinegar. Add to the casserole and stir gently to mix. Place in the oven and bake, uncovered, for 2 hours, or until the meat is very tender and the sauce is reduced and thick.

NOTES TO THE COOK:

✳ Daubes freeze well and thus can be made far in advance. In Provence, leftover daube meat is used to fill ravioli.

✳ In warm weather, the meat is packed with its gelatinous cooking liquid into a terrine and then chilled and served like headcheese, accompanied by pickles, capers, and shallot vinaigrette.

Slow-Cooked Pork with Sage, Mustard, and Tomatoes

SERVES 3 TO 4

Here is a Provençal recipe for an aromatic slow-roasted pork butt cooked in an open clay dish under a layer of charred caramelized tomatoes. The qualities of sweetness and meatiness contrast nicely with pungent mustard and the special combination of sage, thyme, and garlic that lends the sauce an aroma emblematic of the region.

> **PREFERRED CLAY POT:**
>
> An earthenware skillet, such as a French *poêlon de terre*, or an 11- or 12- inch Spanish cazuela or straight-sided flameware skillet
>
> If using an electric or ceramic stovetop, be sure to use a heat diffuser with the clay pot.

1 (1½ pounds) boneless pork butt or shoulder

3 medium Yukon Gold potatoes

¼ cup fresh lemon juice

3 teaspoons fresh thyme leaves

Salt and freshly ground black pepper

2 garlic cloves, bruised and sliced, plus 1 teaspoon chopped

2 large fresh sage leaves, torn into small pieces, plus 1 teaspoon chopped

1 tablespoon Dijon mustard

1 medium tomato, sliced

¼ teaspoon sugar

2 tablespoons extra virgin olive oil

1 teaspoon chopped fresh flat-leaf parsley

1 About 3½ hours before serving, remove the pork from the refrigerator and let stand for 30 minutes. At the same time, peel the potatoes, cut them into quarters, and place in a medium bowl. Add 2 tablespoons of the lemon juice, 1 teaspoon of the thyme leaves, and a pinch each of salt and pepper; let stand for about 30 minutes.

2 Preheat the oven to 275°F. Rinse and dry the pork. Using a thin, sharp knife, butterfly the meat horizontally, opening it up like a book. Season with ½ teaspoon salt and ¼ teaspoon pepper and scatter the sliced garlic, slivered sage, and 1 teaspoon of the remaining thyme leaves over one side of each piece, dividing everything evenly. Fold over to re-form the slices and tie securely with white kitchen string.

3 Place the pork, fattiest part side down, in the oiled cazuela. Brush the mustard over the top of the pork. Cover with a single layer of tomato slices. Season with the sugar and a light sprinkling of salt and pepper. Surround with the potatoes; drizzle the potatoes with the olive oil. Place in the oven and bake, uncovered, for 2 hours without opening the door.

4 Transfer the hot cazuela to a wooden surface or folded kitchen towel to prevent cracking. Tilt the pot and spoon off the extra fat. Toss the potatoes in the pan juices and return to the oven to roast for about 1 hour longer, until an instant-read thermometer inserted in the center of the meat registers 175°F.

5 Transfer the meat to a cutting board and let rest for 10 minutes before slicing. Transfer the potatoes to an ovenproof serving dish and return to the oven to keep warm. Add the remaining 2 tablespoons lemon juice and ½ cup hot water to the pan juices in the cazuela and set over medium heat. Bring to a boil and cook, stirring, to form a sauce. Stir in the chopped garlic, chopped sage, parsley, and remaining 1 teaspoon thyme leaves. Slice the pork across the grain and arrange next to the potatoes, surround with the sauce, and serve at once.

Gratin of Pig's Foot with Vin Jaune and Comté Cheese

SERVES 4 TO 6

My friend Daphne Zepos is a professional cheese maven who now specializes in just one cheese, a Comté, from the Jura region of France. "I decided to fill a need," Daphne recently told me. She hand-selects comté cheeses that are exceptionally strong in flavor, with the aroma of toasted nuts. Comtè is great for gratins and fondues or for just plain nibbling. Moreover, it goes well with dry sherry as well as either red or white wine.

When I discussed this recipe with Daphne, she strongly recommended I use a *vin jaune* made from the Savagnin grape, the "noble" grape of the Jura. Because of the type of natural yeast that forms on the grapes, *vin jaune,* she told me, has a flavor somewhat similar to sherry. Well, *vin jaune* isn't easy to find, and it's rather expensive to use for cooking, so I tried mixing Chardonnay wine with some fino (dry) sherry and a few pinches of ground spices and was extremely pleased with the result.

> **PREFERRED CLAY POT:**
>
> **A small Spanish cazuela or Chinese sandpot for the sauce**
>
> **A 3- or 4-cup earthenware gratin or a stoneware baking dish suitable for use in an oven heated to 400°F**
>
> **If using an electric or ceramic stovetop, be sure to use a heat diffuser with the clay pots.**

2 pig's feet, preferably from the foreleg (2½ pounds total), split lengthwise

2½ cups chopped onion

1½ cups chopped carrot

½ cup chopped leek, white part only

½ cup chopped celery

6 fresh flat-leaf parsley sprigs plus 2 tablespoons chopped

3 fresh thyme sprigs plus 1 teaspoon leaves

1 bay leaf

2 garlic cloves, sliced

Salt and freshly ground black pepper

2 tablespoons extra virgin olive oil

1 large tomato, peeled, seeded, and finely diced

1 cup vin jaune or ¾ cup Chardonnay mixed with ¼ cup fino sherry and ⅛ teaspoon each ground ginger, ground coriander, and curry powder

3 tablespoons unsalted butter

¾ cup fresh bread crumbs

4 ounces (Comté cheese, shredded, 1 packed cup

1 Wash the pig's feet and place in a conventional pot with water to cover. Bring to a boil over medium-low heat, skimming carefully. Add ½ cup each of the chopped onion, carrot, leek, and celery, the sprigs of parsley and thyme, the bay leaf, garlic, and ¼ teaspoon each salt and pepper. Cover and simmer until tender, about 2 hours.

2 Transfer the pig's feet to a cutting board and let stand until cool enough to handle. Measure out and reserve ½ cup of the cooking liquid; discard the remainder. As soon as you can handle the pig's feet, cut off all the skin and meat; chop into a small dice. Discard the fat, bones, and gristle. Season the skin and meat while still warm with 1 teaspoon salt and ½ teaspoon pepper.

3 In the small cazuela, heat the oil over medium heat. Add the remaining 1 cup onion and cook until soft and golden, about 10 minutes. Add the tomato and remaining 1 cup carrot and cook, stirring, for 5 minutes. Add the wine, the reserved pig's foot stock, the chopped parsley, and the thyme leaves. Bring to a boil, reduce the heat, and simmer until the carrot and onions are tender and the liquid is well reduced, about 30 minutes.

4 Preheat the oven to 400°F. Use 1 tablespoon of the butter to grease the gratin dish. Place pig meat and skin in the buttered gratin dish and cover with the sauce. Mix the bread crumbs and grated cheese and spread over the sauce. Dot with the remaining 2 tablespoons butter and set in the upper third of the oven. Bake for 20 to 30 minutes, until bubbling. Serve hot.

Adapted from a recipe provided by the tourist office of the Pays du Lomont.

Estofat of Wild Boar with Almonds and Chocolate Picada

SERVES 8

A Catalan *estofat* differs in technique from a French daube, but the alchemy of long, slow cooking in a clay pot achieves the same desirable tenderness. Boar is perfect for an *estofat* because of its rich taste, and when cooked slowly it develops a luscious flavor. Wild boar is available frozen from D'Artagnan (www.dartagnan.com) or Broken Arrow Ranch (www.brokenarrowranch.com).

As in so many wonderful Catalan recipes, this one calls for final thickening via the addition of a *picada*, a finely pounded blend of toasted almonds and unsweetened cocoa, to produce a luxuriously smooth texture and ethereal flavor.

> **PREFERRED CLAY POTS:**
>
> A 4- or 5-quart deep earthenware or flameware casserole with a tight-fitting lid
>
> A 9- × 13-inch stoneware or earthenware baking dish
>
> If using an electric or ceramic stovetop, be sure to use a heat diffuser with the clay pots.

5 pounds boneless shoulder of wild boar

1 bottle (750 ml) full-bodied dry red wine, such as a Syrah

2 tablespoons cognac or brandy

Salt and freshly ground black pepper

3 tablespoons extra virgin olive oil

2 carrots, sliced

1 onion, thickly sliced

1 tablespoon dried Mediterranean oregano

2 imported bay leaves

2 teaspoons bruised juniper berries

1 teaspoon bruised black and/or white peppercorns

1 head of garlic, halved horizontally

⅓ cup red wine vinegar

Garlic, Almond, and Cocoa Picada (recipe follows)

Chopped fresh flat-leaf parsley for garnish

1 Two days in advance, trim any excess fat from the wild boar and cut the meat into 24 pieces of approximately equal size. Gather all the trimmed fat and set aside.

2 In a flameware casserole, bring the wine and cognac to a boil over medium-low heat. Turn off the heat and ignite, averting your face. When the flames subside, cover the casserole to keep the liquid hot.

3 Generously season the wild boar with salt and pepper. Heat 2 tablespoons olive oil in a large conventional skillet. Sauté the meat in batches over medium-high heat, turning, until nicely browned all over, about 5 minutes. As they are done, add each batch of hot meat to the hot wine in the casserole. Let stand for 1 hour.

4 Meanwhile, add the trimmed fat to the skillet and cook over medium-high heat until golden brown, about 5 minutes. Add the carrots, onion, oregano, bay leaves, juniper berries, peppercorns, garlic, vinegar, and ¼ cup water. Reduce the heat to medium-low and simmer for 10 minutes. Scrape the contents of the skillet into the casserole.

5 Ladle 1 cup of the liquid from the casserole into the skillet and bring to a boil, scraping up any browned bits still clinging to the bottom of the pan. Boil over high heat until reduced and syrupy, about 5 minutes. Ladle another cup of the marinade from the casserole into the skillet and again boil down to a syrup. Return this reduced syrupy liquid to the casserole.

6 Preheat the oven to 250°F. Set the casserole over medium heat and slowly bring to a boil. Cover with a sheet of crumpled parchment paper and a tight-fitting lid and cook over low heat for 30 minutes.

7 Transfer the casserole to the oven and bake for 1½ hours. Remove the lid but not the paper and continue to cook for 2 hours. Transfer to a wooden board or folded kitchen towel to prevent cracking. Discard the paper and use a slotted spoon to transfer the meat to a bowl.

8 Strain the liquid and vegetables through a fine sieve set over a conventional saucepan. Press hard to get every drop of liquid. Skim off some of the fat and boil the juices over high heat until reduced to about 3 cups. Let cool; then cover and refrigerate the sauce and meat separately.

9 A day or two later, remove the meat and sauce from the refrigerator and let stand for about 2 hours to bring the meat and sauce back to room temperature. Meanwhile, brush a shallow baking dish with 1 tablespoon olive oil. Preheat the oven to 350°F.

10 Place the boar in the baking dish. Remove the fat from the surface of the sauce. Set aside 2 tablespoons of the sauce for the picada. Gently reheat the rest of the sauce in a conventional saucepan. Scrape the picada into the sauce and cook over medium-high heat until the sauce thickens slightly, about 2 minutes. Correct the seasoning with salt and pepper and pour over the boar. Place in the oven and bake for 30 minutes. Sprinkle with parsley and serve hot.

Garlic, Almond, and Cocoa Picada

MAKES ABOUT 1 CUP

A clay mortar and wooden pestle are ideal for making a smooth sauce. Otherwise, use a blender or food processor.

24 blanched almonds, toasted

5 garlic cloves, cut up

2 tablespoons chopped fresh flat-leaf parsley

1 slice stale country white bread cut 1 inch thick, toasted, and crust trimmed

1 teaspoon unsweetened cocoa powder

1 tablespoon brandy

2 tablespoons degreased sauce from step 10 of the main recipe

In a mortar, blender, or mini food processor, grind the almonds and garlic to a coarse paste. Add the parsley, toast, cocoa, brandy, and 2 tablespoons of the degreased sauce.

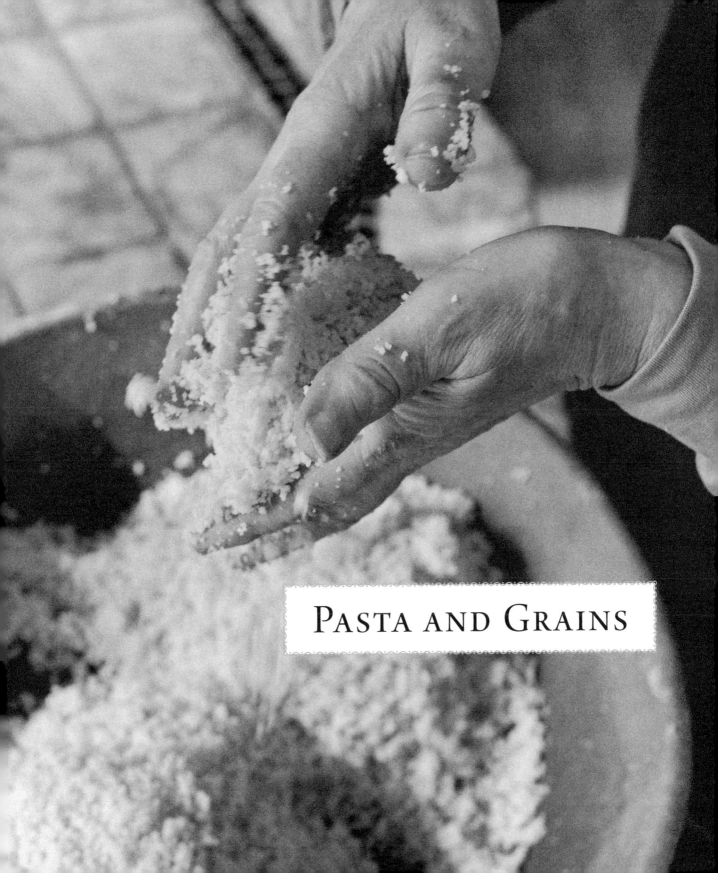

PASTA AND GRAINS

Green Wheat Pilaf with Breast of Chicken

SERVES 6

In this Turkish version of the famous Egyptian dish (*tagin hamam bi-l-frik*, which is made with pigeon), slices of broiled yogurt-marinated chicken are served over a mixture of green wheat cooked with bulgur, ground lamb, and spices in an unglazed earthenware pot.

Green wheat, called *freekah* in the Middle East, is harvested in early spring. After the stores of winter wheat have been exhausted and before the newly planted wheat is ready for harvest, farmers gather piles of this immature wheat from the fields, carefully set them afire, and thresh the charred sheaves. The resulting toasted grain, rich in protein and mineral content, offers a unique earthy flavor with hints of smoke.

Turkish food writer Ayfer Ünsal advises that cooking green wheat in clay is equivalent to cooking beans in a clay pot, in other words "the only way to go."

PREFERRED CLAY POT:

A deep 3-quart glazed or unglazed earthenware casserole or a Turkish *guvec*

If using an electric or ceramic stovetop, be sure to use a heat diffuser with the clay pot.

3 skinless, boneless chicken breasts
(4 to 5 ounces each)

¾ cup yogurt

1 teaspoon crushed garlic

1 teaspoon tomato paste, canned or homemade
(page 317)

Salt and freshly ground black pepper

1 cup baby green wheat (see Note)

4 tablespoons (½ stick) unsalted butter

½ cup chopped onion

8 ounces lean ground lamb or beef

¼ cup coarse bulgur

1 teaspoon Turkish sweet red pepper paste

1½ cups chicken stock or water

2 tablespoons extra virgin olive oil

1 cup frozen baby peas, thawed

½ cup pine nuts

¼ teaspoon Aleppo pepper

2 tablespoons chopped fresh flat-leaf parsley

2 tablespoons chopped fresh mint

1 Trim any fat or gristle from the chicken breasts. In a medium bowl, stir together the yogurt, garlic, tomato paste, ¼ teaspoon salt, and ⅛ teaspoon pepper. Add the chicken and marinate at room temperature for up to 1 hour or, preferably, in the refrigerator for up to 24 hours.

2 Put the green wheat in a coarse sieve and shake over the sink to remove any grit or sand. Rub the cracked wheat kernels between your fingertips and palms vigorously to feel for tiny stones or other foreign matter. Dump the wheat into a finer strainer and set under running water until it runs clear and the kernels feel free of all grit; drain well.

3 In the earthenware casserole set over medium-low heat, melt 2 tablespoons of the butter. Add the onion and meat. Cook, stirring occasionally, cook until the meat is no longer pink, about 10 minutes.

4 Stir in the remaining 2 tablespoons butter, the green wheat, bulgur, red pepper paste, and stock. Cover with a sheet of parchment and a lid and cook for 10 minutes. Season with salt and pepper to taste.

5 Meanwhile, in a large conventional skillet, sauté the chicken breasts in the olive oil, turning once, until just tender and white in the center but still juicy, 2 to 3 minutes per side. Let stand for 5 minutes; then thickly slice crosswise.

6 Use a fork to fluff up the wheat; scoop out and reserve about half. Arrange the chicken slices on the wheat in the casserole. Top with the reserved wheat. Cover with the parchment paper and the lid and cook over medium-low heat for 20 minutes.

7 Add the peas to the casserole and cook for 5 minutes longer. Use a fork to fluff up the wheat and arrange the chicken slices on top. Sprinkle with the pine nuts, Aleppo pepper, parsley, and mint. Serve hot.

NOTES TO THE COOK:

✳ Green wheat is a delicious grain that formerly required tedious cleaning before use. Now, thankfully, it's available "cleaned" in some Middle Eastern grocers as well as on line at www.kalustyans.com. In fact, some green wheat is so clean that the smoky flavor is a bit elusive. Nonetheless, it still needs a good rinsing as described in step 2. If this is the only kind available at your Middle Eastern grocer, revive it by spreading it out on a clean unglazed flowerpot saucer or comal and slowly toast it on top of the stove over low heat, stirring often to avoid burning.

✳ Store green wheat in the freezer if you aren't going to use it right away.

Bulgur and Greens with Pistachios and Yogurt

SERVES 6

This is another recipe from Musa Dağdeviren, my favorite Turkish chef. Musa is an expert on Turkish regional cooking, shares my love for cooking in clay pots, and can talk about bulgur for hours. It is, he maintains, one of the first cultivated grains, which has long been matched with other regional ingredients, such as pistachios, as in this recipe, as well as pomegranate molasses, sumac, hazelnuts, almonds, and spices, to produce numerous stunning Mediterranean dishes.

Fine-grain bulgur need only be soaked, but the coarse-grain variety must be cooked. Here Musa uses it in a subtle dish popularly prepared in the coastal towns that border the Marmara Sea. The grain is combined with spinach, garlic, red pepper, pistachios, and lemon and then finished with dollops of yogurt and a handful of fresh mint. It makes a great accompaniment for lamb kebabs.

PREFERRED CLAY POT:

A 3-quart earthenware casserole, preferably unglazed, such as La Chamba, with a lid, or a Turkish *guvec*

If using an electric or ceramic stovetop, be sure to use a heat diffuser with the clay pot.

---

1 pound fresh large-leaf spinach, preferably bunched, with pinkish stems

4 ounces watercress, thick stems removed

Coarse salt

3 large shallots, minced

3 large garlic cloves, minced

1½ cups coarse bulgur

½ cup extra virgin olive oil

2 tablespoons sun-dried or homemade tomato paste

2 tablespoons Turkish sweet red pepper paste

½ teaspoon ground cumin

½ teaspoon freshly ground black pepper

½ teaspoon Marash or Aleppo pepper, plus more to taste

½ cup shelled pistachio nuts

1 cup fresh mint leaves without stems

2 cups yogurt, drained in a cheesecloth-lined sieve for 2 hours

Lemon wedges for serving

1 Cut away the damaged spinach and watercress leaves; discard any damaged stems from each clump and trim away the roots. Roughly shred the leaves and place in a colander, preferably ceramic or stainless steel. Cut the spinach stems into ¼-inch dice and add to the leaves. Rinse well under cold running water; toss with 2 tablespoons coarse salt and let drain in the colander for about 30 minutes.

2 Rinse the greens again under cold running water and, working in small batches, squeeze in your hands or press against the colander to extract most of the moisture. (It should be damp but not wet.) Chop fine. Toss the greens with half the shallots and garlic.

3 Put the bulgur and greens in the earthenware casserole. Knead with your hand as if making bread dough until well blended, about 10 minutes. (The moisture from the greens will soften the bulgur and infuse it with flavor.)

4 In a small conventional skillet, cook the remaining shallots and garlic in the olive oil over medium-low heat until softened, 2 to 3 minutes. Add the tomato paste and Turkish red pepper paste and cook, stirring, for 1 to 2 minutes. Scrape over the green bulgur mix in the clay pot.

5 Knead until well blended. Season with the cumin, 1 teaspoon salt, black pepper, and Marash pepper. Gradually work in 1⅓ cups water.

6 Set the casserole over low heat and slowly raise it to medium as the pot heats up. Cook, stirring, for 2 to 3 minutes. Cover the bulgur mixture with paper towels, cover the casserole with a lid, turn the heat to the lowest setting, and let the green bulgur steam without uncovering for 45 minutes. Serve hot or cold with a sprinkling of nuts, dollops of yogurt, and a sprinkling of fresh mint leaves. Serve with lemon wedges.

Bulgur Pilaf with Toasted Noodles

SERVES 6

All pilafs cook beautifully in clay; it's as if the grain and the pot were made for one another. This recipe is a personal favorite and one that's remarkably easy to prepare. Please remember, though, that bulgur can turn mushy from overcooking, so measure carefully. Although unglazed clay will wick off some excess moisture, it won't save your bulgur if too much liquid is used.

> **PREFERRED CLAY POT:**
>
> **A 3-quart earthenware casserole with a lid, preferably unglazed, such as La Chamba**
>
> **If using an electric or ceramic stovetop, be sure to use a heat diffuser with the clay pot.**

8 tablespoons (1 stick) unsalted butter

1 cup broken vermicelli or spaghetti in 1-inch pieces

2 cups coarse bulgur

2 teaspoons coarse salt

3 cups boiling chicken or meat broth

½ teaspoon freshly ground black pepper

1 Melt 5 tablespoons of the butter in the earthenware casserole set over medium heat. Add the pasta and fry, stirring often until golden brown, 2 to 3 minutes. Stir in the bulgur and salt and stir until the bulgur is nicely coated in butter.

2 Pour in the hot broth and boil for 2 to 3 minutes. Cover, reduce the heat to low, and simmer for 10 minutes, or until all the liquid is absorbed. Place a kitchen towel or double layer of paper towels over the grains, cover with the lid, and transfer to a wooden surface or folded kitchen towel. Let stand for 10 to 15 minutes.

3 Melt the remaining 3 tablespoons butter in a small conventional skillet. Add the pepper and let sizzle. Drizzle the pepper butter over the bulgur, stir it in, and serve at once.

NOTE TO THE COOK: If using extra-large-grain bulgur, increase the broth to 3½ cups.

Turkish Bulgur and Egg Koftes

MAKES 16 TO 20 KOFTES, SERVING 4 TO 5

I learned this unusual dish in the town of Birecik along the Euphrates River in Turkey. I had gone there to meet an intense young woman named Gulsen Sozmer, who was famous for her codification and preservation of old Turkish dishes from the region. As I waited for her in her living room, I was treated to a special pleasure: a rare sighting of the northern bald ibis just outside the window.

After a while Gulsen came in, holding a notebook filled with handwritten recipes. I was dazzled as she read them off to me, each sounding more interesting than the last. However, the one that struck me most was this fascinating no-cook *kofte* dish in which bulgur is combined with the local sweet, smoky, dark Urfa pepper, after which crumbled fried eggs are folded in lightly. The mix is shaped into kofte balls, which are traditionally served with soft salad greens and a glass of *ayran,* or thinned yogurt (recipe follows).

The kneading works perfectly when done in an unglazed clay bowl, such as a La Chamba baking dish. The porosity of the bowl wicks off excess moisture as you work, resulting in lighter bulgur with a wonderful earthy flavor and aroma.

> **PREFERRED CLAY POT:**
>
> An unglazed flowerpot saucer or a La Chamba shallow baking dish, or a Chilean unglazed wok

8 ounces fine bulgur

4 scallions, white parts plus 2 inches of the green parts, chopped

¼ cup finely chopped fresh flat-leaf parsley

Salt and freshly ground black pepper

1½ teaspoons Urfa, Marash, or Aleppo red pepper

1½ tablespoons Turkish sweet red pepper paste

1½ tablespoons canned or homemade tomato paste

4 tablespoons (½ stick) unsalted butter

4 eggs

Fresh mint leaves and assorted baby greens—such as mustard greens, watercress, or romaine—for serving

1 In the unglazed earthenware dish, moisten the bulgur with 1 cup warm water. Add the scallion, 2 tablespoons of the parsley, 1 teaspoon black pepper, and the Urfa pepper. Knead the mixture with your hands as if you were working bread dough until it is well blended. Add the Turkish pepper paste and tomato paste and continue to knead, adding 1 or 2 tablespoons warm water as necessary, until the mixture is moist but holds together.

2 Melt the butter in a large conventional skillet over medium heat. Crack the eggs and slip them into the pan. Reduce the heat to low and cook until the whites are completely set and the yolks are just beginning to thicken but are still runny. With a fork, break up the yolks and gently stir them into the whites. Season with 1 teaspoon salt and a pinch of pepper. Remove from the heat and let stand for 2 minutes; then scrape the eggs and the butter over the bulgur mixture. Add the remaining 2 tablespoons parsley and mix gently to combine. Handling it lightly, form the bulgur mixture into 16 to 20 finger-shaped koftes and arrange on a large platter lined with fresh mint leaves and other greens. Serve at room temperature.

Ayran

MAKE 8 CUPS, SERVING 4 TO 5

This is the beverage traditionally served with Turkish Bulgur and Egg Koftes. Make sure it is ice cold.

1 quart whole-milk cow's or goat's milk yogurt

1 quart ice-cold water

Sea salt

1 Blend the yogurt, water, and 2 teaspoons sea salt until smooth. Chill for at least 2 hours or preferably overnight.

2 Pour into glasses, add a pinch of salt, and serve at once.

Risotto with Wild Mushrooms and White Truffle Oil

SERVES 3 TO 4 AS A LUNCH DISH OR A FIRST COURSE

Risotto cooks beautifully in clay. Try it in a flameware or La Chamba casserole or in a traditional Italian *umidiera*. I urge you to try your favorite risotto recipe in clay. If you do, you may never go back to a conventional pot. This unusual recipe is especially rich, due to the combination of dried and fresh porcini mushrooms, enriched with a slab of creamy fontina cheese. The effect of the lightly fermented fontina on the mushrooms creates a wonderful earthy flavor and woodland aroma. Yes, fresh porcini are expensive, but they do up the texture and flavor of the dried cèpes. Alternatively, substitute large fleshy shitake mushrooms.

¼ cup dried cèpes or porcini

1 quart chicken broth, simmering

Salt

6 to 8 ounces fresh porcini or shiitake mushrooms

2 tablespoons extra virgin olive oil

¼ cup finely chopped onion

3 tablespoons finely chopped shallot

1 cup risotto rice, preferably Carnaroli

⅓ cup dry white wine

¼ cup diced Italian fontina cheese (2 ounces)

1 tablespoon unsalted butter

½ teaspoon white truffle oil, or more to taste

Freshly ground black pepper

(continued)

> **PREFERRED CLAY POT:**
>
> A 3- to 4-quart casserole such as flameware or La Chamba or an Italian *umidiera*
>
> If using an electric or ceramic stovetop, be sure to use a heat diffuser with the clay pot.

1 Soak the dried cèpes in ½ cup warm water for at least 30 minutes to soften them. Drain, reserving the liquid. Rinse the soaked cèpes under running water to rid them of any grit; chop them into small pieces. Strain the soaking liquid through a paper coffee filter or several layers of damp cheesecloth and add to the simmering broth. Dilute the broth with 3 cups water and add a pinch of salt; set aside.

2 Wipe or brush the fresh porcini mushrooms to remove any dirt. Trim the butt end of the stem. Cut the porcini lengthwise into ¼-inch-thick slices. If using fresh shiitakes, cut off the stems and slice the caps.

3 Set the casserole over medium-low heat., Add the olive oil, onion, and shallot and cook, stirring, until they just begin to turn golden, about 5 minutes. Add the chopped reconstituted dried cèpes and stir once to coat with the oil. Add a pinch of salt and a few tablespoons of the simmering broth. Raise the heat to medium and continue to cook until all the moisture has evaporated, 1 to 2 minutes.

4 Add the fresh porcini or shiitake mushrooms and cook until all moisture has evaporated, about 10 minutes. (The dish can be prepared up to this point up to 3 hours in advance. Set aside at room temperature and turn off the heat under the broth. Slowly reheat the contents of the pot and return the broth to a simmer before proceeding.)

5 Add the rice to the casserole and stir to coat with the oil in the pan. Cook, stirring, over medium-low heat for 2 to 3 minutes to toast the rice lightly without coloring. Raise the heat to medium. Add the wine and cook, stirring, until all the liquid evaporates, about 3 minutes. Add 1 cup of the simmering broth and cook, stirring, until almost all of the liquid has been absorbed. Repeat, adding the stock 1 cup at a time and cooking the risotto for 15 to 18 minutes, until the rice is tender but retains a firm bite. Reduce the heat to low, add the cheese, and stir until it is melted. Remove the risotto from the heat. Add the butter and white truffle oil. Season with freshly grated pepper to taste and serve at once.

Spanish Rice with Blood Sausage, Fava Beans, and Caramelized Lardons

SERVES 4 TO 6 AS A MAIN COURSE

While traveling in Catalonia a few years ago, I came upon a wonderful restaurant called Sant Carles in the town of Tortosa on the Ebro River. The chef, Margarita Nofre, is famous for her fish recipes, but since I was researching rice, I ordered one of her main-course *arros* dishes and was dazzled by its simple elegance.

Black sausage and fresh fava beans are a traditional combination, but Chef Nofre's addition of mint and sweet Muscat wine gave this warhorse a wonderfully fresh élan. Since I purchase precooked black sausages, all I have to do is remove the skins, slice them, and then cook the slices on both sides until lightly crisp.

> **PREFERRED CLAY POT:**
>
> An 11- to 12-inch Spanish cazuela
>
> If using an electric or ceramic stovetop, be sure to use a heat diffuser with the clay pot.

6 ounces salt pork, thickly sliced

1½ pounds fresh fava beans

5 tablespoons extra virgin olive oil

1 cup chopped scallion, white part only

2 cups sliced spring garlic bulbs or ramps or ¼ cup sliced garlic plus 1 more cup chopped scallion

3 tablespoons sweet fortified wine, such as Madeira, Muscat, or muscatel wine

1 bay leaf

2 fresh spearmint sprigs plus 2 tablespoons slivered fresh mint leaves

5 cups hot chicken stock

Salt and freshly ground black pepper

8 ounces Spanish- or French-style blood sausage

1 cup short-grain rice, such as Spanish Calasparra or Bomba, or Italian risotto rice (e.g., Carnaroli)

1 ounce Serrano ham, slivered

1 Blanch the salt pork in a small conventional saucepan of boiling water for 5 minutes; drain and divide into 4 slices. Fill the bottom of a steamer with water and bring to a boil. Add the salt pork and boil for 45 minutes.

2 At the same time, place the steamer basket or rack above the salt pork and, working in batches, steam a handful of fava beans in their pods until tender, 5 to 8 minutes, depending on their age. Rinse under cold running water to cool. Peel off both the pod and the outer skin of each bean. Repeat with the remaining beans. Spread out the peeled beans on paper towels, roll up, and keep in a cool place.

3 Transfer the salt pork to a cutting board and let cool. Thinly slice on the diagonal and pat dry.

(continued)

4 Set the cazuela over medium heat and add 3 tablespoons of the olive oil, slices of salt pork, scallion, garlic, Madeira, bay leaf, and mint sprigs. Cook, stirring, for 5 minutes. Add 1 cup of the hot stock and a pinch each of salt and pepper. Cook, stirring occasionally, for 20 minutes, or until the liquid has evaporated and the pork slices just begin to caramelize.

5 Skin and thickly slice the blood sausages on the diagonal. Add the slices to the cazuela and cook until they develop a slightly crisp crust on each side. Scrape the contents of the cazuela onto a side dish; remove and discard the bay leaf and mint sprigs.

6 Heat the remaining 2 tablespoons oil in the cazuela. Add the rice and stir constantly for 1 minute; then add the remaining 4 cups hot stock and bring to a boil. Simmer for 10 minutes. Arrange the slices of pork and black sausage over the rice, scatter the chopped scallion and spring garlic over the meats, and top with the reserved peeled fava beans. Cover with a paper towel and a lid or a sheet of foil and simmer for 5 minutes. Turn off the heat and let stand for 10 minutes. Scatter the slivered ham and slivered mint over the rice and serve at once.

NOTE TO THE COOK: I used Peregrino's Spanish-style blood sausage (*morcilla*) with rice and onions from www.latienda.com.

Fideos with Clams, Shrimp, and Mussels

SERVES 6

"A dish that contains the essence of the sea," writes Catalan author Manuel Vázquez Montalbán of this unique Catalan fishermen's preparation, which cooks toasted noodles in a flavorful fish broth until they are crispy on top but still soft and juicy underneath. A bowl of garlic mayonnaise is served on the side.

> **PREFERRED CLAY POT:**
>
> An 11- or 12-inch Spanish cazuela
>
> If using an electric or ceramic stovetop, be sure to use a heat diffuser with the clay pot.

8 ounces small clams or cockles

8 ounces small cultivated mussels, scrubbed

1 dried New Mexico red pepper

1 pound medium raw shrimp

Sea salt and freshly ground black pepper

5 tablespoons extra virgin olive oil

3 garlic cloves, gently bruised

1 large onion, thinly sliced

3 red ripe tomatoes, halved, seeded, and grated

1 teaspoon Spanish sweet paprika

18 blanched almonds, toasted

¼ cup fish glaze

⅛ teaspoon saffron threads

1 pound fideos or spaghetti, broken into 1-inch lengths

Garlic Mayonnaise (recipe follows)

1   Scrub the clams and mussels under cold running water. Place in a bowl, cover with lightly salted water, and soak for 20 minutes. Drain, rinse, and keep cool until ready to use.

2   Stem and seed the dried pepper and tear it into pieces. Soak in a small bowl of hot water until soft, about 5 minutes; drain.

3   Peel the shrimp, reserving the shells. Season the shrimp lightly with sea salt, cover with plastic wrap, and refrigerate until ready to use.

4   Place the shrimp shells in the cazuela and set over medium heat. Add 2 tablespoons of the olive oil and 3 of the whole garlic cloves and cook until the shells turn pink and the oil smells aromatic, about 5 minutes. Add the onion, grated tomatoes, and New Mexico red pepper. Cook until all the excess moisture evaporates, about 30 minutes. Season with the paprika, 1 teaspoon sea salt, and ¼ teaspoon black pepper. Press through a sieve back into the cazuela.

5   Place the almonds in a blender or food processor. Add the contents of the cazuela and 1 cup water; puree until smooth. Return to the cazuela. In a medium conventional saucepan, warm the fish glaze with 2 quarts water to make a fish stock. Add 7 cups of this fish stock and the saffron to the cazuela. Bring to a boil over medium heat, reduce the heat slightly, and simmer for 15 minutes.

6   Preheat the oven heat to 350°F. On a jelly roll pan, toss the fideos in the remaining 3 tablespoons olive oil. Bake for 5 minutes, or until golden brown. Remove the noodles from the oven and toss them to keep from browning too much.

7   Raise the oven temperature to 400°F. Add the toasted noodles to the cazuela; press them down gently until they are submerged. Scatter the clams, mussels, and shrimp on top. Set the cazuela in the middle of the oven and bake until the shellfish are open wide and the fideos crusty on top and moist and tender within, about 10 minutes. Remove from the oven and let stand for about 5 minutes before serving right from the cazuela. Pass a bowl of garlic mayonnaise on the side.

Garlic Mayonnaise

MAKES ABOUT 2 CUPS

5 garlic cloves, crushed

Sea salt and freshly ground black black

1¼ cups extra virgin olive oil

2 egg yolks, at room temperature

3 tablespoons fresh lemon juice

1   In a mortar, crush the garlic into a fine puree; add 1 teaspoon salt and a few drops of olive oil to make a paste. Add the egg yolks and beat until thick and smooth.

2   Gradually work in the remaining oil drop by drop in a slow, steady stream, stirring in one direction only until you obtain a thick, creamy emulsion that resembles a very thick mayonnaise. Season with salt, pepper, and lemon juice. Cover with plastic wrap and keep in a cool place until ready to serve.

Baked pasta dishes such as lasagne, cannelloni, and pasticci, referred to as *al forno,* all come out beautifully when cooked in shallow earthenware and stoneware vessels. And if you've seen the movie *The Big Night,* you know about the elaborate Neapolitan baroque-style timpano, a summit of baked pasta achievement.

In fact, almost all pasta dishes can profit from a final baking in a clay vessel, even after boiling. (The only exceptions are dishes made with the thinnest pastas.) A good example is *paglia e fieno* ("straw and hay"), the famous combination of yellow and green tagliatelle or fettuccine, which I've included here.

Italian potters have created wonderful vessels for this purpose. Some are elaborately decorated; others, such as the Vulcania brand, are plain brown. For baked pasta, I also use artisanal stoneware, which is handsome and often covered with bright colors.

It has been said: "Hot pasta waits for no man." In fact, pasta prepared *al forno* actually *will* wait for any man or any woman, allowing you more time to prepare the rest of the meal.

Straw and Hay al Forno

SERVES 2 TO 3

The Napa Valley restaurant Bistro Don Giovanni is just twenty minutes by car from my home. Here Chef Scott Warner produces marvelous food for vintners and tourists alike, including great pizzas and pasta dishes baked in his wood-fired ovens. When I asked him for a good clay pot–driven recipe for this book, he suggested this rich version of Straw and Hay. Scott boils his green and white pasta, tosses it with baby artichokes, wild mushrooms, ham, and just enough cream and cheese to create an evenly balanced dish. Then he finishes it off in his wood-fired oven, baking the pasta in the gratin dish in which it is served at table.

Not having a wood-fired oven, I've tried this dish in my ordinary oven and also in my double clay–slabbed oven. It worked well both ways. Use a Spanish cazuela to cook the vegetables; then toss in the pasta, cream, and cheese and bake until bubbly.

You can easily find the half plain egg, half spinach pasta shaped into nests or in long strips packaged together in good food shops. Note that steps 1 and 2 can be done several hours in advance.

3 baby artichokes (4 to 5 ounces total)

2 to 2½ ounces fresh wild mushrooms, preferably small chanterelles or trumpet mushrooms

2 tablespoons extra virgin olive oil

Salt and freshly ground black pepper

2 tablespoons finely chopped white onion

2 garlic cloves, mashed

2 ounces flavorful cooked ham, cut into ½-inch dice

¾ cup heavy cream

¾ cup milk

⅛ teaspoon freshly grated nutmeg

⅓ cup plus 2 tablespoons freshly grated Parmigiano-Reggiano cheese

4 ounces dried egg noodles—half green spinach tagliatelle and half plain

1   Wash the artichokes; trim the stems and remove the tough outer leaves. Boil or microwave in salted water until just tender, about 10 minutes. Immediately drain, cool, and gently press out excess moisture. Wrap in paper towels and set aside.

2   To clean the mushrooms, simply toss them in a deep sieve and shake vigorously to release any surface dirt. Trim the ends and use a water spray to rinse them quickly; drain and blot dry. Coat the bottom of the cazuela with 1 tablespoon of the olive oil and set it over low heat. When the oil is warm, add the mushrooms. Cover with a lid or foil, and steam for 3 to 4 minutes. Then uncover, raise the heat to medium, and sauté until the mushrooms express all their moisture and begin to caramelize. Transfer the mushrooms to a side dish. Set the hot cazuela aside on a wooden surface or folded kitchen towel to prevent cracking; do not wash it.

3   About 30 minutes before serving, preheat the oven to 400°F. Gently press down on each cooked artichoke and thinly slice lengthwise. Season lightly with salt and pepper.

4   Add another tablespoon of olive oil to the cazuela and set it over medium heat. Add the onion and cook until it is soft and lightly caramelized, 10 minutes. Add the garlic, ham, artichokes, and cooked mushrooms. Continue to cook until the garlic is lightly toasted, about 3 to 5 minutes.

5   In a small conventional saucepan, heat the cream and milk until hot. Season with the nutmeg and salt and pepper to taste. Pour the seasoned milk and cream into the cazuela and bring to a boil. Turn off the heat, stir in ⅓ cup of the cheese, and let the sauce stand until you're ready to add the pasta.

6   In a large conventional pot of boiling salted water, cook the pasta until just tender, 9 to 10 minutes. Meanwhile, if necessary, reheat the sauce in the cazuela until hot. Drain the pasta and add to the cazuela, stirring to coat with the sauce. Scatter the remaining 2 tablespoons cheese on top.

7   Transfer the cazuela to the top third of the oven. Bake until the top is lightly browned and the dish is bubbling, 15 to 20 minutes. Serve at once.

Pasta con le Sarde al Forno

SERVES 4 GENEROUSLY

Pasta with sardines and fennel has been one of my favorite Sicilian pasta recipes ever since I first tasted it in Palermo many years ago. The sauce, which is as green as pesto but a little bit more lumpy, does not always cling well to the pasta. For this reason I like to mix the sauce and pasta together in an attractive glazed baking dish and finish it in the oven. It's delicious this way—hot, lukewarm, or even cold.

In Sicily the dish is made with fresh sardines and wild fennel, but I have devised a way of using canned sardines. And if you can't find wild fennel (easy to find here in northern California, where I often spot it growing along the sides of roads), I've come up with a substitute combination of fennel seeds and fresh fennel bulb.

Like most fish and seafood pasta dishes, *pasta con le sarde* does not get a cheese topping, though some Sicilian cooks will add texture by sprinkling on toasted bread crumbs or crushed almonds.

> **PREFERRED CLAY POT:**
> A 10-inch Spanish cazuela

2 tablespoons dried currants

⅛ teaspoon saffron threads

Coarse salt and freshly ground black pepper

8 ounces young wild fennel fronds with tender stalks or 1 small sliced bulb fennel plus 1 teaspoon fennel seeds

¼ cup plus 3 tablespoons extra virgin olive oil

⅓ cup fresh bread crumbs

¾ cup finely chopped onion

5 flat anchovy fillets, rinsed and chopped

¼ cup tomato paste, canned or homemade (page 317)

2 tablespoons pine nuts

2 cans (4 ounces each) top-quality sardines (see Note), drained, bones removed

8 ounces hollow spaghetti—bucatini, penne rigate, maccheroncini, or perciatelli

1 Soak the currants with the saffron in ¼ cup hot water. At the same time, fill a pasta pot with water, salt it generously, and bring to a boil while you prepare the wild fennel greens. Trim off any thick, heavy fronds; keep only the small tender fronds. Peel the stalks with a swivel-bladed vegetable peeler to remove the stringy outer layer. Chop the stalks into 2- or 3-inch lengths. Add the tender fronds and cut stalks of the wild fennel to the boiling water, cover, and cook until the fennel is tender, 15 to 20 minutes. (If using the store-bought sliced fennel bulb and fennel seeds, cook the bulb the same way.) Scoop out and drain the fennel; reserve the fennel water for cooking the pasta and moistening the sauce. Squeeze the fennel in your hands to remove as much moisture as possible. Chop fine to make about 1½ cups.

2 Heat 2 tablespoons of the olive oil in a large conventional skillet set over medium-low heat. Add the bread crumbs and toss until lightly toasted, 2 to 4 minutes. Scrape into a dish.

3 Add ¼ cup of the remaining olive oil to the skillet along with the onion. Cook over medium heat until the onion is soft and golden, about 5 minutes. Add the anchovies and crush them well with a fork. Stir in the tomato paste, chopped fennel, currants with their saffron soaking water, and pine nuts. Cook, stirring, for a few minutes to blend the flavors.

4 Add 1½ cups of the reserved fennel-cooking water and the canned sardines. Crush a few of the sardines into the liquid. Simmer for 2 to 3 minutes. Season with salt and pepper to taste. There will be about 3 cups of sauce. Scoop out and reserve about 1 cup.

5 Preheat the oven to 350°F. Bring the remainder of the fennel-cooking water to a boil. Add the pasta and cook according to the package directions. Immediately drain the pasta and toss with the sauce remaining in the skillet.

6 Oil the cazuela and sprinkle half the toasted bread crumbs over the bottom. Scrape the pasta into the dish. Spread the reserved 1 cup sauce over the pasta, and scatter the remaining bread crumbs on top. Drizzle the remaining 1 tablespoon olive oil over the crumbs. Bake in the oven for 10 minutes, or until the top is nicely browned. Serve hot, warm, or at room temperature.

NOTES TO THE COOK:

❋ Look for sardines packed in olive oil, preferably French, Italian, or Portuguese.

❋ To substitute fresh sardines, purchase 8 to 12 silver sardines. Cut off the head from each of the fish. Slit each belly lengthwise; turn back the fillets and pull out the bones. Trim the tails. Wipe away the guts with a paper towel. Sprinkle the flesh with salt and pepper. Add the fresh sardines to the sauce along with the onion in step 3.

STEAMING COUSCOUS IN A CLAY COLANDER

Though a ceramic colander is not on my list of must-have clay pots, it's one of the items used most frequently in my kitchen—one I employ to steam greens, drain eggplant and other salted foods, and steam couscous and other grains.

For years I made couscous in a metal couscousier. Now I only steam it in clay, the traditional method in Tunisia and Sicily. I like the way my clay colander conducts and distributes heat, and I truly believe it produces better-tasting couscous while preserving the delicate texture of the grain.

The trick is to obtain a good snug fit between the high-sided metal pot of boiling water and the clay colander filled with couscous set above. To do this I use a couple of old linen napkins tied together or wet cheesecloth to create a tight seal between metal bottom and ceramic top. I also make certain there's at least an inch of space between the level of the boiling water and the bottom of the colander—room for the steam to rise through the holes of the colander and not leak out the sides where bottom vessel and colander meet.

As soon as the water boils, I quickly brush the insides of the colander with butter or oil, add the wet couscous, and steam as directed in the recipe. Don't worry about grains falling through the holes; they won't. And don't listen to those who tell you to line your colander with cheesecloth. If there's a full boil below, nothing will fall through.

A trick: Add a nickel coin to the water. During steaming you'll hear it bouncing around. If and when you stop hearing it, it's time to add more boiling water.

Sicilian Fish Couscous

SERVES 8

This Sicilian dish, a famous specialty of Trapani, is totally clay oriented. First the grain is seasoned with salt, pepper, bay leaf, sliced onion, and a heavy, rich olive oil and allowed to stand for one to two hours in a wide, shallow clay dish with sloping sides called a *mafaradda*. I usually use an unglazed flowerpot saucer or the bottom of a tagine. Then it's transferred to a clay colander, steamed over boiling water, and served with a rich tomato-based fish stew also cooked in a clay vessel.

Years ago, when I was demonstrating Moroccan couscous at Macy's in New York, two women stayed after class. They were Sicilian-born residents of Long Island, and one, Vita Coppolo Poma, offered to teach me her native Trapani version of the dish, on which the following recipe is based. One major difference between the Sicilian method and the North African method for cooking couscous is that while in North Africa the grain is steamed several times, in Sicily, where only fine-grade couscous is used, it is subjected to a single long steaming.

The accompanying fish stew is absolutely delicious. I cook the tomato sauce base for it in a glazed earthenware casserole for an hour, allowing it to develop a dark and sticky richness, an almost "meaty" background, before adding chunks of fresh fish. In fact, you can make the sauce a few days in advance.

PREFERRED CLAY POTS:

An unglazed flowerpot saucer to "season" the couscous (optional)

A ceramic colander or steamer

A 4- or 5-quart earthenware casserole for the fish broth and stew

If using an electric or ceramic stovetop, be sure to use a heat diffuser with the clay pots.

Tomato Sauce with Parsley and Garlic (recipe follows)

1½ pounds fine-grain couscous

2 medium onions, sliced

2 imported bay leaves

2 small cinnamon sticks

Sea salt and freshly ground black pepper

¾ cup extra virgin olive oil

2 pounds assorted mixed white-fleshed fish fillets—snapper, cod, monkfish, bass, or halibut—rinsed and drained

2 celery ribs, coarsely chopped

3 garlic cloves, chopped

¼ cup dry white wine

1 cup almond meal (about 3 ounces)

2 lemons, quartered

1 jarred roasted red bell pepper, sliced

2 tablespoons chopped fresh flat-leaf parsley

(continued)

1   Make the tomato sauce up to 3 days in advance and refrigerate. Reheat before using in step 5.

2   At least 4 hours before serving, spread out the couscous in an even layer on a large dish, preferably of unglazed earthenware and gradually stir in 1 cup of tepid water and half the chopped onion, bay leaves, cinnamon sticks, 1½ teaspoons sea salt, 1 teaspoon freshly ground black pepper, and 3 tablespoons of the olive oil. Sprinkle the seasonings evenly over the couscous and gently toss to mix. Spread out the couscous in an even layer again and cover with a damp kitchen towel. Let rest for at least 2 hours, tossing the couscous with wet fingers from time to time to break up any lumps.

3   Rinse the fish fillets briefly under cold running water. Drain well and pat dry. Divide the fillets into 12 or 18 chunks approximately the same size. Season lightly with additional salt and pepper. Drizzle 2 tablespoons of the olive oil over the fish. Cover and refrigerate until ready to add to the fish stew.

4   About 2 hours before serving, bring plenty of water to the boil in a deep metal pot over high heat. Put a nickel in the water to act as an alarm for you if the water gets too low. When the water is boiling rapidly, put the ceramic colander in place, setting it on top of a long strip of cloth to seal and fasten it in place., Reduce the heat to medium. Add the couscous to the colander, cover the colander with a clean kitchen cloth—preferably terrycloth folded in two to best absorb the excess moisture—cover with a lid, and steam for 1 hour without disturbing it. (If the coin stops clicking, carefully remove the cloth, use mitts to lift off the ceramic cooker, and add more boiling water to the kettle.)

5   Meanwhile, prepare the fish stew. Put the olive oil in the earthenware casserole over medium heat. Add the remaining onion, the celery, and the garlic. Cook until softened and golden, about 10 minutes. Add the wine and bring to a boil. Stir in half of the tomato sauce and 1 quart of water and bring to a boil. Reduce the heat to low and simmer for 1 hour, stirring occasionally.

6   After an hour, uncover the couscous and use a long fork or a whisk to fluff up the grain and break up any lumps. Cover again and steam for another 30 minutes.

7   Dump the couscous into a large shallow serving dish. Toss again to break up any lumps; discard the cinnamon sticks and bay leaves. Dilute the remaining tomato sauce with 1 cup water. Sprinkle over the couscous. Use a whisk to toss with the grains; let stand until swollen, about 15 minutes. Set aside in a warm place.

8   Meanwhile, add the reserved fish chunks to the simmering fish stew, cover, and poach gently until fully cooked, about 10 minutes. Carefully transfer the fish to a side plate. Stir the almond meal into the fish poaching liquid. Adjust the seasoning with the juice of one of the lemon quarters, salt and plenty of ground black pepper. Add 1 to 2 cups of the stew to the couscous if it seems a little dry. Sicilian couscous should be moist but not soupy. You may not need all the liquid. Pour the remainder into a bowl. Decorate the top of the couscous with the fish. Garnish with the roasted red pepper, chopped parsley, and remaining lemon wedges. Pass the reserved sauce for those who like their couscous very moist.

Tomato Sauce with Parsley and Garlic

MAKES ABOUT 1 QUART

6 tablespoons extra virgin olive oil

1 medium onion, finely chopped

¼ cup fish glaze or 4 fish bouillon cubes

¼ teaspoon ground cinnamon

1 bay leaf

1 small carrot, sliced

1 tablespoon coarse sea salt

2 teaspoons freshly ground black pepper

¼ teaspoon cayenne pepper, or more to taste

2 cans (28 ounces each) plum tomatoes, drained
   through a colander, seeds discarded

¾ cup fresh flat-leaf parsley sprigs, stems removed

6 garlic cloves, halved

1 In a 4-quart flameproof earthenware casserole, cook the onions in the olive oil over medium heat until softened but not browned, about 5 minutes. Add the fish glaze, cinnamon, bay leaf, carrot, salt, black pepper and cayenne, and saute over medium heat for 5 minutes. Add the tomatoes and simmer, uncovered, until dark and thick, 30 minutes.

2 Pass the sauce through a sieve or the large blade of a food mill, pressing on the vegetables to extract all their juices. There should be about 3 cups.

3 In an electric blender or food processor, combine the parsley and garlic with 1 cup of the tomato sauce and blend until smooth. Stir back into the remaining tomato sauce. Reserve half of the tomato sauce for step 5 above. Reserve the remainder for step 7.

Mhamas with Extra Virgin Olive Oil and Sun-Dried Tomatoes

SERVES 6

My Tunisian culinary friend, Abdelmajid Majoubi, producer of what I consider the finest artisanal North African olive oil, tells me that *mhamas,* a type of a large Tunisian couscous, was developed by Berber tribespeople as a way to preserve their grain for use long after the wheat harvest.

Mhamas is made by crushing peeled durum wheat, mixing it with salt and olive oil, sun-drying it, and then storing it in earthenware jars. Tunisian cooks steam or boil the couscous, which causes it to double in size. Then it's doused with rich buttermilk and served with preserved butter *(smen)* and honey.

At Abdelmajid's home, the *mhamas* jars are stored in the coolest part of the house along with stores of olive oil, pickled vegetables, and *kadide.* If the grain is not used within the year, the jars are opened and the grain is spread out on cloths in the open air to sun-dry again. Scatterings of dried whole hot red peppers are added, and then the grain along with the peppers is repacked into earthenware jars until needed.

For a recent birthday, instead of olive oil, Abdelmajid sent me several jars of *mhamas,* along with his mother's recipe for preparing it with raisins, spiced and preserved meat (called *kadide*), olive oil, and sun-dried tomatoes. This *mhamas* is larger than the couscous imported from France or North Africa and tiny compared to commercial Lebanese and Israeli varieties. It also has a more complex flavor and feels richer and more buttery in the mouth than the larger, firmer "couscous" grain from the Middle East.

In the olden times, Abdelmajid told me, without these stores of grain, Berber people wouldn't have been able to survive bad harvest years. Jars of *mhamas* were also secreted away in the fields and in caverns in the mountains to keep them from falling into the hands of marauding enemy Berber tribesmen.

These days, Majoubi brand *mhamas* is available in small glass jars (see Sources), with a few peppers added out of respect for tradition. You don't use the peppers in the mhamas in the following recipe.

> **PREFERRED CLAY POT:**
>
> **A 3-quart earthenware casserole, preferably unglazed, such as La Chamba**
>
> **If using an electric or ceramic stovetop, be sure to use a heat diffuser with the clay pot.**

8 sun-dried tomato halves

5 tablespoons extra virgin olive oil

1 large onion, chopped

**4 pieces kadide at room temperature or
    2 ounces imitation kadide (recipes follow)**

2 teaspoons finely chopped garlic

⅔ cup raisins

1 jar (1 pound) hand-rolled mhamas

Salt

1. Soak the sun-dried tomatoes in hot water for 20 minutes, until soft. Drain and cut into thin slices.

2. Meanwhile, put 2½ tablespoons of the olive oil in the earthenware casserole set over low heat. When the oil begins to sizzle, add the onion and cook, stirring often, until it is golden, 4 to 5 minutes.

3. Remove the kadide and 1 tablespoon of the oil from the jar. (Reserve the remaining oil in the jar, if you like, for cooking highly seasoned dishes.) Add the slices of kadide or the beef jerky alternative and 1 tablespoon of the preserving oil to the casserole. Add the garlic and 2½ to 3 cups hot water, or enough to cover the onions and meat by about 1 inch. Raise the heat to medium and bring to a boil.

4. Slowly scatter the raisins and mhamas over the boiling liquid without losing the boil. Reduce the heat to medium-low and continue to cook, stirring with a wooden spoon, until all the liquid is absorbed and the couscous is swollen and tender but still al dente, about 5 minutes.

5. Season with salt to taste. Gently scrape the bottom of the casserole to release any mhamas stuck to the bottom. Cover and cook for 1 to 2 minutes longer. Remove from the heat and stir in the remaining 2½ ½ tablespoons olive oil and the slivered sun-dried tomatoes. Serve at once.

Kadide: Tunisian Spiced and Preserved Lamb

MAKES 15 TO 20 PIECES

When Tunisian country people make *kadide,* they spice their lamb strips, leave them overnight, wipe them dry, and then hang them out on a line to dry in the sun for several days. Opting for safety and omitting the flies, I dry my strips on racks in a slow oven. Tunisian cooks insist that *kadide* will keep for a year if well stored, but I've never kept mine for more than a few months.

As you remove pieces of *kadide,* add fresh oil to keep all remaining pieces from being exposed to air. Always soak *kadide* in water to remove excess salt before cooking, about 15 minutes. The leftover preserving oil, called *dhen,* is especially good for cooking beans, vegetables, and meat with North African spicing.

> **PREFERRED CLAY POT:**
> **A glazed earthenware mixing bowl**

1¼ pounds boned lamb shoulder chops

⅓ cup coarse sea salt

6 garlic cloves, crushed

1 teaspoon crushed hot red pepper or
   1 tablespoon harissa

½ teaspoon ground caraway

½ teaspoon ground coriander

½ teaspoon dried mint, pressed through a sieve

3 cups olive oil, or more as needed

(continued)

1 Cut each chop into 3 or 4 long strips. Rub the meat with the salt and garlic. Stack the strips of meat, sandwiching them between strips of paper towels in a deep bowl. Cover and refrigerate overnight.

2 The following day, preheat the oven to 150°F. Dry the meat well with paper towels. Mix together the hot pepper, caraway, coriander, and mint and rub all over the lamb. Set the strips on cake racks and place in the low oven to dry, about 8 hours. The meat is ready when it is dry to the touch but still supple enough to bend slightly.

3 In a deep skillet or saucepan, heat the olive oil over medium heat to slow bubbling. Add the dried lamb meat and fry until a light brown crust forms all over, 4 to 5 minutes. Remove from the heat and let the meat cool in the oil.

4 Divide the meat between 2 Mason jars (1 pint each). Ladle the frying oil over the meat. Then add enough fresh olive oil to completely cover the strips by 1 inch. Store in the refrigerator for at least 2 weeks before opening.

Imitation Kadide

Here's a quick shortcut substitute for kadide made with packaged all-natural beef jerky. Look for a package that states it contains no pepper, Asian spices, preservatives, antibiotics, or hormones. Cut 2 ounces into 12 to 18 thin slabs. Soak in a small saucepan with ¼ cup hot water, ½ teaspoon crushed hot red pepper or 1 tablespoon harissa, and 2 tablespoons extra virgin olive oil for at least 10 minutes. Simmer, uncovered, over low heat until the water has evaporated, the oil is sizzling, and the jerky feels soft enough to cut with a wooden spoon, about 10 minutes.

Chard Stuffed with Toasted Corn and Hazelnuts in the Style of the Black Sea

SERVES 6

This recipe is from the Turkish town of Trabzon on the Black Sea coast, where dried sweet corn and anchovies are the two most popular staples in the local diet. Here this form of corn is used as the basis of stuffings as well as to make bread and to enrich egg dishes. The sweet, milky, fresh-picked corn is toasted and dried in stone ovens for about 8 hours while still on the cob; then the kernels are scraped off and dried a while longer. The resulting toasted corn has a delicious sweet, earthy flavor.

It's combined here with toasted hazelnuts and slow-cooked onions to provide a lush melting filling for rolled chard leaves. And, like all stuffed vegetable dishes, this one is particularly well suited for clay pot cooking.

¾ cup toasted corn kernels, about 4 ounces (see Note)

Salt and freshly ground black pepper

¼ teaspoon sugar

12 large chard leaves (from about 2 bunches)

3 tablespoons unsalted butter

1 medium onion, chopped

8 ounces pastrami or basturma, shredded

1 tablespoon tomato paste, canned or homemade (page 317)

½ teaspoon Turkish or Aleppo pepper or ¼ teaspoon crushed hot red pepper

2 ounces soft cheese such as crescenza, mozzarella, Teleme, or cream cheese

⅓ cup whole hazelnuts (1½ ounces), toasted

2 tablespoons fresh flat-leaf parsley leaves

2 tablespoons fresh mint leaves

1 Rinse and drain the dried corn kernels. Place 3 cups water in a saucepan and bring to a boil, add the corn, and soak for 2 hours. Then add 1 teaspoon salt, ½ teaspoon pepper, and the sugar. Reheat to boiling and cook for 10 minutes. Drain well.

2 Cut off the stems from the chard; coarsely chop them and set aside. Blanch the leaves in a large pot of boiling water for 1 minute. Drain immediately and rinse under cold running water. Squeeze gently to remove excess moisture. Pull back on the tough central rib to remove it from the leaf, but do not tear. Pile the chard shiny side down. Cut large leaves into approximately 5-inch squares. You should have 4 dozen leaves.

3 In a 10-inch conventional skillet, melt the butter over medium heat. Add the onion, pastrami, tomato sauce, and Aleppo pepper and cook for 5 minutes, stirring often. Remove from the heat.

4 Transfer the contents of the skillet to a food processor. Add the corn kernels, cheese, half of the hazelnuts, the parsley, and the mint. Pulse until gritty textured and well combined. Season generously with salt, pepper and additional Turkish or Aleppo pepper to taste.

5 Line the bottom of the casserole with the chopped chard stems. Put one leaf in the palm of one hand, top with a tablespoon of filling, and then roll it up like an egg roll, squeezing gently to enclose. Arrange the stuffed leaves close together, seam side down, on top of the chopped stems. Season lightly with salt. Cover the rolls with a flat plate, pressing down gently, and add 1 cup boiling water. Cover the casserole with a lid and cook over low heat for 40 minutes.

6 Transfer the hot casserole to a wooden surface or folded kitchen towel to prevent cracking and let rest for 20 minutes. Transfer the chard rolls to a shallow serving dish. Coarsely chop the remaining hazelnuts and sprinkle them on top. Serve the dish warm.

NOTE TO THE COOK: Toasted sweet corn is one of the earliest American food products. In pre-Revolutionary times, settlers set out corn kernels to dry in the sun and then used them in creamed corn dishes. This product is now available from www.copefoods.com in Lancaster County, Pennsylvania, where John Cope's family has been making it for over one hundred years.

Oven Polenta in a Clay Pot

SERVES 6

*H*ere's a great way to produce perfect polenta without a lot of work, using a well-greased earthenware cazuela. The method described in the recipe coaxes extra flavor from the coarse cornmeal by allowing it to toast as it cooks, resulting in soft, tender polenta with a lovely glossy sheen.

> **PREFERRED CLAY POT:**
>
> **A 12-inch Spanish cazuela**

2 cups medium- or coarse-ground organic stone-ground cornmeal

2 tablespoons unsalted butter or extra virgin olive oil

2 teaspoons salt

1 Preheat the oven to 350°F. In the cazuela, stir together the cornmeal, 8 to 10 cups cool water, the butter, and the salt. Bake, uncovered, for 1 hour and 20 minutes.

2 Stir the polenta and bake for 10 minutes longer.

3 Remove the cazuela from the oven and set on a wooden surface or folded kitchen towel to prevent cracking. Let the polenta rest for 5 minutes before spooning it into a buttered bowl. Serve hot.

NOTE: The consistency of the polenta is a factor in deciding how much liquid to use. For soft polenta, use 5 parts liquid to part cornmeal and for firm polenta 4 parts liquid to 1 part cornmeal.

Sautéed Polenta Slices

Prepare the polenta through step 2. Immediately transfer the hot polenta to a greased loaf pan or bowl. Let cool until set; then turn out and slice with a taut string or an oiled knife. Brush the bottom of a large cast-iron skillet with about 2 teaspoons olive oil, butter, or drippings from roast beef, pork, or chicken. Slip in a leaf of sage or a sprig of rosemary and heat slowly until fragrant. Add 2 halved garlic cloves and cook, stirring, until just golden; remove and discard the garlic. Add the polenta slices and fry, turning once, until crisp, puffed, and golden, about 5 minutes on each side. Serve as an accompaniment to Fonduta Valdostana (page 15), grilled poultry, or roast meat.

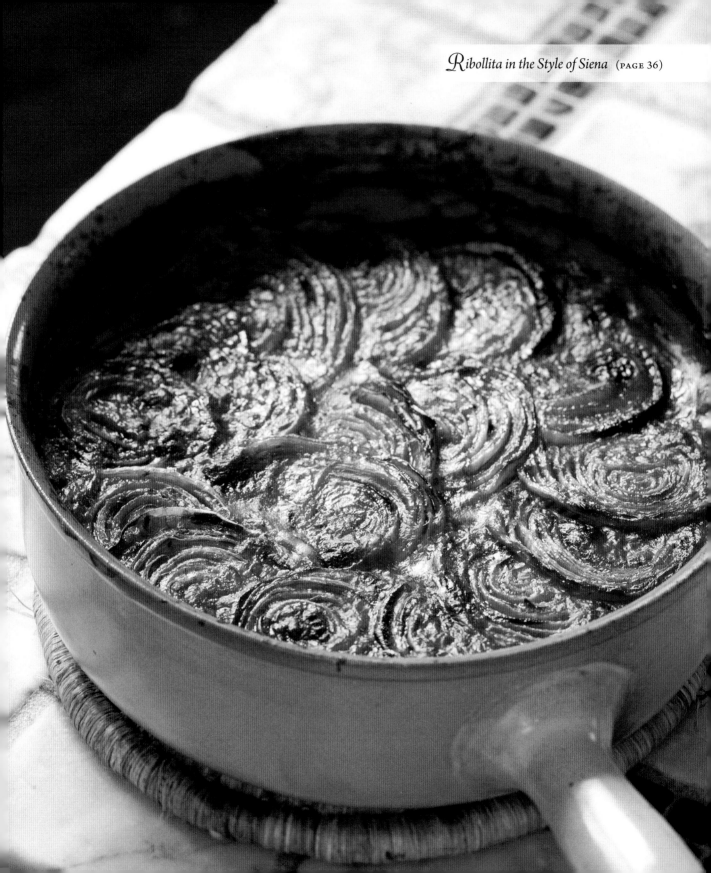

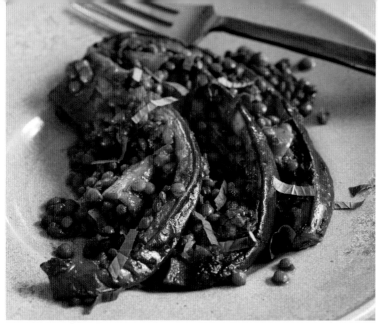

LEFT

Casserole of Lentils, Eggplant, and Mint
(PAGE 240)

BELOW

*Charentaise Daube of Beef with Red Wine
and Cognac* (PAGE 153)

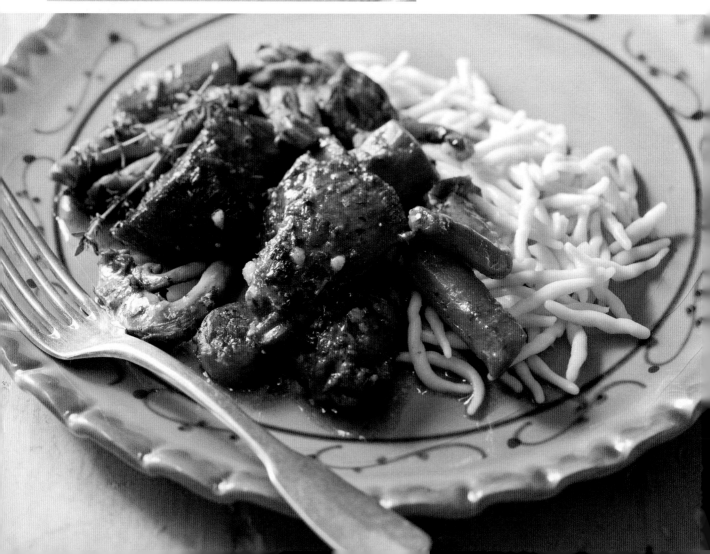

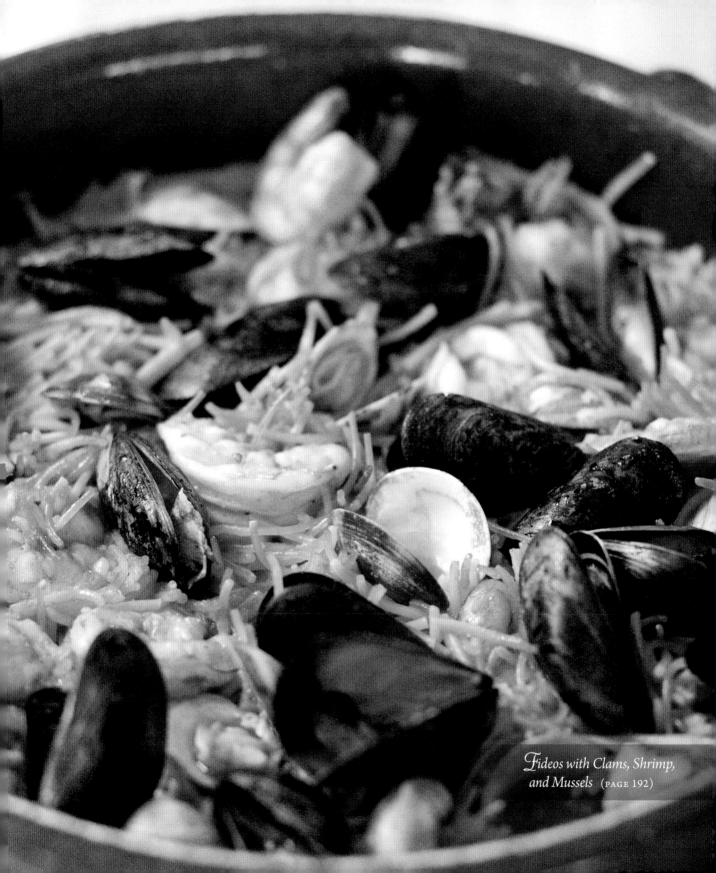

Fideos with Clams, Shrimp, and Mussels (PAGE 192)

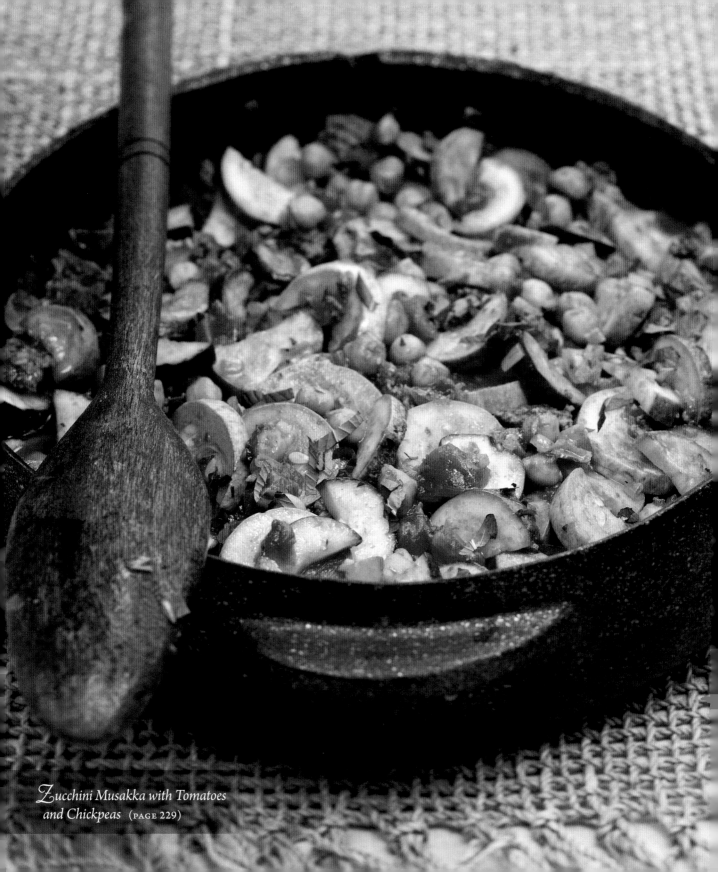

Zucchini Musakka with Tomatoes and Chickpeas (PAGE 229)

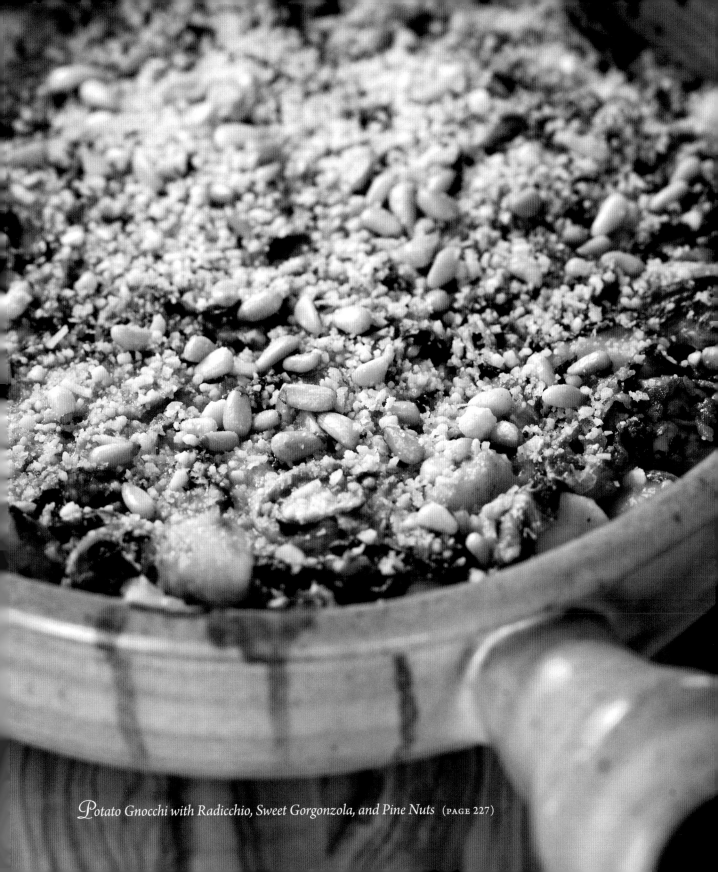

Potato Gnocchi with Radicchio, Sweet Gorgonzola, and Pine Nuts (PAGE 227)

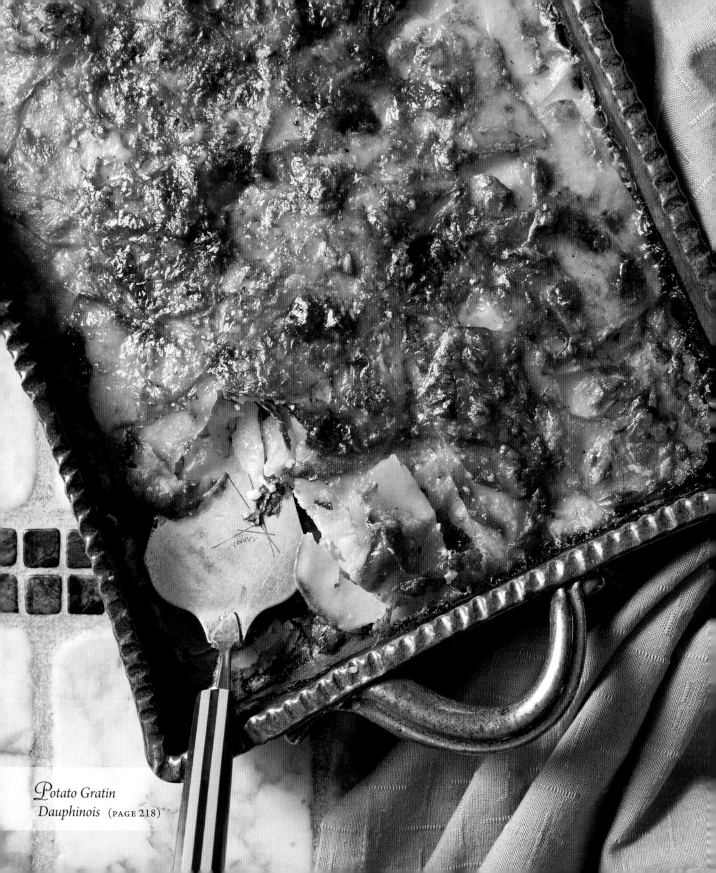

*Potato Gratin
Dauphinois* (PAGE 218)

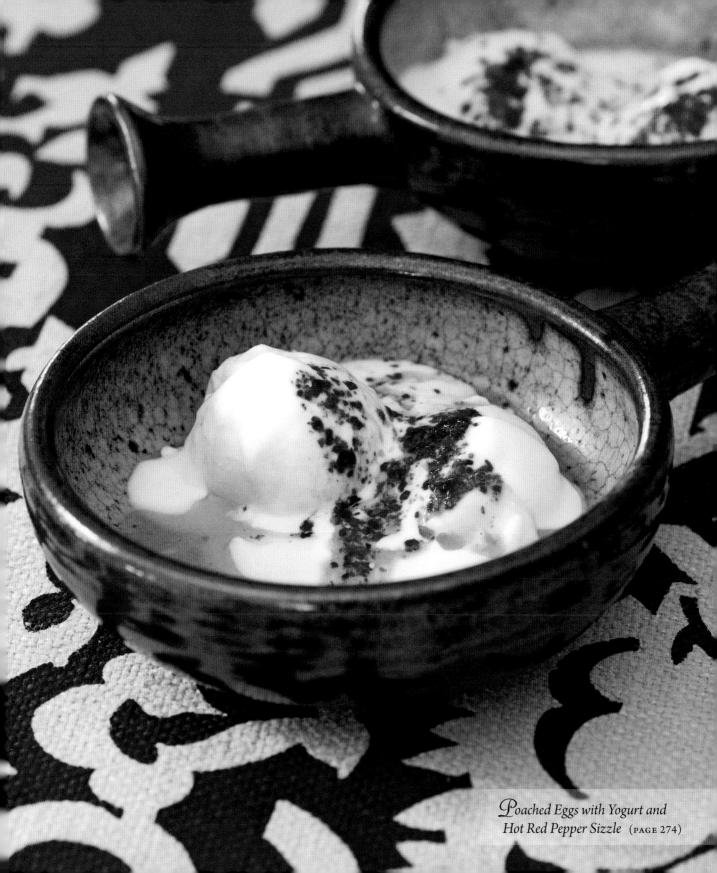

*Poached Eggs with Yogurt and
Hot Red Pepper Sizzle* (PAGE 274)

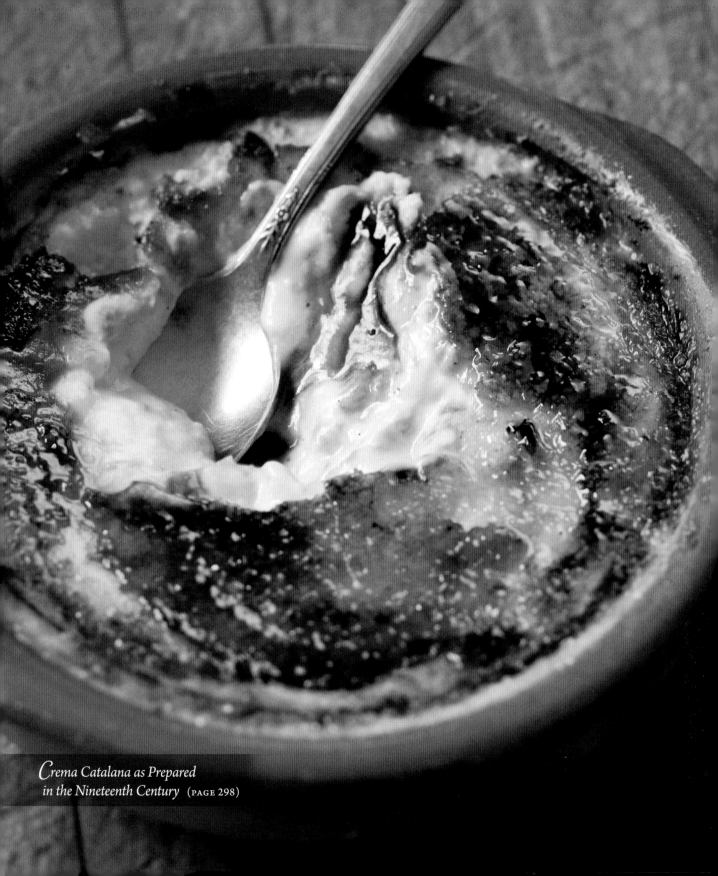

*Crema Catalana as Prepared
in the Nineteenth Century* (PAGE 298)

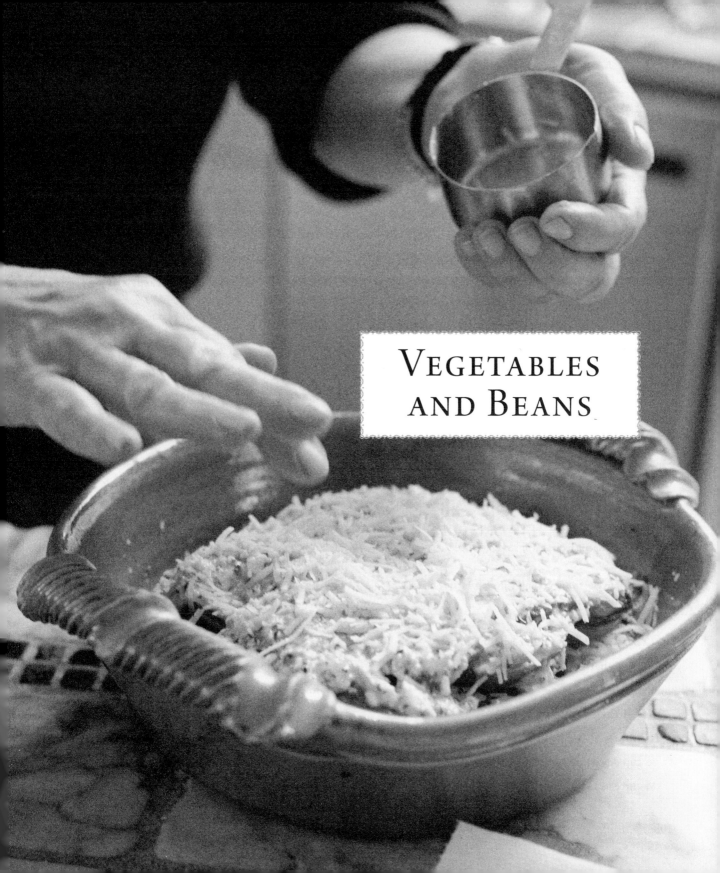

VEGETABLES
AND BEANS

Artichokes à la Provençale

SERVES 4

*A*rtichokes are stunning cooked in earthenware, as exemplified in this tempting vegetable ragout, a variation on the more famous *artichauts barigoule de Provence*. Here young, very tender artichokes with undeveloped chokes simmer slowly in a cazuela in seasoned olive oil accompanied by pancetta and sweet spring onions until meltingly tender.

Look for artichokes that measure roughly 1¼ inches in diameter and weigh about 1 ounce each. The lack of chokes makes them easy to clean.

I prepare this dish early in the day and then leave it out on the counter to allow the flavors to mellow. Serve it at room temperature as a vegetable dish to accompany your favorite roast or pan fried fish. A final splash of good French truffle oil will make it sublime.

PREFERRED CLAY POT:

A 10-inch Spanish cazuela or straight-sided flameware skillet

If using an electric or ceramic stovetop, be sure to use a heat diffuser with the clay pot.

---

12 baby artichokes (about 1 pound total)

1 lemon, halved, plus a few drops juice

1 cup chicken stock

3 fresh thyme sprigs

2 imported bay leaves

½ cup dry white wine

¼ cup extra virgin olive oil

1½ ounces thinly sliced pancetta, shredded

3 or 4 spring bulb onions, bunching onions, large scallions, or shallots, chopped (½ cup)

1 garlic clove, chopped

Salt and freshly ground black pepper

2 to 3 drops French black truffle oil (optional)

2 tablespoons chopped fresh flat-leaf parsley

1 Rinse and clean the artichokes one at a time: Remove the thick outer leaves until you arrive at the delicate light green center. Slice off about one-third of the pointy top. Use a swivel-bladed vegetable peeler to trim away the tough stem on the bottom and around the base of the artichoke. Then place in cold water with the juice of the lemon half.

2 Put the trimmed artichokes in a small conventional saucepan, preferably stainless steel, with the stock, thyme, and bay leaves. Bring to a boil, reduce the heat, and simmer for 10 minutes, or until the hearts are half cooked. Scoop out the artichokes and drain on paper towels. Boil the stock until it is reduced to ⅓ cup. Add the wine to the stock and boil again until reduced by half to ⅓ cup.

3 Meanwhile put 3 tablespoons of the olive oil, the pancetta, onions, and garlic in the cazuela and set it over medium heat. Cook, stirring, for 15 minutes, or until the onion is soft and golden.

4 Add the warm artichokes to the cazuela and cook, stirring until they develop a lovely golden glaze, about 10 minutes. Strain the reduced stock and wine over the artichokes and season lightly with salt and pepper. Cover with a piece of crumpled wet parchment and a lid or foil and cook over medium-low heat for 15 minutes, until the liquid is absorbed and the artichokes are plump and shiny. Test for doneness by piercing with a thin bamboo skewer. Transfer the cazuela to a wooden surface or folded kitchen towel to prevent cracking.

5 Mix the remaining tablespoon of olive oil with a few drops of lemon juice and the truffle oil and sprinkle over the artichokes. Gently shake the cazuela and let stand for a few hours. Scatter the parsley on top just before serving.

Summer Carrots Cooked in a Clay Pot

SERVES 4

*I*n this easy recipe, young organic or farmstand carrots are cooked very slowly in a few tablespoons of liquid in a closed clay pot, causing them to steam in their own moisture and ultimately glaze in their naturally released sugars. The carrots turn melt-in-your-mouth tender while retaining their structure, and the slower the cooking, the sweeter they will be.

PREFERRED CLAY POTS:

A 2- or 3-quart Chinese sandpot or earthenware saucepan with a tight-fitting lid

If using an electric or ceramic stovetop, be sure to use a heat diffuser with the clay pot.

1 pound slender organic carrots

3 tablespoons unsalted butter

Pinch of salt

Pinch of sugar

1 Trim and peel the carrots; then cut them diagonally into 1-inch pieces. Place in the sandpot with the butter, salt, sugar, and 2 tablespoons water.

2 Cover with a sheet of crumpled parchment and a lid. Cook over low heat until the carrots are tender, about 20 minutes, shaking the pot after about 10 minutes to ensure that the carrots glaze all over. Serve hot.

NOTE TO THE COOK: If you don't have access to organic or farmstand carrots, you can make this dish with grocery store carrots so long as you add another tablespoon of water and an extra pinch of sugar.

Corsican Chestnut Gnocchi with Wild Mushrooms

SERVES 4 TO 6

A subtle addition of chestnut flour to the gnocchi recipe adds a pure, faintly sweet, and earthy flavor and results in slightly darker color. In Corsica, in the high Alps of Provence, and in Liguria, chestnut flour is used to achieve these effects. This flour is available online or at high-end Italian groceries. It stales quickly, so remember to stock up when it's fresh in autumn and keep it frozen until you're ready to use it.

For Chestnut Gnocchi, prepare the recipe for Potato Gnocchi as directed on page 226, but substitute ⅓ cup chestnut flour for the cake flour.

> **PREFERRED CLAY POT:**
>
> **A 10-inch Spanish cazuela or a straight-sided flameware skillet**

3 to 4 fresh porcini or small chanterelle mushrooms (about 3 ounces total)

2½ tablespoons extra virgin olive oil

1 large shallot, finely chopped

1 large garlic clove, peeled and bruised

4 ounces fresh oyster mushrooms, trimmed and sliced

¼ cup dry white wine

½ cup heavy cream

½ cup chicken stock

1 tablespoon chopped fresh flat-leaf parsley

1½ teaspoons fresh thyme leaves

Salt and freshly ground black pepper

Chestnut Potato Gnocchi (page 226)

2 tablespoons dried bread crumbs

1½ ounces Parmigiano-Reggiano cheese, shaved

1 Preheat the oven to 350°F. Separate the porcini caps and stems. Wipe clean with a damp cloth. Trim away any soft parts. Remove any spongy parts underneath the caps. Cut the mushroom caps and stems into slices about ⅜ inch thick.

2 Heat 2 tablespoons of the olive oil in the cazuela over medium-low heat. Add the shallot and garlic and cook until softened, about 4 minutes. Raise the heat gradually until the oil sizzles. Add the porcini and cook, stirring, until lightly browned, about 10 minutes.

3 Scoop up the mushrooms and set aside. Add the oyster mushrooms to the cazuela and cook, stirring, for 5 minutes. Add the wine and boil until it is absorbed by the mushrooms, about 5 minutes. Return the porcini to the dish, add the cream and stock, and bring to a boil, stirring. And the parsley and thyme and season with salt and pepper to taste. Add the cooked chestnut gnocchi and toss gently to coat with the mushrooms and sauce. Scatter the Parmigiano-Reggiano cheese on top.

4 Bake for 15 minutes; then switch the heat to broil. Slide the baking dish under the broiler about 6 inches from the heat and broil until bubbling and golden brown on top, about 3 minutes. Serve at once, while the sauce is still bubbling.

NOTE TO THE COOK: If using frozen gnocchi: Brush 1 tablespoon olive oil over a large heavy skillet and set over medium-high heat. Add the partially defrosted gnocchi and brown on one side only, about 2 minutes. Use a spatula and a few tablespoons of water to loosen the gnocchi, carefully transfer them to the cazuela, and coat with the sauce. Finish baking and broiling as described.

Compote of Fennel with Onion, Pancetta, and Currants

SERVES 4

The technique for making vegetable compotes is old-fashioned and marvelously simple. All the vegetables are thinly sliced using a mandoline or food processor for precision. Then they are cooked together very slowly in their own exuded juices inside a glazed earthenware pot. An occasional stirring encourages the slices to break down and merge into a sumptuous vegetable jam studded with tender bits of pancetta and sweet currants. This compote makes an excellent accompaniment to grilled fish or lamb.

> **PREFERRED CLAY POT:**
>
> A 3-quart Chinese sandpot or a glazed earthenware or flameware casserole
>
> If using an electric or ceramic stovetop, be sure to use a heat diffuser with the clay pot.

2 medium-firm fennel bulbs

1 medium onion

2 tablespoons extra virgin olive oil

1½ ounces thinly sliced pancetta, shredded

¼ cup dried currants or raisins

Salt and freshly ground black pepper

1 Use a fine blade on a mandoline or the 2 millimeter blade on a food processor to cut the fennel and onion into very thin slices.

2 Place the fennel, onion, olive oil, pancetta, currants, ¾ teaspoon salt, and ¼ teaspoon pepper in the sandpot. Cover with a sheet of crumpled parchment and a lid, and cook, stirring occasionally, over low heat for 1 to 2 hours, or until the contents are reduced to about 1 scant cup.

3 Remove the cover, raise the heat to medium, and gently fry the mixture until it is golden brown and lightly caramelized, about 10 minutes. Season with additional salt and pepper to taste. Let the compote stand at room temperature for a few hours to further blend the flavors. Reheat the compote to lukewarm just before serving.

Inspired by a recipe created by Chef Christian Etienne of Restaurant Christian Etienne in Avignon, France.

Cazuela Roasted Garlic

MAKES 8 TO 10 HEADS

Roasted garlic shows up all around the Mediterranean, adding flavor to stews, soups, and pastas. It is used to flavor mashed potatoes, as a condiment with cooked root vegetables, as a spread for toasted country bread along with peppered cheese, in mayonnaise for grilled shrimp, or as simply something marvelous to be devoured on its own along with the *diable* (devil) potatoes on page 223. The aroma of slowly roasting garlic will fill your kitchen and arouse the appetites of anyone who passes through.

The best time to make this dish is in late spring, when plump young tender white garlic bulbs become available. A good way to store uncooked fresh garlic is in a ceramic garlic jar, a small glazed perforated jug with a cover. The holes in the sides enhance air flow. A simple ceramic strawberry jar from your local garden center will work well too. Cover with cloth secured by a rubber band.

Serve as a vegetable accompaniment for meat, fish, or chicken.

> **PREFERRED CLAY POT:**
> A small earthenware baking dish or Spanish cazuela just large enough to hold the garlic heads snugly

8 to 10 heads of fresh garlic (about 1 pound)

2 tablespoons unsalted butter

5 ounces thinly sliced fatty prosciutto, shredded

½ teaspoon sea salt

¼ teaspoon freshly ground black pepper

1 teaspoon sugar

½ cup simmering water

1 Preheat the oven to 325°F.

2 In a conventional saucepan, cover the garlic with cold water and bring to a boil. Cook for 2 minutes; drain. Remove the upper outer skin of each garlic head, leaving the bottom skin intact to hold the garlic cloves in place. Trim off the tips of each clove with a pair of scissors or a paring knife. Avoid removing the papery skin between the cloves.

3 Lightly grease the baking dish with 1 teaspoon of the butter. Scatter half of the prosciutto over the bottom of the baking dish. Arrange the heads of garlic in a single layer and tuck the remaining prosciutto in between the heads. Cut the remaining butter into bits and scatter on top along with the sea salt, black pepper, and sugar. Cover with foil and bake the garlic for 1 hour.

4 Remove the foil, gradually pour in the simmering water to prevent any shock to the pan, baste with the juices, and return to the oven. Bake, uncovered, for 30 more minutes, or until the garlic is glazed. Serve the garlic right from the cazuela.

NOTE TO THE COOK: Any leftover roasted garlic can be stored in a closed jar in the refrigerator for 2 to 3 days. To store it longer, press the garlic out of the skin, mix 2 tablespoons olive oil with 2 tablespoons crushed garlic, season with pinches of salt and pepper, and mash to a smooth paste. Pack in a small jar, cover, and store in the refrigerator for up to a week.

Garlic Custard

SERVES 4

*M*any recipes for garlic flans and custards call for cooking the garlic cloves until soft and creamy. That method works well but in my view doesn't take full advantage of the flavor potential of this fine ingredient. In this recipe, given to me by the late great Gascon chef Jean-Louis Palladin, whose Washington, D.C., restaurant Jean-Louis at the Watergate was regarded as the finest in the capital for many years, the garlic is cooked twice. First the cloves are lightly caramelized in their cooking juices. Then they are crushed to a paste, blended with a custard base, and baked in porcelain ramekins set in a water bath. The result is a gentle, rich custard with melt-in-your-mouth texture, an extraordinary deep flavor, and marvelous heady aroma.

Serve with roasted meats or poultry.

> **PREFERRED CLAY POTS:**
>
> **4 ceramic ramekins (4 ounces each)**
>
> **A 2- or 3-quart Spanish cazuela or Chinese sandpot**
>
> **If using an electric or ceramic stovetop, be sure to use a heat diffuser with the clay pot.**

1 tablespoon plus 2 teaspoons unsalted butter

8 ounces garlic heads, cloves separated but not peeled

1 cup chicken stock

½ teaspoon white wine vinegar

⅛ teaspoon sugar

½ teaspoon salt

¼ teaspoon finely ground white pepper

2 whole eggs and 1 egg yolk at room temperature, lightly beaten cup milk, warmed

½ cup heavy cream, warmed

1 Preheat the oven to 300°F. Use 2 teaspoons of the butter to grease the ramekins.

2 Put the garlic cloves in a small conventional saucepan and cover with cold water. Bring to a boil, cook for 2 minutes, and drain. Repeat; peel the garlic.

3 Place the peeled garlic in the cazuela and add the stock, vinegar, sugar, salt, white pepper, and remaining tablespoon butter. Simmer over medium-low heat for 30 minutes, or until the liquid is reduced to a golden glaze.

4 Crush the garlic into the glaze with a fork to make a puree. Whisk in the whole eggs, egg yolk, warm milk, and warm cream; strain through a sieve. Ladle the mixture into the buttered ramekins.

5 Place the ramekins in a small baking pan and set in the center of the oven. Add enough simmering water to the pan to reach halfway up the sides of the ramekins. Bake for 45 minutes, or until the custards puff lightly and barely shimmer when prodded lightly with two fingers. Since different-shaped molds and materials require different cooking times, you may need to cook them for 5 minutes longer. If the custards are not set, turn off the heat and leave them in the oven for 5 to 10 minutes longer. Remove the baking pan from the oven and let the molds stand in

(continued)

the hot water for 10 minutes. Then take the molds out of the water bath. (The custards can be prepared to this point up to 2 hours ahead. They can be reheated in a warm oven for 5 minutes before unmolding.)

6 To unmold, place a wide spatula over the mold and invert onto a plate. Slip the spatula from underneath, leaving the custard and mold in place. Lift off the mold.

Slow-Cooked Sandpot Mushrooms

SERVES 4

When you slow-cook cultivated white mushrooms in a closed clay pot, such as a Chinese sandpot, an extraordinary alchemy takes place. These ordinary mushrooms, which normally taste quite bland, acquire an earthy flavor, almost as deep as that of wild ones.

I never cease to be amazed at the transformation, which I attribute to the clay vessel. My theory, stated earlier in this book, is that wonderful flavor can often be developed when there is no interference between earth—that is, the clay—and food. I think this simple recipe proves my point.

> **PREFERRED CLAY POT:**
>
> **A 3-quart Chinese sandpot**
>
> **If using an electric or ceramic stovetop, be sure to use a heat diffuser with the clay pot.**

1 pound white mushrooms

6 garlic cloves, sliced

1½ tablespoons extra virgin olive oil

Salt and freshly ground black pepper

1 Clean the mushrooms, either by brushing them off or by wiping the caps with wet paper towels. Cut off the very ends of the stems.

2 Place the mushrooms in the dry sandpot. Add the garlic and olive oil and toss to mix. Cover with a crumpled sheet of parchment, which will keep in all moisture and aroma, and the lid and set over low heat for 45 minutes, shaking the pot from time to time so they cook evenly. Season with salt and pepper and serve hot or warm.

Green Beans with Tomatoes and Garlic

SERVES 4

*L*ebanese food writer Anissa Helou has kindly given me permission to include this recipe from her superb cookbook *Lebanese Cuisine: More than 250 Authentic Recipes from the Most Elegant Middle Eastern Cuisine.* The dish, made with seasonal green string or snap beans, is wonderful whether served warm, at room temperature, or cool. The garlic cloves, are creamy, buttery, and soft—to die for!

An unglazed Lebanese clay pot for this dish is called a *qudrat,* and it is traditionally used to cook either beans or lentils. An unglazed La Chamba casserole makes a fine substitute.

Here are Anissa's instructions for serving and eating this dish the "village way": "Take one pita bread, tear it open at the seams, and lay one half, rough side up, on a plate. Spoon some beans and tomato sauce onto the bread, spreading the vegetables evenly across it, and serve hot with trimmed spring onions or peeled and quartered normal ones. Eat with your hands by using a torn piece of bread from the other half to scoop up a few beans and with each mouthful take a bite of onion and suck a garlic clove out of its skin. Once you finish eating the beans, arrange a few pieces of onion in a line in the middle of the tomato-soaked bread, roll it up, and eat like a sandwich. Then lock yourself up for the next twenty-four hours as no one will want to be anywhere near your breath!"

> **PREFERRED CLAY POT:**
>
> A 2- or 3-quart earthenware casserole, preferably unglazed, such as La Chamba, or a glazed Chinese sandpot
>
> If using an electric or ceramic stovetop, be sure to use a heat diffuser with the clay pot.

1 pound green beans

½ cup extra virgin olive oil

1 medium onion, finely chopped

8 to 10 large garlic cloves, unpeeled

Salt

3 medium tomatoes, peeled and chopped

1 Trim the green beans by "topping and tailing" them. Cut the beans into 1-inch lengths. Rinse, drain, and set aside.

2 Put the olive oil, onion, and garlic cloves in the earthenware casserole set over medium-low heat. Cook, stirring, for 2 to 3 minutes. Slowly raise the heat to medium and cook until the onion turns golden, 3 to 5 minutes.

3 Add the green beans, sprinkle with a generous pinch of salt, and sauté, stirring occasionally, until they become glossy and turn a brighter green, 3 to 4 minutes.

4 Add the tomatoes and bring to a boil. Cover, reduce the heat to medium-low, and cook for 30 minutes. Turn off the heat and let stand, covered, for 10 minutes longer. The sauce should be thick, the beans tender, and the aroma just wonderful.

Spring Greens Marmalade with Pecorino Sardo Cheese

SERVES 6 TO 8

*H*ere's a variation on a favorite southern Italian greens marmalade, which I first published years ago in my book *World of Food.* Later, when I wrote *Mediterranean Grains and Greens,* I learned a lot more about mixing different greens and cooking them in combination. My new recipe here reflects this knowledge. In southern Italy, greens mixtures such as this are cooked inside doughy calzones. I prefer to serve this mix on toasted bread rounds, which I sprinkle with cheese and run under the broiler. They are best eaten as soon as they are cooked.

> **PREFERRED CLAY POT:**
>
> **A 10-inch Spanish cazuela**
>
> **If using an electric or ceramic stovetop, be sure to use a heat diffuser with the clay pot.**

10 ounces spinach leaves

5 ounces Swiss chard leaves or young arugula

5 ounces watercress leaves

Coarse salt and freshly ground black pepper

12 oil-cured black olives, pitted

¼ cup dried currants or golden raisins

¼ teaspoon crushed hot red pepper flakes

3 tablespoons extra virgin olive oil

1 garlic clove, chopped

4 large flat anchovy fillets, rinsed, drained, and crushed to a paste with a fork

12 capers, drained and rinsed

2 to 3 dozen grilled or fried thin round slices of Italian or French bread

2 ounces pecorino cheese, preferably Sardinian pecorino Medora, coarsely grated (about ½ cup)

1 Bring a large pot of water to a boil. Meanwhile, swish the spinach, chard, and watercress around in a large bowl of water; then transfer to a colander and let drain. Remove any tough leaves and stalks.

2 When the water is boiling, add about 1 tablespoon salt per quart. Working in batches, add a handful of the greens to the boiling water. Cook for 7 to 8 minutes. Scoop out the greens to a bowl of cold water to stop the cooking and then transfer to a colander to drain. Repeat with the remaining greens; then press down on all the greens to remove moisture and squeeze dry.

3 With a large stainless-steel knife, finely chop the greens. Add the olives, currants, and pepper flakes and coarsely chop them into the greens.

4 Brush the cazuela with oil and set over medium-low heat. Add the garlic, anchovies, and capers and cook, stirring, for 1 minute. Add the chopped mixed greens and cook for 2 minutes longer. Season with salt and pepper to taste. (The greens can be prepared to this point up to 2 days in advance. Transfer the hot cazuela to a wooden surface or folded kitchen towel to prevent cracking. Let cool, then cover and refrigerate.)

5 Shortly before serving, preheat the broiler. Finely chop the greens mixture again. Spread onto the bread rounds. Sprinkle the cheese on top and run under the broiler until glazed, about 2 minutes. Serve warm or at room temperature.

Peas with Pancetta Lardons

SERVES 4

*H*ere is my friend Barbara Wilde's recipe for an old favorite French dish immortalized in the popular song "Petits Pois Lardons," by the French singer Julien Clerc. Clerc's song tells the story of a young man with peas who finds a young woman with lardons and how, having found one another, they make the kitchen "swirl!"

Barbara prepares her version in an earthenware saucepan. Note that it's made with peas, pancetta, spring onions, and a little butter but not a single drop of water. This is contrary to the way we usually cook peas. Remember to stir constantly as instructed until the peas turn bright green. Continue cooking without adding even a single drop of water and you'll produce a stellar dish that goes beautifully with shellfish or poultry.

> **PREFERRED CLAY POT:**
>
> A wide 2-quart glazed earthenware saucepan, stovetop-safe ceramic fondue pot, or a Chinese sandpot
>
> If using an electric or ceramic stovetop, be sure to use a heat diffuser with the clay pot.

2 pounds fresh green peas in the pods

3 large spring bulb onions, green onions, or bunching onions or 6 large scallions

1 tablespoon unsalted butter

3 ounces very lean pancetta, diced

Sea salt and freshly ground black pepper

2 tablespoons chopped fresh flat-leaf parsley

1 Shell the peas. Quarter the bulb part of the spring onion; discard the tops.

2 In the earthenware saucepan, combine the butter and pancetta and set over medium-low heat. Cook, stirring occasionally, for 5 minutes. Add the onions and cook until soft, 5 to 7 minutes longer.

3 Add the peas and cook, stirring constantly, until they all turn bright green. Cover with a tight-fitting lid or a sheet of foil, reduce the heat to low, and cook until the peas and onions are very tender, about 15 minutes. (No water is necessary.) Gently shake the pan from time to time, but do not stir, or the peas will turn mushy. Season with salt and pepper to taste, sprinkle the parsley on top, and serve.

Potato Gratin Dauphinois

SERVES 6 TO 8

*J*ust as every Provençal cook has his or her own way of preparing bouillabaisse, so will every Dauphiné home cook have his or her version of this most famous of all French potato gratins. On the website www.gratindauphinois.com, there are more than two hundred recipes deemed acceptable to the residents of the Rhône-Alpes region of France where Dauphiné is located.

In my version, thinly sliced potatoes are bathed in an egg-enriched cream and then piled into a gratin dish. A tip I learned from the website: Bake the gratin, let it stand for at least fifteen minutes, and then reheat it before serving. The second heating makes the gratin taste even better.

PREFERRED CLAY POT:
A 9- × 12-inch gratin or shallow baking dish (10- to 12-cup capacity)

SUGGESTED CLAY ENVIRONMENT:
Double slabs of pizza stones or food-safe quarry tiles set on the upper and lower oven racks

1 garlic clove, halved

2 tablespoons butter

1½ cups whole milk or half-and-half

1½ cups heavy cream

1 egg

1 cup shredded Emmenthaler, Gruyère, or Comté cheese (about 3½ ounces)

1½ teaspoons salt

½ teaspoon freshly ground black pepper

¼ teaspoon grated nutmeg

2½ pounds Yukon Gold potatoes, peeled, thinly sliced, rinsed, and patted dry

1 Preheat the oven to 350°F. Rub the inside of the gratin with the garlic clove. Use 1 tablespoon of the butter to grease the dish.

2 Heat the milk and ¾ of the cream in a large conventional saucepan until bubbles just begin to appear around the edge of the pan.

3 In a medium bowl, beat the egg lightly. Gradually whisk in the hot creamy milk in a thin stream to temper the egg. Add ¾ cup of the cheese, return to the saucepan, and cook over medium heat, stirring, for 3 to 4 minutes to melt the cheese. Season with salt, pepper, and nutmeg.

4 Add the potato slices to the sauce and stir to coat. Transfer to the buttered gratin and spread out in an even layer. Sprinkle the remaining ¼ cup cheese on top and dot with the remaining 1 tablespoon butter. Set in the oven. Raise the heat to 400°F and bake for 1 hour.

5 Transfer the gratin to a wooden surface or folded towel to prevent cracking; let cool for 15 minutes. Loosen the sides of the gratin with a flat knife and, brush the top of the gratin with the remaining ¾ cup heavy cream. Return the baking dish to the oven to bake for 15 minutes. Turn off the heat and let the gratin finish browning in the receding heat for 30 minutes longer.

Gratin Dauphinois in the Style of the French Alps

Some cooks, particularly in the Vercors near the Drôme in eastern France, make this dish differently. There the potatoes are simmered in milk—with no cream—until they are just tender but still quite firm a day in advance.

They are then left to soak in the hot milk overnight. The next day the milk is drained off and the potatoes are arranged in a gratin dish, covered with cheese and butter, and baked quickly in a hot oven until golden brown.

Potato Gratin with Cauliflower

SERVES 4 TO 6

PREFERRED CLAY POT:

A 10- or 11-inch Spanish cazuela or straight-sided flameware skillet

If using an electric or ceramic stovetop, be sure to use a heat diffuser with the clay pot.

SUGGESTED CLAY ENVIRONMENT:

Double slabs of pizza stones or food-safe quarry tiles set on the upper and lower oven racks

Salt

1 small cauliflower, trimmed

1 pound small red potatoes, peeled

3 tablespoons unsalted butter

1 tablespoon all-purpose flour

1 cup milk, warmed

1 bay leaf

⅛ teaspoon freshly ground black pepper

⅛ teaspoon freshly grated nutmeg

3 ounces Cantal or Comté cheese, finely shredded (about 1 cup)

2 tablespoons heavy cream

1 Fill a saucepan with water and salt. Peel the potatoes and place in the water. Set a colander or a steamer basket on top and add the cauliflower, stem end down. Cover tightly and steam over medium-high heat for 20 minutes.

2 Preheat the oven to 400°F. Melt half of the butter in the cazuela over low heat. Sprinkle on the flour, raise the heat to medium-low, and cook, stirring, for 3 or 4 minutes without allowing the flour to color. Whisk in the warm milk. Add the bay leaf and season with ¼ teaspoon salt, the pepper, and the nutmeg. Bring to a boil, reduce to a simmer, and cook, stirring often, for 5 minutes.

3 Transfer the steamed cauliflower to a cutting board. Drain the potatoes. Thickly slice both vegetables. Add them to the milk mixture and spread out in an even layer. Scatter the cheese and heavy cream on top and dot with the remaining butter.

4 Bake the gratin for 30 minutes, or until golden brown and bubbly. Turn off the heat and let cook in the receding heat for 20 to 30 minutes. Serve hot.

Potato Gratin with Julienne of Mushrooms and Comté Cheese

SERVES 6

I'm especially fond of this potato gratin since it employs two of my favorite ingredients: mushrooms and cheese. For depth of flavor I use a mix of fresh meaty oyster mushrooms and dried morels, which contribute a lovely smoky undertone. Mildly sweet and slightly nutty, Comté cheese is the first choice for this dish, but Gruyère makes a fine substitute. The cheese is shredded and mixed into the milk with the mushrooms and just a little cream to produce a lovely sauce with no added flour. This gratin goes beautifully with roast beef or leg of lamb.

> **PREFERRED CLAY POT:**
>
> A 10- or 11-inch Spanish cazuela or straight-sided flameware skillet
>
> If using an electric or ceramic stovetop, be sure to use a heat diffuser with the clay pot.
>
> **SUGGESTED CLAY ENVIRONMENT:**
>
> Double slabs of pizza stones or food-safe quarry tiles set on the upper and lower oven racks

½ ounce dried morels

4 tablespoons (½ stick) unsalted butter

3 spring onions, wild leeks, or ramps, quartered lengthwise, or 6 fat scallion bulbs, halved

10 ounces large fresh oyster mushrooms, thinly sliced lengthwise

Salt and freshly ground black pepper

2 tablespoons minced fresh chives

1 tablespoon chopped fresh flat-leaf parsley

3 tablespoons heavy cream

5 ounces Comté or Gruyèr cheese, shredded (about 1⅓ cups)

2 cups milk

2 pounds Yukon Gold potatoes, peeled and thinly sliced

1 Soak the dried morels in a small bowl filled with 1 cup warm water for 30 minutes. Remove the morels and squeeze them gently over the bowl to catch all the liquid. Cut each morel in half lengthwise. Strain the soaking water through a paper coffee filter or several layers of damp cheesecloth and reserve.

2 Melt 1½ tablespoons of the butter in the cazuela over medium-low heat. Add the spring onions, cover with a sheet of foil or a loose-fitting cover and cook slowly for 10 minutes. Add the remaining 2½ tablespoons butter and the oyster mushrooms and cook, covered, for 5 minutes longer. Turn off the heat.

3 Add the morels to the cazuela along with their reserved soaking water. Slowly raise the heat to medium and boil until the mushrooms absorb all the liquid, about 5 minutes. Season the mushrooms lightly with salt and pepper. Add the chives, parsley, cream, and half of the shredded cheese. Stir until the cheese melts and the mushrooms are nicely coated with sauce. Scoop into a side dish and set aside. Do not wash the cazuela. (The recipe can be prepared to this point up to 2 to 3 hours in advance. Set aside at room temperature.)

4 About an hour before you plan to serve the dish, preheat the oven to 400°F. Stir the milk into the cazuela and set over medium heat. Stir in the remaining cheese and when it is melted, season with salt and pepper to taste. Reduce the heat to low.

5 Add half the potato slices to the cazuela. Cover with all the sauced mushrooms and top with the remaining potatoes. Press down with a spatula lightly to make sure all the potatoes are submerged in the cheese sauce. Cover the cazuela with foil.

6 Bake for 1 hour. Uncover and bake until the potatoes are tender and the top is golden brown, about 30 minutes longer. Without opening the door, turn off the oven and let cook in the receding heat for 15 minutes. Transfer to a wooden surface or folded kitchen towel to prevent cracking and let stand for 5 to 10 minutes before serving right from the clay pot.

Cazuela Potatoes

SERVES 1

*H*ere is a lighter, crisper version of the classic French potato gratin, made with a lot less butter and cream and with the potato slices arranged in a thin layer. This dish is easy to make and goes well with a steak. It is a favorite of my husband's when he dines alone.

A Spanish cazuela is the perfect clay vessel for this gratin. Nothing else quite provides the proper evaporation of moisture and the slow, even cooking necessary to produce a golden, crisp round of potatoes.

> **PREFERRED CLAY POT:**
>
> A 12- to 14-inch Spanish cazuela
>
> If using an electric or ceramic stovetop, be sure to use a heat diffuser with the clay pot.
>
> **SUGGESTED CLAY ENVIRONMENT:**
>
> Double slabs of pizza stones or food-safe quarry tiles set on the upper and lower oven racks

12 ounces waxy potatoes, such as Yukon Gold or red

1 garlic clove, halved

4 tablespoons (½ stick) unsalted butter, melted

2 tablespoons whole milk

1 tablespoon heavy cream

Pinch of coarse sea salt

Freshly ground white pepper

1 Preheat the oven to 375°F. Peel the potatoes and cut them into thin slices. Rinse in cold water; pat them dry between paper towels.

2 Rub the inside of the cazuela with the cut garlic. Brush with 2 tablespoons of the melted butter. Arrange the potato slices, overlapping in concentric circles, in the cazuela. Brush with the remaining melted butter.

3 Bake for 30 minutes, or until the edges of the potatoes are just beginning to brown. Raise the oven temperature to 450°F.

4 Mix the milk and cream and spoon over the potatoes. Bake until the moisture is absorbed and the potatoes are golden brown and crisp, about 15 minutes longer. Serve at once, sprinkled with salt and white pepper.

DRY-COOKED POTATOES

In France, the *diable* is a potbellied unglazed earthenware pot traditionally used to cook potatoes or chestnuts. The idea is to dry-cook the potatoes without any water or fat, a method that develops a crusty charred skin, creamy interior, and wonderful earthy aroma and flavor.

The method is simple: You place one or two layers of washed and thoroughly dried potatoes inside, add a few tablespoons sea salt, cover, and cook over low heat for fifteen minutes, or until the clay turns quite hot. Then raise the heat to medium and cook the potatoes for another forty-five minutes, shaking the pot occasionally to ensure uniform cooking. It is critical never to open the lid, even for a quick peek inside. The process is a bit like steam-cooking, only the steam doesn't derive from soaking the pot but from the natural moisture of the potatoes, which is slowly released and recycled.

After you've finished cooking, place the hot *diable* on a wooden surface or folded kitchen towel to prevent cracking. Nothing cold should ever touch or be added to the hot pot. Also, the pot should never be washed. To clean, simply wipe out the interior with dry paper towels. The inside of the pot will darken with each use and will produce even better-tasting potatoes. (There are other types of potato devils beside the unglazed Charentais model, some of which can be washed without a detergent.)

Always allow the *diable* to heat up slowly in the coals of a wood fire in your fireplace or over a heat diffuser set over a gas or electric burner for about fifteen minutes. Then raise the heat and cook, shaking the pot often, until the potatoes are done Lacking a true *diable,* please do not substitute the sort of unglazed pot that is soaked. Instead, you can substitute a Chinese sandpot or a La Chamba casserole and obtain a good result, but you won't get the earthy burned-embers aroma. The Romertopf company has recently offered a stovetop nonsoak potato pot, which can be washed.

The best potatoes for potato-devil cooking are creamers.

Baby Creamer Potatoes Cooked in the Devil's Pot

SERVES 4 TO 6

*I*t takes about an hour and a half to prepare these potatoes on top of the stove. Please remember to shake the pot every fifteen minutes to ensure uniform crusting.

In the Charentes, the home cook will accompany these potatoes with thin slices of the best-cultured butter.

> **PREFERRED CLAY POT:**
>
> A 3-quart *diable Charentaise*, a Chinese sandpot, or a La Chamba casserole
>
> If using an electric or ceramic stovetop, be sure to use a heat diffuser with the clay pot.

1½ to 2 pounds small waxy potatoes, such as creamers, fingerlings, or baby Yukon Golds, rinsed, scrubbed, and dried

1 garlic clove, halved

1 tablespoon sea salt

1 About 1½ hours before serving, rinse the potatoes and scrub them well, but do not peel them. Dry the potatoes thoroughly.

2 Rub the garlic all over the inside of the *diable*. Place the dry potatoes in the clay pot and toss them with the salt. Cover with a round of parchment and the lid, set on a heat diffuser over medium-low heat, and cook for 15 minutes.

3 Without opening the pot, shake it to roll the potatoes so they don't stick. Slowly raise the heat to medium. Cook for 30 minutes longer, shaking the pot 2 more times. After a total of 45 minutes, open the pot and test for doneness by poking the potatoes with a bamboo skewer. If they are not completely tender, cover and cook for 10 to 15 minutes longer.

4 Transfer the hot clay pot to a wooden surface or folded kitchen towel to prevent cracking. Let stand for 10 minutes; then serve directly from the pot.

NOTE TO THE COOK: If you obtain a true *diable* and must wash it, wipe it out with a wet cloth and be sure to air-dry it for a few days before using. Otherwise, it will crack when heated. When new, do as the Charentais do and rub with garlic to season the pot all over to inhibit rancidity and strengthen the pot.

Slow Cooker Potatoes

If you want to cook a large amount of medium-size potatoes in a manner similar to the *diable*, use an electric slow cooker. Make a bed of about 1 inch of sea salt on the bottom of the pot. Rinse the potatoes and dry well. Prick each potato once or twice. Lightly oil the inside of the pot, add 3 or 4 bay leaves, pack in the potatoes, and cook until tender, about 6 hours on low or 3 hours on high.

POTATO GNOCCHI

Great potato gnocchi should be tender, ethereally light, and able to carry most any kind of sauce. In addition, the taste of the potato should be noticeable. So why does this marvelous dish, composed of just a handful of ingredients, frequently turn out heavy and tasteless?

Though I've been writing about food for forty years, it's only this year that I entered what I call the "gnocchi sphere." I spent a month experimenting in the kitchen, figuring out how to create gloriously tender, cloudlike gnocchi. From my explorations I've come up with the following ten-step method. At each step, there's a fork in the road. If you take the wrong turn (as I often did), you'll end up with poor results. But if you follow the correct path, you'll arrive at a delightful destination.

Step 1: Choose the right variety of potato. Most commentators recommend russets. They'll do, but if you use Yukon Gold, you'll come a lot closer to the old-fashioned yellow-fleshed potatoes used by cooks in Italy and the south of France where the dish originated.

Step 2: Don't boil the potatoes. Boiling activates water absorption, and water is the enemy of good gnocchi dough. I cook my potatoes by piercing them and baking them on an inch-thick bed of coarse salt to draw out moisture as they cook. At this stage, if you mix a handful of sea salt with the coarse salt, you gain a lovely briny fragrance as well.

Step 3: Don't mash or puree the potatoes; rice them. As soon as the potatoes are cooked, slash them to release the steam, slip off the skin, and pass them through a fine potato ricer or, better, a 10- to 12-inch drum sieve, called a *tamis*. The latter produces tiny crumbles of potato and releases more moisture, thus producing extra-light gnocchi.

Step 4: Use the correct type of flour. A proportion of two-thirds all-purpose flour to one-third cake flour is ideal. All-purpose flour isn't milled finely enough to be completely absorbed into the potato crumbles. Plus, it has too much protein, or gluten. High-protein wheat results in chewy gnocchi. If you want to "go Italian," look for imported Italian flour marked *00 tenero*, which is milled from soft wheat with a low protein content and can be used in place of the two-flour combination.

Step 5: Use the correct amount of flour. To calculate how much flour to use, weigh the potato *after* it is baked and riced; do not use the raw weight. This is crucial, as the potatoes will lose almost half their weight! Once I understood this, my gnocchi started becoming wondrous. Figure about 1 cup of flour for every pound of sieved potato. Note that some of the riced potato is reserved in case you need it in step 8.

Step 6: Do not add any egg. Despite what many cookbooks say, if you use the right flour, the extra moisture of an egg is superfluous and will simply add more weight to your gnocchi.

Step 7: Combine the potato and flour properly. Most books instruct you to sprinkle the cooked potatoes with flour, gather the mass together, and knead until smooth. Kneading is too harsh an action for this light dough. My advice is to use a bench scraper to blend in about three-quarters of the flour. Later use the remainder of the flour to roll out and shape the dough. Moisture content, age of the potatoes, and even the weather will determine the proper amount of flour.

Step 8: Test the dough first. Check for balance and tenderness by forming a single ¾-inch gnocco (a single dumpling). Boil it in a pot of salted water until it floats to the surface; then scoop it out. If you've used too little flour, the gnocco will have broken apart or may even dissolve; fix simply by adding a little more flour to your dough and test again. If there's too much flour, the dumpling will be hard; in which case, work in a little more reserved potato.

Step 9: Shape the gnocchi according to your whim. Divide the dough into manageable portions and with your hands roll out into ropes ½ to ¾ inch in diameter. Cut into ¾-inch lengths. Then shape.

Step 10: Cook the gnocchi in batches as directed in the recipe. At this point your gnocchi are ready to be sauced and served.

Potato Gnocchi

SERVES 4 TO 6

There are all sorts of wonderful things you can do with these gnocchi. Try dressing them in an unheated pesto sauce as the Ligurians do or tossing them with grated cheese, a bit of foaming butter, and slivered sage leaves as they do in the Piedmont. You can mix them with a chunky tomato sauce or smother with a wild boar ragu. In fact, you can dress up gnocchi in as many ways as you can dress pasta.

PREFERRED CLAY POT:
A 10-inch Spanish cazuela

2 pounds Yukon Gold potatoes

1 to 1½ cups plus 3 or 4 tablespoons coarse salt

About ⅔ cup all-purpose flour

⅓ cup cake or pastry flour

Pinch of fine salt

1 teaspoon extra virgin olive oil

1 Scrub the potatoes and prick all over with a thin skewer or the tip of a knife. Place on a 1-inch bed of salt in the cazuela. Place in the oven and set the temperature at 400°F. Bake for 1½ hours, or until the potatoes are tender. Alternatively, you can pile the potatoes into a dry electric slow cooker and bake them on a ¼-inch bed of salt on the high setting until they are tender, about 3 hours.

(continued)

2 Remove the potatoes and immediately slash open to release the steam. This will allow excess moisture to escape. Slip off the skins while still hot and press the potatoes through a drum sieve or ricer, letting the potato fall onto a large tray or board lined with paper towels. Let rest for at least 30 minutes to dry out and cool down. Weigh the shredded potato. Measure out 1 pound. Reserve the remainder.

3 Sift together the all-purpose flour, cake flour, and a pinch of salt. Turn out the 1 pound of sieved potato onto a pastry board or other work surface. Sprinkle the flour over the potatoes and drizzle with the olive oil. Using a pastry scraper, gently fold the potatoes over the flour, working repeatedly, until it forms a smooth ball with no visible flour.

4 Test the gnocchi dough: Bring a small saucepan of salted water to a boil. Using your hands, form one ¾-inch round—a single gnocco. Boil the gnocco until it floats to the surface, about 1 minute. Using a slotted spoon, transfer it to a plate and let cool. The dumpling should be light and tender but still hold together. If the gnocco breaks apart in the boiling water, the dough has too little flour; work in a little more, 1 to 2 tablespoons at a time. If the gnocco is tough and chewy, the dough has too much flour; cut in a little more of the reserved riced potatoes.

5 Divide the dough into 4 equal pieces. With your hands, roll each into ½-inch-thick ropes. Cut each rope into ¾-inch pieces. Roll each piece against the tines of a fork to flatten slightly and create light ridges. Transfer the gnocchi to a paper towel–lined baking sheet and let stand, uncovered, at room temperature for 1 hour to dry. (This allows the gnocchi to develop a thin skin, which helps them hold their shape when boiled.)

6 Bring a large pot of water to a boil over high heat. Add 1 tablespoon coarse salt for each quart of water. You don't need to be exact; just be sure there is plenty of salt. Fill a large bowl with ice water. Add about 12 gnocchi at a time to the boiling water. Cover the pot immediately to return the water to a boil quickly; then uncover and boil until the gnocchi rise to surface. Wait about 15 seconds until they turn over; then immediately scoop them out with a long-handled strainer; "shock" them by dipping them into the bowl of ice water to stop the cooking. Drain on paper towels. Repeat with the remaining gnocchi. (The gnocchi can be prepared to this point up to 3 hours in advance. Set aside at room temperature. Or freeze as described in the Note. Then sauce and bake as suggested in the recipe that follows.)

NOTE TO THE COOK: In *Bouchon,* chef Thomas Keller provides the following tip for freezing potato gnocchi after they are cooked. After they are shocked and drained, arrange the gnocchi on large sheet pans or baking trays. Freeze them on the pans, uncovered, until they are hard. Then portion into freezer bags or storage containers and freeze for up to 6 weeks. When you are ready to cook them, partially defrost, sauté on one side only in hot butter in a large skillet for about 2 minutes, and arrange in a buttered cazuela. Cover with a sauce and bake in a preheated 350°F oven for about 20 minutes.

Chestnut Potato Gnocchi

Prepare the recipe for Potato Gnocchi as directed, but substitute ⅓ cup chestnut flour for the cake flour.

Potato Gnocchi with Radicchio, Sweet Gorgonzola, and Pine Nuts

SERVES 4 TO 6

I usually bake and serve gnocchi in a ceramic gratin, relieving me of the stress of last-minute cooking. These pillowy light gnocchi can take a really lush sauce like this one from the Emilia-Romagna region of Italy, which balances the sweetness and sharpness of Gorgonzola cheese with the smoky bitterness of radicchio.

Gorgonzola comes in three grades: *dolce* ("sweet"), *medio* ("medium"), and *piccante* ("piquant"). For this sauce, the sweet, which is often labeled *Gorgonzola dolce latte,* is best. Serve this dish as a first course or for lunch.

PREFERRED CLAY POT:

A large rectangular earthenware or stoneware baking dish, about 9 × 13 inches

---

2 tablespoons unsalted butter

Potato Gnocchi (page 225)

1 tablespoon extra virgin olive oil

2 ounces thinly sliced lean pancetta, shredded

2 garlic cloves, minced

1 medium head of radicchio (8 ounces), cored and slivered

⅓ cup heavy cream

⅓ cup milk

4½ ounces Gorgonzola dolce latte, crumbled

Salt and freshly ground black pepper

½ cup grated freshly grated Parmigiano-Reggiano cheese

3 tablespoons dried bread crumbs

3 tablespoons pine nuts

1 Preheat the oven to 350°F. In a large nonstick skillet, melt the butter. Add the gnocchi and cook over high heat until browned on the bottom, about 2 minutes. Transfer to the baking dish.

2 In the same skillet, heat the olive oil over medium heat. Add the pancetta, garlic, and radicchio and cook until soft and glazed, about 5 minutes. Add the cream, milk, and Gorgonzola cheese. Simmer, stirring, until the cheese is melted and the sauce is smooth. Season with salt and pepper to taste.

3 Spoon the sauce over and around the gnocchi in the baking dish. Top with the Parmigiano-Reggiano cheese, bread crumbs, and pine nuts. Bake for 30 minutes, or until the gratin is golden. Serve while still bubbling.

NOTES TO THE COOK:

☀ Gorgonzola will continue to age under refrigeration, increasing in piquancy as it does. To slow this process, wrap the cheese tightly in plastic wrap and store in the coldest part of your refrigerator.

☀ If the pancetta is fatty, fry it alone in step 2 for 5 minutes. Remove excess fat and continue cooking as directed.

Slow-Roasted Tomatoes with Rosewater

SERVES 6

*H*ere is an unusual salad from the famed Hotel Mamounia in Marrakech—unusual because it is not made this way anywhere else. The hotel manager, Robert Bergé, kindly gave me the recipe and told me it was a brilliant variation by a French chef inspired by Moroccan salads and vegetable accompaniments. "And who was this brilliant chef?" I asked. He turned out to be the very famous Daniel Boulud.

Slices of moist, charred sweet tomatoes, caramelized with raw sugar and cinnamon, are baked, drizzled with floral water, and finally topped with toasted sesame seeds or pine nuts.

Rosewater is the condiment of choice in Marrakech, a city famous for its roses.

Preferred Clay Pot:

A 10-inch stoneware or earthenware baking dish

Suggested Clay Environment:

Double slabs of pizza stones or food-safe quarry tiles set on the upper and lower oven racks

7 or 8 red ripe medium tomatoes

Coarse sea salt

1 tablespoon turbinado sugar

Pinch of ground cinnamon

1 tablespoon extra virgin olive oil

2 tablespoons rosewater

2 tablespoons pine nuts or sesame seeds, toasted

1 Cut each tomato in half horizontally and squeeze gently to extract the seeds. Lightly salt the tomatoes, turn them upside down on paper towels, and let drain for 30 minutes.

2 Gently squeeze the tomatoes again to rid them of any excess moisture. Arrange in a single layer in the lightly oiled stoneware baking dish. Mix 1 teaspoon coarse salt with the sugar and cinnamon; sprinkle a pinch over each tomato half. Drizzle with the olive oil.

3 Place the tomatoes in the oven and set the temperature at 250°F. Bake for 3 hours.

4 Raise the oven temperature to 400°F and continue to bake for 30 minutes. Turn off the oven and let the tomatoes finish baking in the receding heat; they will be wrinkled and slightly charred.

5 Remove the roasted tomatoes from the oven. Splash with the rosewater and scatter the toasted nuts on top. Let stand until cooled to room temperature.

Zucchini Musakka with Tomatoes and Chickpeas

SERVES 6

The word *musakka* (spelled *moussaka* in Greece, and *mussak'a* in Lebanon and Syria) describes different dishes in different countries. This southern Turkish version has been popularized by Musa Dağdeviren, a tall, talkative, playful Turkish chef who does more miraculous things with vegetables than anyone else I know. His restaurant, Ciya, on the Asian side of Istanbul, is a national treasure house of Turkish regional food. Every foodie in Istanbul raves about Musa's cooking and the opportunity he provides to taste regional specialties never before served in the city.

His *musakka* is an assembly of summer vegetables (tomatoes and zucchini) packed into a thick, deep Turkish clay pot called a *guvec,* covered with a thin veil of mashed garlic and lemon juice and garnished with some warmed mint-scented olive oil just before being set in the oven. The dish bakes until the vegetables are fully cooked and the oil has browned the top lightly. After baking the musakka is left to cool, to be served at room temperature with a good spoonful of yogurt mixed with garlic and parsley.

> **PREFERRED CLAY POT:**
>
> A 3- or 4-quart *guvec,* La Chamba or flameware casserole, or deep cazuela
>
> If using an electric or ceramic stovetop, be sure to use a heat diffuser with the clay pot.

Kosher salt and freshly ground black pepper

2 pounds medium zucchini, halved lengthwise and sliced crosswise ¾ inch thick

¼ cup extra virgin olive oil

8 ounces ground lamb

2 medium onions, finely chopped

2 cups crushed tomatoes or 1 can (14 ounces) fire-roasted crushed tomatoes

3 tablespoons Turkish sweet red pepper paste

1 cup cooked chickpeas

1 tablespoon mashed garlic

1 tablespoon fresh lemon juice

2 teaspoons dried mint, finely crushed

2 cups plain yogurt

3 tablespoons chopped fresh flat-leaf parsley

1 Preheat the oven to 375°F.

2 In a large bowl, combine 6 cups water and 2 tablespoons kosher salt and stir until dissolved. Add the zucchini and soak for 15 minutes. (This ensures that the skin will remain green and the white flesh will remain crisp during cooking.) Drain and pat dry, pressing gently to remove as much moisture as possible.

3 In the guvec, heat half of the olive oil with the lamb over medium-low heat. When everything is hot, raise the heat to medium and cook, stirring often, until the meat loses its redness, 3 to 4 minutes. Add the onions and cook, stirring occasionally, until the onions are softened, about 5 minutes.

(continued)

4 Stir the crushed tomatoes and the pepper paste into the meat. Add the zucchini and cook, stirring, until well coated with the tomato. Stir in the chickpeas and season with salt and pepper. Mix the garlic and lemon juice to a smooth paste and brush over the contents of the guvec. Quickly heat the remaining olive oil in a small conventional skillet. Add the crushed mint; stir for an instant. Sprinkle over the vegetables. Place in the oven and bake for 30 minutes.

5 Serve at room temperature with an accompanying bowl of yogurt mixed with the chopped parsley.

FRENCH VEGETABLE TIANS, CASSOLOS, AND GRATINS

When we hear the words *gratin* and *au gratin,* we rightly think of wonderful, luscious clay pot–cooked dishes with burnished crusty tops. In fact, the word *gratin* literally means to "scratch" or scrape. Some pundits believe this is a reference to the procedure by which bits of food, clinging to the sides of the cooking vessel, are loosened and stirred back into the meld.

The recipes that follow are named after one or another of the various ceramic baking dishes in which they're cooked and served: the tian, the *cassolo,* or the plain old gratin dish. These traditional heartwarming recipes are rarely found on restaurant menus. Rather, they represent true French family-style farmhouse cooking. Traditionally the dishes were assembled at home in earthenware vessels, which were then carried to a communal village wood-burning bread oven for slow, even baking in the receding heat. In the recipes that follow I encourage you to simulate this bread oven effect by altering your home oven environment (see page xviii). If you do so, you'll be able to replicate these French country gratins at their best.

Spinach, chard, eggplant, zucchini, leeks, and potatoes are mainstays of these dishes. Herbs, oil and/ or butter, cream, bread crumbs, and cheese are often added for flavor and to encourage the formation of a good top crust. Eggs, bits of meat, poultry, salt cod, or anchovies are also sometimes added to the mix.

A typical ceramic gratin dish, such as the Provençal tian, tends to be round with flared edges. On the other hand, *cassolos,* popular in France's Camargue and Languedoc regions, tend to be deep and range in size from very small to a full gallon. This large size is used to cook cassoulets. You can substitute any earthenware or stoneware baking dish—whether square, rectangular, oval, or round, straight sided or flared—for these traditional vessels.

These ceramic dishes retain heat, thus encouraging slow, even cooking. The object is to create dishes that are soft and moist below and glazed and crusty on top. They are also perfect for serving the finished dish, whether hot from the oven or at room temperature.

Cassolo of Spinach and Artichokes

SERVES 6

I came across this method for preparing spinach and artichokes in an old cookbook, *Vielles Recettes de Cuisine Provençale*, which I purchased in Marseille in the early 1980s. The recipe comes from the Camargue, an area lying on the coast between the Languedoc-Roussillon and Provence.

What attracted me to the recipe was, first, the name of the specified pot. I had always thought of a *cassolo* as a gallon-size flared clay pot used to cook cassoulet. Now I learn that in the Camargue it can also refer to a very small flared dish used to cook vegetables.

The second thing that struck me was the instruction to add chopped raw spinach to the *cassolo* without blanching it first. Similarly, the thinly sliced artichoke rounds were to be added to the dish without a preliminary bathing in acidic water. Reading this, I worried that the dish might turn out somewhat bitter and the artichokes turn a nasty brown color. In fact what emerged was an unusual velvety, mellow blend in which the thinly sliced artichokes seemed to have dissolved into the spinach. This dish is stunning and is even more delicious the following day.

To remove excess moisture from spinach (or, for the matter, any type of leafy green) I use an eastern Mediterranean method, stemming and shredding the leaves, salting them lightly, and allowing them to wilt for a short while before rinsing and squeezing out as much excess water as possible. For this recipe I recommend using large leafy spinach rather than the tiny baby leaves.

PREFERRED CLAY POT:

A 3 to 4 cup shallow earthenware baking dish

SUGGESTED CLAY ENVIRONMENT:

Double slabs of pizza stones or food-safe quarry tiles set on the upper and lower oven racks

3 to 4 bunches of large fresh spinach (about 3 pounds)

Coarse salt

3 large globe artichokes

2 garlic cloves

8 fresh flat-leaf parsley sprigs, stems removed

½ teaspoon freshly ground black pepper

2 tablespoons all-purpose flour

½ cup milk

3 tablespoons fresh fine bread crumbs

2 tablespoons grated Gruyère or Comté cheese

Extra virgin olive oil

1 About 2 hours before serving, remove the stems from the spinach, discarding any blemished or yellow leaves. Rinse and drain the spinach. Coarsely shred the leaves, put them in a colander set over a bowl, and toss with 1½ teaspoons coarse salt. Let wilt and drain for 15 minutes; be sure to keep the spinach water that collects underneath.

(continued)

2 To prepare the artichokes, cut the top quarter off 1 artichoke and snip the pointy tips that remain. Remove the tough outer leaves by snapping them back. Trim the bottom to remove any tough dark green exterior with a small paring knife or a swivel-bladed vegetable peeler. Remove the hairy choke in the center with a melon scoop, then scrape along the inside wall of the artichoke bottom until smooth. Drop the trimmed artichoke into the bowl of spinach water collected in step 1 to prevent it from darkening. Repeat with the remaining artichokes. One by one, thinly slice the artichoke bottoms horizontally into rounds and return to the spinach water.

3 Preheat the oven to 350°F. Rinse the spinach. Gently squeeze the spinach in your hands to remove excess moisture; finely chop it with a mezzaluna or a large sharp knife. Finely chop the garlic and parsley. Mix the spinach with the parsley, garlic, pepper, flour, and milk.

4 Spread one-third of the spinach mixture over the bottom of the baking dish. Cover with a layer of artichoke slices, then another layer of spinach. Repeat ending with a layer of artichoke slices. Scatter the breadcrumbs and cheese on top. Drizzle the olive oil over the casserole and set in the oven.

5 Bake for 40 minutes. Transfer the hot casserole to a wooden surface or folded towel to prevent cracking. Serve warm, right from the dish.

Tian of Eggplant, Tomato, and Fresh Cheese

SERVES 4 TO 5

Here is a personal favorite, a tian of ripe summer vegetables at their peak—layers of small heirloom tomatoes, sweet bulb onions, thin-skinned eggplant, and fresh salty cheese such as ricotta or chèvre. I like to prepare this tian in the morning and serve it no sooner than 6 hours after it has emerged from the oven, allowing time for the flavors to meld. It should be left at room temperature; refrigeration diminishes the taste.

My method of setting the tian in a preheated clay-lined oven and then, at the appropriate time, turning the oven off and allowing the tian to set for an additional thirty minutes in the receding heat simulates the way food cooks in a traditional wood-burning oven. That is, first the food is cooked in the hottest part over the wood fire; then the tian is moved to the coolest part of the oven to finish the development of its topping.

PREFERRED CLAY POT:
A 9- or 10-inch round earthenware baking dish or pie dish

SUGGESTED CLAY ENVIRONMENT:
Double slabs of pizza stones or food-safe quarry tiles set on the upper and lower oven racks

1¼ pounds long, slender eggplants

Coarse salt

6 small ripe tomatoes (about 1½ pounds)

½ cup soft cheese, such as ricotta or fresh goat cheese, at room temperature

1½ tablespoons all-purpose flour

⅓ cup milk

1 egg

½ teaspoon freshly ground black pepper

¼ teaspoon freshly grated nutmeg

3 tablespoons extra virgin olive oil

1 bay leaf

2 fresh thyme sprigs

¼ cup chopped fresh flat-leaf parsley

½ cup chopped spring bulb onion, green or bunching onion, or fat scallions

2 garlic cloves, peeled and bruised

1½ ounces Parmigiano-Reggiano cheese, grated (⅓ cup)

2 pinches of sugar

1 Trim and peel the eggplants. Cut lengthwise into slices about ½ inch thick. Sprinkle both sides with salt and drain in a colander for 30 minutes. Rinse the eggplant slices and pat dry.

2 Use a serrated swivel-bladed vegetable peeler to skin the tomatoes or dip them briefly in a pot of boiling water and slip off the skins. Slice the tomatoes and spread them out on paper towels. Dust lightly with coarse salt.

3 In a mixing bowl, mash the soft cheese with the flour and milk until smooth. Beat in the egg. Season with ½ teaspoon salt, the pepper, and the nutmeg. Set the cheese mixture aside.

4 Heat 1 tablespoon of the olive oil in a medium conventional skillet. Add the bay leaf, thyme, parsley, spring bulb onion, and one of the garlic cloves. Cook over medium-low heat until the onion is soft and golden, about 10 minutes. Remove from the heat and discard the bay leaf.

5 Preheat the oven to 400°F. Set a ridged grill pan over medium-high heat; lightly brush with olive oil. When the pan is hot, grill the eggplant, in batches as necessary, turning once, until lightly browned, about 2 minutes on each side.

6 Rub the earthenware baking dish with the second garlic clove and brush with oil. Layer about half of the eggplant slices over the bottom. Combine the onion and cheese mixture and spread on top. Cover with a layer of half of the tomatoes. Add another layer of eggplant slices, sprinkle with the Parmigiano-Reggiano cheese, and top with the remaining tomato slices. Sprinkle the sugar and remaining oil on top and bake for 1 hour.

7 Turn off the heat and leave the tian in the oven for another 45 to 60 minutes, or until the tomatoes acquire a lovely charred edge but remain shiny on top. Serve directly from the dish at room temperature. Do not refrigerate.

Gratin of Leeks and Pancetta

SERVES 4

This luscious tian of skinny leeks is out of the ordinary. Rather than simply boiling and baking the leeks and topping them with the standard Gruyère or Swiss cheese, here baby leeks are blanched briefly and pressed to remove as much moisture as possible. Then they are baked atop a bed of flavorful pancetta and smothered with Gorgonzola *dolce latte* or a soft goat cheese.

> **PREFERRED CLAY POT:**
>
> **A 9-inch Spanish cazuela, or La Chamba or flameware skillet**
>
> **If using an electric or ceramic stovetop, be sure to use a heat diffuser with the clay pot.**
>
> **SUGGESTED CLAY ENVIRONMENT:**
>
> **Double slabs of pizza stones or food-safe quarry tiles set on the upper and lower oven racks**

8 to 12 baby leeks (about 2½ ounces each)

½ teaspoon salt

2 large eggs

3½ ounces Gorgonzola dolce latte or a natural soft goat cheese, at room temperature

⅓ cup heavy cream

2 tablespoons freshly grated Parmigiano-Reggiano cheese

3 ounces sliced pancetta, slivered

1 tablespoon extra virgin olive oil or unsalted butter

2 tablespoons fresh bread crumbs

1 Trim the leeks to remove the hairy roots. Remove the thick outer dark green leaf. Rinse the leeks well. Place them in the cazuela, cover with water, add the salt, cover with a sheet of foil or a cover, and gradually bring the water to a boil. Turn off the heat and let the leeks soak in the hot water for 15 minutes. Drain the leeks and pat dry on a kitchen towel. Press to remove as much moisture as possible; fold each in half so they are doubled. Wipe out the cazuela.

2 Preheat the oven to 350°F. In a medium bowl, beat the eggs with the Gorgonzola until fairly well blended. Whisk in the cream and half of the Parmigiano-Reggiano cheese.

3 Add the pancetta and olive oil to the cleaned cazuela and set it over low heat. When the pan is hot, slowly raise the heat to medium and cook until the pancetta is golden, about 4 minutes. Arrange the folded leeks on top, spread out like the spokes of a wheel. Dollop the cheese and cream mixture over the leeks and sprinkle the bread crumbs and remaining Parmigiano-Reggiano on top. Press down with the back of a spatula to spread into a thin layer.

4 Set on the middle shelf of the oven. Raise the heat to 400°F and bake for 40 minutes, or until the tian is bubbling and the top is golden brown. Turn off the oven and let bake in the receding heat for 20 minutes longer. Serve directly from the cazuela.

Roasted Late Summer Vegetables from the Island of Corfu

SERVES 6

I learned this quintessential clay pot vegetable dish on the island of Corfu. In typical fashion, it was a female cook who presided over a type of restaurant called a *koutoukian,* a small eating place with just eight to ten tables, situated in the garden of a private home. *Koutoukians* are one-woman shows; people come because they know the cook personally, and they know her food is honest. Only the freshest ingredients are used, and the olive oil in which they're cooked is locally pressed.

A Corfu-style vegetable mélange is called a *tourlou.* My recipe is for a late-summer version made with tomatoes, zucchini, eggplant, and onions strewn with fresh herbs and a good dousing of fragrant extra virgin olive oil. This is Greek food at its best— simple, honest, without any pretension, and baked in clay in a wood-burning oven.

PREFERRED CLAY POT:

A large earthenware or stoneware baking dish such as a lasagna pan

SUGGESTED CLAY ENVIRONMENT:

Double slabs of pizza stones or food-safe quarry tiles set on the upper and lower oven racks

1½ pounds red ripe tomatoes, peeled, cored, and sliced

1 pound zucchini, cut into ½-inch slices

1 pound eggplant, peeled, cut into 1¼-inch chunks

Coarse sea salt

¼ cup fruity extra virgin olive oil

1½ pounds Yukon Gold potatoes, peeled and cut into 6 wedges each

1 pound medium red or yellow onions, cut into 6 wedges each

2 celery ribs, cut into 1¼-inch chunks

4 minced garlic cloves

1 teaspoon sugar

½ teaspoon fresh ground black pepper

½ cup chopped fresh flat-leaf parsley

1½ tablespoons chopped fresh dill

1 teaspoon chopped fresh mint or marjoram

1   Preheat the oven to 400°F. Lay out the tomato, zucchini, and eggplant slices on separate trays or sheets of wax paper and salt them lightly. Let stand for 10 to 15 minutes. Pat dry with paper towels.

2   Brush the gratin with 1 tablespoon of the olive oil. Alternating the tomatoes, zucchini, and eggplant, arrange half of the slices on the bottom of the dish. Scatter the potatoes, onions, and celery on top. Lay the remaining zucchini and tomatoes over these vegetables. Sprinkle with the garlic, 2 teaspoons salt, the sugar, pepper, parsley, dill, and mint. Drizzle the remaining 3 tablespoons olive oil over all.

3   Bake, uncovered, for 30 minutes. Stir carefully to redistribute the vegetables and bake for another 30 minutes. Turn off the oven heat and let the vegetables bake without disturbing for 15 minutes longer. Serve hot, warm, or at room temperature.

PEELING CHICKPEAS

If peeling chickpeas sounds daunting, please don't be put off by the task. Keep in mind that it's always an optional step. But getting rid of that fibrous, tasteless outer skin endows the chickpeas with more intense flavor, creamier texture, and greater digestibility and makes the dishes feel lighter.

There are numerous ways to peel chickpeas. The fastest is to submerge hot, partially or fully cooked, peas a handful at a time in a deep bowl of cool water, plunge your hands into the water, and gently rub the peels off. As the peels rise to the surface, remove and discard them. Drain the chickpeas when you're through.

The last time I was in Morocco, an old friend took me to lunch at the home of Saad Hajouji, grandson of El Glaoui, the legendary pasha of Marrakech. The food was lavish and included pigeons smothered in raisins with huge amounts of peeled chickpeas and peeled green grapes in a sauce seasoned with onions, nutmeg, saffron, ginger, black pepper, cubed lamb's liver, and a touch of vanilla. This was Moroccan palace cookery at its finest, highly labor intensive and reproducible only if one has a staff of old women cooks, called *dadas*.

In Israel, I met a Palestinian restaurateur famous for his hummus. He told me his secret was to pound cooked chickpeas in a stone mortar and then press them through a very fine sieve to catch the skins while allowing the inner flesh to pass through.

Chef Fulvio Pierangelini of the Gambero Rosso restaurant in San Vincenzo in Livorno, Italy, shared his technique in the recipe for Chickpea Puree with Shrimp. He's adamant that the chickpeas not be processed first, lest the skins become blended with the flesh. He soaks chickpeas overnight in very salty water, washes off the salt in the morning, and then cooks them in a clay pot with flavorings until tender. After cooking, he peels them and then presses them through a fine sieve.

What intrigued me most about this chef's method was his use of excessive salty water, since I'd always been taught that too much salt will turn beans mealy. To understand his method I contacted the Salt Institute, where I spoke to its technical director and molecular biologist, Dr. Morton Satin. A lover of Italian food, he immediately understood my question and gave me an excellent answer.

Dr. Satin told me that, first, salt helps dissolve the protein layer that holds the skin to the bodies of chickpeas. Second, it brings out their natural sweetness by moderating their mildly bitter flavor. And third, due to the salt soaking, when rinsed and subsequently cooked in fresh water, the bodies of the peas expand and split right out of their skins.

I now use this method for preparing the smoothest and most digestible hummus (page 237).

My Best Hummus

MAKES ABOUT 1⅓ CUPS

This is the best recipe I know for preparing hummus. I use an electric blender to achieve the smoothest and glossiest version. Peeling and sieving the chickpeas takes about ten minutes.

PREFERRED CLAY POTS:

A 3-quart Chinese sandpot or beanpot

If using an electric or ceramic stovetop, be sure to use a heat diffuser with the clay pot.

---

1 cup dried chickpeas

Coarse sea salt

¼ cup tahini, preferably organic

2 garlic cloves, crushed

¼ cup fresh lemon juice

1 to 2 tablespoons extra virgin olive oil

Ground cumin and/or crushed hot red pepper for garnish

1 In a large bowl, soak the chickpeas with 3 cups water and 3 tablespoons coarse salt for at least 12 hours.

2 Drain the chickpeas, rinse them well, and put them in a 3-quart sandpot or other earthenware casserole. Add enough fresh cold water to cover by about 3 inches. Set over medium-low heat and bring the water to a boil. Reduce the heat to a simmer and cook, partially covered, until the chickpeas are very tender, about 2 hours. Add more boiling water if the water evaporates.

3 Drain the chickpeas, reserving about ¼ cup of the cooking liquor. Working by the handful, submerge the chickpeas in a deep pot or bowl of cold water and rub the chickpeas between your hands to rub and pinch off the skins. The skins will rise to the surface; remove and discard them. Repeat with the remaining handfuls of chickpeas. Set aside about ¼ cup peeled chickpeas for garnish.

4 Stir up the tahini in its jar with the oil until well blended. Place tahini in blender jar and blend the tahini, garlic, and lemon juices until the mixture "whitens." With the machine running, add the reserved liquor. Add 1¾ cups peeled chickpeas and process until smooth and glossy. Correct the seasoning with salt and lemon juice. Allow the hummus to mellow at room temperature for 1 to 2 hours.

5 To serve as a dip, spread the puree on a shallow serving dish. Use the back of a spoon to make a well in the center, drizzle with olive oil, and sprinkle with cumin and/or hot pepper, and scatter the reserved chickpeas on top.

Chickpea Puree with Shrimp

SERVES 4

I'm indebted to my good friend, cookbook author Faith Willinger, who has lived in Florence for more than three decades, for obtaining and publishing this wonderful modern Italian recipe in her cookbook *Adventures of an Italian Food Lover: With Recipes from 254 of My Best Friends*. One of Faith's numerous "best friends" is Chef Fulvio Pierangelini of the Gambero Rosso restaurant in San Vincenzo in Livorno, Italy, who works, Faith tells me, with a full complement of the latest kitchen equipment—except when it comes to chickpeas. These, he insists, must be cooked the old-fashioned way, which means, of course, in a clay pot.

The chef bills this dish as a soup, and serves it in small warmed individual ramekins with four to five shrimp on top of each serving. The taste and texture of the chickpeas are heavenly—deliciously nutty and wonderfully silky.

As noted in the box on page 236, this recipe requires peeling the chickpeas and sieving them through the finest strainer to obtain a silky puree.

PREFERRED CLAY POTS:

A 3-quart Chinese sandpot or beanpot

4 ramekins (6 ounces each)

If using an electric or ceramic stovetop, be sure to use a heat diffuser with the clay pot.

---

1 cup dried chickpeas

Sea salt and freshly ground black pepper

1 garlic clove

1 fresh rosemary sprig

¼ cup extra virgin olive oil

3 tablespoons heavy cream

1 pound medium shrimp, in their shells

Zest of 1 lemon

1 In a large bowl, soak the chickpeas in 3 cups water with 3 or 4 tablespoons of sea salt for at least 12 hours and up to 24 hours.

2 Drain the chickpeas, rinse them well, and put them in the sandpot with the garlic and rosemary. Add enough fresh cold water to cover by about 3 inches. Set over medium-low heat and bring the water to a boil. Reduce the heat to low and cook, partially covered, until the chickpeas are very tender, about 2 hours.

3 Drain the chickpeas, reserving about 1 cup of the cooking liquid. Working by the handful, submerge the chickpeas in a deep pot or bowl of cold water and rub the chickpeas between your palms and fingers to rub or pinch off most of the skins. The skins will rise to the surface; remove and discard. Repeat with the remaining handfuls of chickpeas.

4 Place a flat fine-mesh sieve or tamis over a mixing bowl. Working in batches, use a dough scraper to press the peeled chickpeas across the sieve. Repeat with the remaining chickpeas. You should have about 1¼ cups pureed chickpeas.

5 Stir in the cream, 2 tablespoons of the olive oil, and ¼ cup of the chickpea-cooking liquor. Season to taste with salt and pepper and keep warm.

6 Preheat the oven to 400°F. Meanwhile, clean and peel the shrimp. Season them lightly with salt and pepper and toss with the lemon zest and 1 tablespoon olive oil. Place the shrimp close together on a sheet of aluminum foil. Cover with a second sheet of foil and crimp the edges to seal. Place on a baking sheet and slide into the oven. Bake for 3 to 4 minutes, until just cooked.

7 Fill each of 4 ramekins with one fourth of the warm puree, top with 4 or 5 of the shrimp, drizzle with remaining 1 tablespoon olive oil, and sprinkle with a little freshly ground pepper and a pinch of salt. Serve at once.

SPICED WHEAT AND BEAN BREAKFAST DRINK

One of the oldest methods for handling and preserving grains is still alive and well on the Tunisian island of Djerba. Every morning, while staying in a home there, I was served the family breakfast of *zommita,* a drink made with beans and grains that had been toasted in a dry unglazed earthenware skillet similar to a Mexican *comal.* After toasting, the beans (dried split favas and chickpeas), grains (skinned wheat berries), and aromatics (ground cumin, ground caraway, ground red pepper, ground fennel seeds, crushed aniseed, oregano, dried orange peel, and salt) were milled into a spicy flour—perhaps one of the earliest forms of instant cereal!

A Tunisian woman typically makes her *zommita* with forty pounds of grain, spending an entire day toasting, grilling, and grinding. This flour, stored in clay jars, is quickly turned into a breakfast drink by the addition of a little olive oil and cold water.

Casserole of Lentils, Eggplant, and Mint

SERVES 4 TO 6

*H*ere's a delicious summer recipe from the coastal town of Senköyon on the Bay of Iskenderun near the Turkish Mediterranean coast. In every home in this town there's a small iron wood-burning stove called a kuzine that's kept lit all day long, even in summer. These stoves are perfect for clay pot cooking—just what's needed for this outstanding summer lentil dish.

What makes this dish stellar is the special technique used to prepare the eggplant slices. They are not merely salted but immersed in heavily salted water, which removes any bitter juices but keeps them plump. Another distinguishing trick is the way the slices that line the bottom of the dish are notched along their sides. These indentations ensure that any liquid that seeps down from above will be absorbed fully. Slow, steady cooking keeps this bottom layer from burning—and, in fact, transforms it into a lovely skin.

I like to make this dish early in the day and allow it to rest. It's served at room temperature accompanied by bowls of garlic-spiked yogurt.

> **PREFERRED CLAY POT:**
>
> A 10- inch Spanish cazuela
>
> If using an electric or ceramic stovetop, be sure to use a heat diffuser with the clay pot.

2 pounds long, slender eggplant

Coarse salt

¾ cup dried green lentils (4 ounces)

2 pounds ripe tomatoes, halved, seeded, and grated

1 small onion, finely chopped

6 garlic cloves, chopped

⅓ cup loosely packed coarsely chopped fresh mint leaves

1 mild green chile, preferably Anaheim or Italian frying pepper, stemmed, seeded, and chopped

1 tablespoon Turkish sweet red pepper paste

1 tablespoon tomato paste, preferably homemade (page 317)

¼ teaspoon Marash or Aleppo pepper

¼ teaspoon freshly ground black pepper

⅓ cup extra virgin olive oil

3½ tablespoons imported pomegranate molasses or California pomegranate concentrate plus 1 teaspoon fresh lemon juice

1 At intervals, peel 3 lengthwise strips of skin from each eggplant, leaving it striped; cut each eggplant lengthwise into 6 slices. In a large bowl, dissolve ¼ cup coarse salt in 2 quarts water. Add the eggplant, push it down to submerge it, and soak for at least 30 minutes. Rinse and drain the eggplant and pat dry. With the point of a knife, make a series of small slits along the edges of half of the eggplant slices.

2 Meanwhile, put the lentils in a small conventional saucepan, add enough water to cover by at least 2 inches, and bring to a boil. Reduce the heat to medium and simmer until the lentils are about half cooked, 15 to 20 minutes. Drain the lentils and set aside.

3 In a mixing bowl, combine the grated tomatoes, onion, garlic, 2 tablespoons of the mint, the green chile, red pepper paste, tomato paste, Marash pepper, 1 tablespoon coarse salt, and black pepper.

4 Brush the cazuela with 1 tablespoon of the olive oil Arrange the snipped eggplant slices over the bottom in a single layer. Top with half of the lentils and half of the tomato mixture; repeat with the remaining eggplant, lentils, and tomato. In a small bowl, whisk together the pomegranate molasses and remaining olive oil; drizzle over the top.

5 Cover and bring to a boil; remove the cover and cook over low heat for 1½ hours. Remove from the heat and let cool for at least 2 and up to 6 hours. Serve at room temperature, with the remaining shredded mint scattered on top.

With thanks to Musa Dağdeviren and Ayfer Ünsal for sharing this recipe.

MEDITERRANEAN BEAN POTS

A bean pot is one cooking vessel that *must* be made of clay, whether it's produced in Boston, Italy, Egypt, Mexico, Spain, or China. There's just a special affinity between earthenware and beans. Shape matters too. In Spain, earthenware bean pots, called ollas, are tall and straight. The Greek *yiouvetsis* and Turkish *comleks,* with unglazed exteriors and glazed interiors, are also straight sided and short. Yankee bean pots, like the Italian *coccio* are squat and potbellied. The Italians also have a tall, straight-sided bean pot, called a *pignata.*

When I lived in Tangier, Morocco, Fatima Ben Lahsen Riffi, my housekeeper, showed me one day how to use a *gedra,* a potbellied clay bean pot from her native village. She cooked dried fava beans in it and then used a smaller clay bowl to crush them against the sides until they turned smooth, at which point she worked in garlic and olive oil to create a dip she served with anise-flavored bread. (See my *Slow Mediterranean Cooking* for a Marrakech version of this dish.)

Red Beans with Chorizo, Blood Sausage, and Piment d'Espelette

SERVES 4

The basis of this great pepper- and vinegar-scented Basque stew textured with pork sausages is the purplish *alubia de Tolosa,* one of the most coveted beans in Spain. Since alubias are difficult to find, I've substituted the earthy scarlet runner or the creamy red nightfall bean, in both cases achieving superb results.

It's best to prepare this stew a day in advance and serve it after a gentle reheating. If you love beans as much as I do, you will not be disappointed.

> **PREFERRED CLAY POTS:**
> A 4-quart Spanish olla, bean pot, or earthenware casserole
> A 10-inch Spanish cazuela
> If using an electric or ceramic stovetop, be sure to use a heat diffuser with the clay pots.

1½ cups dried small red beans, preferably red nightfall or scarlet runner

Coarse salt

4 or 5 ounces pork belly or salt pork

¼ cup extra virgin olive oil

2 medium onions, chopped

2 teaspoons chopped garlic

4 ounces fresh mild chorizo sausage

6 ounces blood sausage, preferably Spanish morcilla con cebolla

2 carrots, cut into 1-inch chunks

1 green bell pepper, peeled and cut into ½-inch squares

¼ teaspoon sugar

Salt and freshly ground black pepper

½ teaspoon *piment d'Espelette* (Spanish paprika)

2 tablespoons chopped fresh flat-leaf parsley

1 teaspoon red wine vinegar

1 Rinse and pick over the beans. Soak in plenty of lightly salted water to cover overnight. The following day, drain the beans, reserving the soaking water. Put the beans in a large conventional saucepan; add just enough of the reserved soaking water to cover and bring to a boil, skimming often.

2 Meanwhile, blanch the pork belly for 10 minutes in a conventional pot of boiling water. Drain, rinse, and pat dry. Cut the pork belly into 1-inch cubes.

3 Heat half of the olive oil in the bean pot over medium heat. Add the onions and the garlic; cook until soft, about 5 minutes. Add the whole chorizo and the cubes of pork belly and sauté for 3 minutes. Add the beans and just enough of the bean-cooking liquid to cover. Place a round of parchment directly on the beans and cover the pot. Cook over very low heat for 1½ to 2 hours, or until the beans are tender but not mushy. (The recipe can be prepared to this point up to 2 days in advance.)

4 About 1 hour before serving, preheat the oven to 350°F. Bring the beans to room temperature. Scoop out the chorizo and cut it into bite-sized pieces. Peel the blood sausage and cut into 6 slices. Heat 1 tablespoon of the remaining olive oil in the cazuela, add the chorizo and blood sausage, and slowly fry until crisp on both sides. Scrape into the beans and stir gently to combine.

5 Add the carrots, bell pepper, sugar, remaining 1 tablespoon olive oil, and salt and pepper to taste. Cook over medium heat for 5 minutes. Add the piment d'Espelette and continue to cook, stirring, until the vegetables are glazed evenly, 2 to 3 minutes.

6 Scoop out ½ cup of the cooking liquid; stir in the parsley and vinegar and set aside. Transfer the beans, sausages, and remaining cooking liquid to the cazuela. Cover with a sheet of foil and place in the oven. Bake for 30 minutes to blend the flavors. Serve hot with a light sprinkling of vinegary bean pot liquor.

SOAKING AND SALTING BEANS

Contrary to popular lore, you can soak and cook beans in the same water without changing it, provided the beans have been sorted and rinsed well beforehand. Also, the water can be salted lightly to boost the flavor without toughening the beans, assuming they are less than two years old and have been stored properly. If in doubt, omit the salt.

Steve Sando of Rancho Gordo Beans told me, "If you know the source of the beans and they're within two years old and properly stored, you can soak or not, salt or not. It's hard to ruin them, and salting does add flavor. In a side-by-side study, soaked beans have a better texture. On the other hand, I just hate to speak in absolutes about beans because there are so many variables, and there are a lot of bad, poorly stored beans out there."

"If you haven't soaked," he added. "don't fret. Go ahead and cook them, knowing it will just take longer."

Two beans that must be soaked are the popular Mediterranean Old World favorites, fava beans and chickpeas, which require at least eight to twenty-four hours. New World beans, such as cannellini, and all white and red beans that come from America, such as lingots and pintos, need about four hours, but an overnight soak won't damage them. If your tap water is heavily chlorinated, use filtered water to cook any dried beans. The timing, texture, and flavor will be much better.

Red Lentil and Bulgur Koftes

SERVES 6

My Turkish friend Filiz Hösukoğlu likes these lentil *koftes* so much that she makes a batch of them for her family and friends at least twice a month. When I first met her in Gaziantep, Turkey, twenty years ago, she was still experimenting with this recipe, working to perfect it. The method she finally came up with to control the moisture is to knead and shape the finger-shaped *koftes* in an unglazed clay pot.

Serve cold, as Filiz does, with pickles, chopped parsley, green onions, and glasses of *ayran*, yogurt thinned with water and seasoned with a pinch of salt.

> **PREFERRED CLAY POT:**
>
> **A large unglazed clay bowl or new flowerpot saucer, scrubbed and dried**

1 cup dried red lentils

1 tablespoon tomato paste, canned or homemade (page 317)

1 tablespoon Turkish sweet red pepper paste

1 cup fine bulgur

½ cup extra virgin olive oil

2 medium onions, finely chopped

3 garlic cloves, chopped

1 to 1½ tablespoons Marash or Aleppo red pepper

1 teaspoon salt

3 spring onions or scallions, chopped

2 green garlic shoots, trimmed, or 2 garlic cloves, chopped

1 cup chopped fresh flat-leaf parsley

½ cup chopped fresh tarragon or 1 teaspoon dried

Romaine lettuce and fresh mint leaves for garnish

1 Rinse and drain the lentils. Place in a medium conventional saucepan, add 5 cups water, and bring to a boil, skimming off any foam that rises to the top. Reduce the heat and simmer until the lentils are soft and creamy, about 30 minutes. Add the tomato paste and sweet red pepper paste and continue to cook, stirring, for 3 minutes longer. Remove from the heat. Add the bulgur and mix together. Set aside to cool.

2 Meanwhile, in a small conventional skillet, heat the olive oil. Add the onions and garlic and sauté over medium-high heat until pale golden, about 3 minutes. Add the Marash pepper and salt. Remove from the heat and let cool.

3 When the lentil mixture is cool enough to handle, turn it out into a clay bowl and knead with your hands for 5 minutes. Mix in the chopped spring onions, garlic shoots, parsley, and tarragon. Add to the lentil mixture and continue kneading for about 5 minutes. Add the sautéed onion with all of its oil. Shape the mixture into finger-length oval patties and arrange on a serving dish lined with romaine and mint leaves.

SOURCING AND SEASONING A TUSCAN BEAN POT

As a clay pot enthusiast, I set out to find an authentic Tuscan bean pot: a clay *coccio* or a *fiasco*. I checked first with friend and fellow food writer Dana Jacobi, author of *The Best of Clay Pot Cooking*. She told me she had one but had never used it because she wasn't sure what sort of tempering it needed.

Through the Internet I found several Italian artisans who specialized in *coccios* handmade from redware clay. The pot I bought from one of them was beautiful—a lightly glazed, two-handled terra-cotta vase with a narrow neck and a mouth just large enough so I could shake out swollen cooked beans.

It was suitable, too, for use in the fireplace, in the oven, or, with a heat diffuser, directly on a gas stovetop.

If you have a Chinese sandpot, it makes a fine stand-in for the *coccio,* either in a wood-burning fireplace or in a 250°F oven. In fact, that's the pot used to cook Tuscan-style beans at the famous Rose Pistola restaurant in San Francisco's North Beach district. But if you do order a *coccio* or purchase one in Italy, be sure to follow any accompanying recommendations for curing the pot and ridding it of its "new clay" flavor.

If there are no instructions, please use my method: Add 2 cups milk and 1 cup water to the pot. Gently warm on a heat diffuser on your stovetop over low heat until the liquid comes to a boil. Transfer the pot to a wooden surface or folded kitchen towel and let stand until completely cool before pouring out the liquid. Finally, rinse the pot thoroughly, scrub with a nonmetal-bristle bottle brush using water but no soap or detergent to remove any milk solids; then set upside down to drain until dry.

On your new pot's maiden voyage, slowly cook either soaked or unsoaked beans for at least 3 hours. These beans will be fine to eat, but the next batch will be even better. As with any clay bean pot, the more you use it, the more flavorful and aromatic the dish.

And please remember that if you place your *coccio* in embers in the fireplace rather than cooking on the stovetop or in a low oven, you'll need to double the cooking time: you're in for an all-day adventure.

In her absorbing cookbook *The Classic Cuisine of the Italian Jews,* Edda Servi Machlin describes the Tuscan bean pots in the Italian town of Pitigliano:

"When the hearth was not only a source of heat, but also the only way to cook meals, a *pignatto* was used to cook beans. A *pignatto* was a tall earthenware pot with a very small bottom, a large belly, and a small opening on the top. It had only one handle. Beans were placed inside the pot with hot water; then the pot was placed at the edge of the hearth with a few red coals very close, under the belly, on the side opposite the handle. The beans cooked to a gentle, even simmering."

Tuscan White Beans with Sage and Garlic

SERVES 4

Tuscany is known for many things: the purity of its spoken Italian, the genius of its artists, the marvelous simplicity of its cuisine. Tuscans are also known as the great bean eaters of the peninsula. Italian slow-cooked bean dishes are famous for their deep flavor and great tenderness as well as for the fabulous thick cooking juices in which they're enrobed.

The most popular dried white beans in Tuscany are cannellini. In some areas, borlotti and small marrow beans are also served. No matter the variety, the basic preparation remains the same: First the beans are soaked overnight. Then they are dropped into a cooking pot, which might be a glazed potbellied earthenware bean pot called a *coccio* or an earthenware chianti wine–shaped bottle called a *fiasco*. Good olive oil, garlic, sage, and bay leaf are added along with enough water to cover the beans by about an inch. The pot is sealed with a lid or knot of kitchen toweling and then nestled in the smoldering embers of a fireplace to cook slowly through the night. The following day, the tender beans are poured out along with their thickened cooking liquid. Some fresh olive oil is poured on top, and the beans are ready to be served or added to other dishes.

Here's the basic recipe for Tuscan white beans. Once these are prepared, you can go on to make many famous Tuscan bean specialties, such as *fagioli con tonno* (white beans with tuna) and *fagioli con pomodoro* (white beans with tomato and sage), page 247.

> **PREFERRED CLAY POT:**
>
> A Tuscan *coccio*, a ceramic bean pot, or a Chinese sandpot
>
> If using an electric or ceramic stovetop, be sure to use a heat diffuser with the clay pot.

1¼ cups dried white or speckled beans, preferably heritage or heirloom beans

Coarse salt

4 garlic cloves, peeled

3 large fresh sage leaves

2 imported bay leaves

¼ cup extra virgin olive oil

Freshly ground black pepper

1 Pick over the beans to remove any grit. Rinse the beans under cold running water; then place them in a large bowl with enough lightly salted water to cover by at least 2 inches, about 6 cups. Soak for a minimum of 4 hours, preferably overnight.

2 The following day, drain the beans, reserving the soaking water. Put the beans in the coccio and season with 2 teaspoons coarse salt. Add just enough of the reserved soaking water to cover the beans by 1 inch. Slowly bring to a simmer over medium heat. Add the garlic, sage, bay leaves, and half of the olive oil. Cover and reduce the heat to low. Cook as slowly as possible for about 3 hours, until the beans still hold their shape but squash easily when pressed between 2 fingers.

3 Drain the beans. Pick out and discard the garlic, sage, and bay leaves. Season with salt and pepper to taste and serve at once.

NOTES TO THE COOK:

※ Though it's true that some varieties of dried beans don't require soaking before cooking, I always soak white beans overnight for *this* recipe.

※ If you prefer to cook the beans in the oven rather than on top of the stove, preheat the oven to 225°F. Cooking time is the same, about 3 hours, but it may well vary depending on the age of the beans. If you wish, turn off the oven after 3 hours and let the beans continue cooking in the receding heat.

※ Try cooking heirloom dried white bean that are no more than two years old for 3 hours at a steady simmer (165°F to168°F). The beans will swell very slowly while absorbing the aromatics, reaching their ultimate size without crumbling.

※ If you plan to store the cooked beans, do not drain them in step 3. Let cool; then transfer the beans and their cooking liquid to a glass or ceramic container, cover, and refrigerate for up to 3 days. Use cooked beans for soups and salads.

White Beans with Tuna

SERVES 4

1½ cups (about half the recipe) cooked and drained Tuscan White Beans with Sage and Garlic (page 246)

1 small red onion, thinly sliced

¼ cup extra virgin olive oil

1 tablespoon strained fresh lemon juice

Salt and freshly ground black pepper

7 ounces oil-packed tuna

1 small ripe tomatoes, diced

1 lemon, cut into wedges

Use 2 forks to toss the beans gently with the red onion, olive oil, lemon juice, and salt and pepper to taste. Mound on a platter. Top with the tuna, broken into small pieces, and the diced tomato. Serve at room temperature, with wedges of lemon on the side.

White Beans with Tomatoes and Sage

SERVES 4

2½ tablespoons extra virgin olive oil

1 teaspoon chopped garlic

4 large fresh sage leaves, slivered

2 medium tomatoes, peeled, seeded and diced

1½ cups (half of the recipe) cooked and drained Tuscan White Beans with Sage and Garlic

Salt and freshly ground black pepper

Heat the olive oil in a large conventional skillet over medium heat. Add the garlic and sauté until golden, about 3 minutes. Add the slivered sage leaves and diced tomatoes. Cook for 10 minutes, stirring occasionally, to make a sauce. Add the beans and cook for 5 minutes longer. Season with salt and pepper to taste and serve hot.

White Beans with Spiced Beef

SERVES 4 TO 6

Basturma is an eastern Mediterranean spicy air-dried meat flavored with a special spice mixture that features sweet and pungent fenugreek. You'll find two types available at Middle Eastern groceries: the Turkish or Armenian type has lots of flavor and also contains more fat, and the Egyptian, which is lean though less tasty. For this dish, please be sure to purchase the fattier variety. The secret to this famous Turkish bean dish is to fry the *basturma* before adding it to the bean pot. The salt and spices will melt into the fat, making the dish exceptionally flavorful and aromatic.

> **PREFERRED CLAY POT:**
>
> A 2½- to 3-quart bean pot or Turkish *guvec*
>
> If using an electric or ceramic stovetop, be sure to use a heat diffuser with the clay pot.

1 cup dried white kidney beans

1 medium onion, chopped

½ large red bell pepper, diced

3 to 4 ounces *basturma,* shredded

3 tablespoons extra virgin olive oil

1 tablespoon tomato paste

3 green cardamom seeds, bruised

1 teaspoon Marash or Aleppo pepper

Salt and freshly ground black pepper

1 Pick over the beans to remove any grit. Rinse the beans under cold running water; then place them in a large bowl with enough lightly salted water to cover by at least 2 inches, about 6 cups. Soak for at least 4 hours or overnight.

2 The following day, drain the beans, reserving the soaking water. Put the beans, onion, and red bell pepper in a 2½- to 3-quart bean pot. Stir in 1¾ cups of the reserved soaking water; reserve the remainder. Cover the pot, set it on a heat diffuser over low heat, and slowly bring to a boil; this can take up to 45 minutes.

3 Boil for 5 minutes, reduce the heat to medium-low, and continue to cook, covered, for 1½ hours, removing the lid from time to time to keep the beans at a constant simmer. If the beans begin to dry out, heat the remaining soaking water and add as necessary.

4 In a small conventional skillet, cook the *basturma* in the olive oil over medium heat until it just begins to crisp, about 3 minutes. Stir in the tomato paste and cook for 30 seconds. Add the cardamom seeds, Marash pepper, a pinch each of salt and pepper, and ¼ cup water. Bring to a boil; then add to the beans. Stir gently, cover, and cook over low heat for 1 hour. Serve hot.

With thanks to Ayfer Ünsal for sharing her recipe.

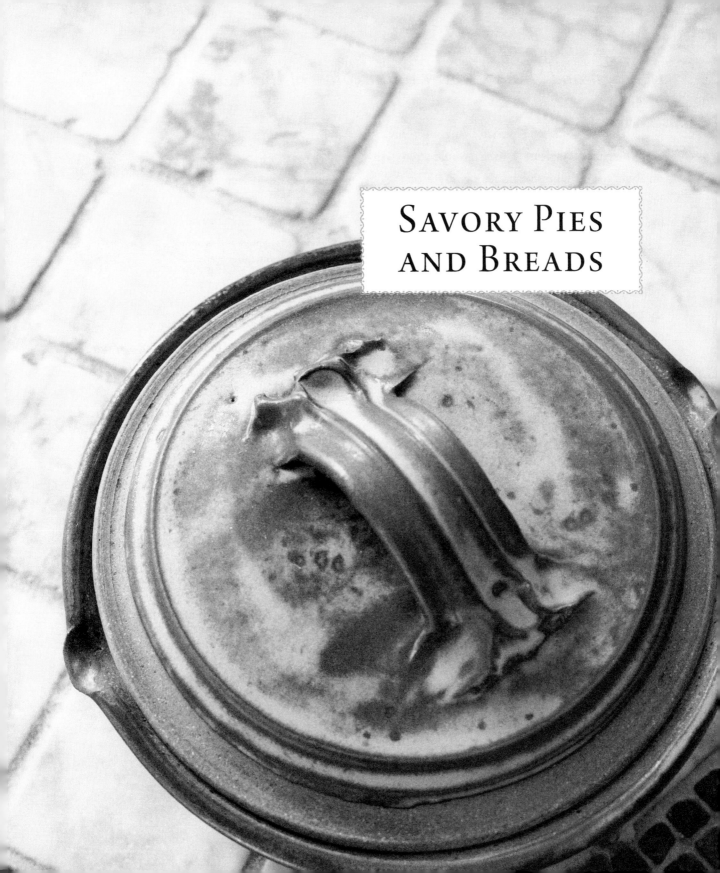

SAVORY PIES
AND BREADS

Chicken and Pork Tourte in the Style of the Languedoc

In the 1960s, when I lived in Paris, one of my neighbors, Vivienne Foucart, would often gush on about the dishes of her hometown, Sète, on the French Mediterranean coast. Eventually she moved back there, and when I moved down to Tangier, it was a simple matter to take the ferry over to visit and watch her cook. Vivienne taught me many recipes, including this chicken and pork pie, which she prepared in the fireplace by heaping coals on top of a thick ceramic *tourtière* she inherited from her grandmother. The solid clay held the heat evenly and created a crust that was flaky and crisp.

I adapted her recipe for a metal cake pan and published it in the original edition of my *Mediterranean Cooking*, but I always felt that I hadn't produced a good enough copy though all my friends and family loved it! Now I am presenting it again, this time using a terra-cotta baking pan. Reworking the recipe for this book, I was amazed at how much better it came out, the bottom crust remaining wonderfully crisp despite the wet filling.

Note that the leaf lard and butter pastry for this recipe must be prepared at least several hours and preferably a day in advance, so plan accordingly.

PREFERRED CLAY POT:

A 10- or 11-inch flameware pie plate, an unglazed terra-cotta saucer, or a Hess pottery pie plate (see Sources)

SUGGESTED CLAY ENVIRONMENT:

Double slabs of pizza stones or food-safe quarry tiles set on the upper and lower oven racks

1 ounce dried cèpes

Salt and freshly ground black pepper

1 tablespoon unsalted butter, duck fat, extra virgin olive oil, or lard

½ cup chopped onion

3 ounces thinly sliced meaty pancetta, finely diced

1 pound skinless, boneless chicken breasts

1 pound lean ground pork

1 tablespoon dark rum or cognac

½ teaspoon quatre épices or pinches of freshly ground white pepper, ground cinnamon, freshly grated nutmeg, and ground cloves mixed together

Leaf Lard and Butter pastry (recipe follows)

2 tablespoons finely chopped fresh flat-leaf parsley

1 tablespoon chopped fresh thyme leaves or 1 teaspoon dried

Egg yolk glaze: 1 egg yolk beaten with 1 tablespoon cream or milk

1   Soak the cèpes in water to cover for at least 1 hour. Strain the soaking liquid into a conventional skillet. Add the mushrooms after rinsing and chopping along with a pinch of salt and pepper. Bring to a boil and simmer for a few minutes. Add the butter and onion and cook slowly until the onions are soft and the liquid has evaporated. Scrape the mushrooms and onions into a side dish to cool. Do not wash the skillet.

2   Add the pancetta to the skillet and allow it to soften and release some fat. Add the chicken pieces and brown gently on all sides. Scrape the pancetta and chicken onto a work surface. Cut the chicken pieces into 1-inch chunks; toss with the pancetta and leave to cool.

3   Season the ground pork with the rum, quatre épices, ½ teaspoon salt, and ¼ teaspoon pepper. Mix thoroughly; then fold in the mushrooms and onions and set aside.

4   Remove the pastry from the refrigerator. Roll out the larger piece of dough between sheets of floured wax paper to make a large, thin round less than ⅛ inch thick. Remove the top sheet of paper, flip the dough over into the pie plate, and peel off the bottom sheet of paper. Fit the pastry into the pie plate. (If the pastry is too soft at this point, simply let it chill in the refrigerator for 10 minutes before lifting off the paper.) Repair cracks or tears with overhanging pieces of pastry; trim off the excess with a thin-bladed knife or by rolling the rolling pin over the edge. Let the pastry rest for 1 hour longer in the refrigerator.

5   About 2 hours before serving, preheat the oven to 375°F. Remove the pastry from the refrigerator. Prick the bottom in 2 or 3 places with the tines of a fork. Add a layer of the pork and top with the chunks of browned chicken, pancetta, and chopped parsley and thyme. Quickly roll out the smaller piece of dough, moisten around the edges with water, cover the tourte, and crimp to seal. Make a small opening in the center of the tourte and insert a small funnel or large plain pastry tip to allow steam to escape during baking. Brush the top with the egg yolk glaze and set in the oven to bake for 1½ hours. Transfer the pie dish to a wooden surface or folded kitchen towel to prevent cracking. Serve hot, using a serrated knife to cut into wedges.

Leaf Lard and Butter Pastry

MAKES ENOUGH PASTRY FOR A DOUBLE-CRUST 10- TO 12-INCH DEEP-DISH *TOURTE*

The combination of lard and butter here ensures a crust that is both crisp and very tender. For best results, this pastry should be prepared a day in advance. Allow to chill for at least 3 to 4 hours.

2¼ cups unbleached all-purpose flour (11 ounces)

1 teaspoon salt

Pinch of sugar

3 ounces rendered leaf lard (see Note), chilled and crumbled

8 tablespoons (1 stick) plus 6 tablespoons unsalted butter (7 ounces total), chilled and diced

1 tablespoon dark rum, cognac, mild vinegar, or strained fresh lemon juice, chilled

2 to 3 tablespoons ice water

(continued)

1   A day in advance or at least 3 or 4 hours before baking, prepare the dough. Place the flour, salt, and sugar in a food processor fitted with the plastic dough blade. Sift by pulsing once. Scatter the lard and butter over the flour. Pulse the machine 4 or 5 times, or until the mixture resembles coarse oatmeal. Combine the rum and ice water; with the machine on, add the liquid to the flour mixture. Process only briefly; be sure to stop before the dough forms a ball.

2   Turn the dough out onto a work surface covered with a sheet of wax paper. It should not be too crumbly; if it is, sprinkle with droplets of ice-cold water, adding just enough so the dough masses together but is not damp.

To make the dough by hand: mix the flour with the salt and sugar; rub in the lard and the chilled butter. Mix in the rum and ice water and form a ball of dough; knead until smooth.

3   Divide the dough into 2 parts, one a few ounces heavier than the other. Wrap both parts tightly in plastic wrap; refrigerate overnight.

NOTE TO THE COOK: To render leaf lard, grind the lard with ½ cup cold water in a food processor. Scrape into a small saucepan and cook over low heat until the fat is completely melted, about 1 hour. Strain and cool, discarding any hard bits of gristle and fat.

Torta with Mortadella, Cabbage, and Pork

SERVES 6

Most everyone loves Ligurian *tortas*—savory, double-crust, main-course southern Italian pies. The most famous is the Easter specialty, torta Pasqualina, which is stuffed with artichoke hearts, eggs, and ricotta. There are many other tortas from the Lungiana region, including one made with pumpkin, rice, and wild greens, which you can find in my *Mediterranean Grains and Greens*. Here is another favorite from the same region—a hearty torta of cabbage, ground pork, and mortadella.

A century ago these pies were cooked in the fireplace in a *testo,* a covered clay pan made with a local gray clay that didn't crack when set in the middle of a bed of embers or when a layer of hot coals was shoveled onto its lid.

Note that the pastry for this recipe must be prepared at least several hours and preferably a day in advance, so plan accordingly.

I suggest baking the torta in a 12-inch pizza pan in a clay oven environment Placing the torta directly on a heated pizza stone imparts instant, even heat and produces a very fine bottom crust. At the same time, the heated stone above will crisp the top.

> **SUGGESTED CLAY ENVIRONMENT:**
> Double slabs of pizza stones or food-safe quarry tiles set on the upper and lower oven racks

1 large green cabbage (2 pounds), quartered and cored

Salt and freshly ground black pepper

½ cup chopped onion

2 tablespoons extra virgin olive oil

4 tablespoons (½ stick) unsalted butter

8 ounces ground lean pork

½ cup peeled, seeded, and chopped tomatoes

2 tablespoons chopped fresh flat-leaf parsley

1 teaspoon chopped fresh marjoram or ½ teaspoon dried

1 garlic clove, finely chopped

2 cups milk

3½ tablespoons all-purpose flour

¼ teaspoon freshly grated nutmeg

1 cup ricotta cheese, drained

⅓ cup grated Parmigiano-Reggiano cheese

Olive Oil Pastry (recipe follows)

5 ounces mortadella, thinly sliced

1 egg, beaten with 1 tablespoon water

1 Boil the cabbage in a large pot of salted water until just softened, about 5 minutes. Drain, separate the leaves, and rinse under cold running water. Drain again and squeeze out as much moisture as possible with your hands. Coarsely chop the cabbage.

2 In a large conventional skillet, sauté the onion in the olive oil and 2 tablespoons of the butter over medium heat until soft and golden, about 5 minutes. Add the ground pork. Cook, stirring to break up any lumps of meat with a fork, until the pork is browned, about 5 minutes.

3 Add the tomatoes, parsley, marjoram, and garlic. Cook, uncovered, for 5 minutes over medium heat. Stir in the cabbage, mixing well. Raise the heat to high and cook, stirring often, until all the liquid in the pan has evaporated and the cabbage begins to brown, about 10 minutes. Season with salt and pepper to taste. Remove from the heat and let cool.

4 Preheat the stone or tile-lined oven to 400°F for 1 hour. Meanwhile, heat the milk to simmering in a small conventional saucepan. Melt the remaining 2 tablespoons butter in a heavy medium conventional saucepan over medium-low heat. Stir in the flour. Off the heat, whisk in the milk, ½ teaspoon salt, ¼ teaspoon pepper, and the nutmeg. Return to medium heat and bring to a boil, stirring until thickened and smooth. Reduce the heat to low and simmer for 2 to 3 minutes. Remove the sauce from the heat and let cool for 30 minutes. Whisk the ricotta and grated Parmigiano-Reggiano cheese into the sauce until well blended. Set the cheese sauce aside.

5 Roll out half the dough into a thin round a little larger than the pizza pan. Put the dough in the pan and prick all over with the tines of a fork. Arrange half the mortadella slices over the pastry. Spread the cabbage and pork mixture on top, patting it down evenly. Pour the cheese sauce over all and cover with the remaining slices of mortadella. Quickly roll out the second pastry to a 12-inch round. Moisten the edges with water, cover the pie, and crimp to seal all around.

6 Cut a small opening in the center and insert a metal pastry tip or small metal funnel to allow steam to escape. Brush the top of the torta with the egg and set in the oven. Bake for 45 minutes. Let stand for at least 15 minutes before cutting into wedges. Serve warm.

Olive Oil Pastry

MAKES A 12-INCH DOUBLE-CRUST PIE

2 cups all-purpose unbleached flour (10 ounces)

½ teaspoon salt

3½ tablespoons extra virgin olive oil

1 Place the flour and salt in a food processor fitted with a plastic dough blade. Sift by pulsing once or twice. Sprinkle the olive oil and ⅔ cup cold water over the flour and pulse quickly 4 or 5 times, until the mixture resembles cornmeal. If necessary, add additional water 1 tablespoon at a time, mixing well after each addition until a dough just begins to form; do not process into a ball.

2 Turn out the dough onto a work surface and gather into a ball, pushing any loose crumbs into the dough with the heel of your hand. Knead until just smooth. Divide in half; flatten each half into a 1-inch-thick round. Dust the rounds lightly with flour, wrap them in plastic wrap, and refrigerate for at least 3 hours and preferably overnight.

PISSALA

The Greeks and Romans all preserved small Mediterranean fish, such as sardines and anchovies, in a fermented paste called *garum*. *Pissala* is similar and unique to Nice, France; I've been told that the Niçois still make it at home, but I've yet to find it sold in shops. Basically, the fish are layered in small earthenware crocks with one pound of sea salt (seasoned with peppercorns, cloves, bay leaves, and thyme) for each four pounds of fish. After a week, the blood and oil rises to the surface and is discarded. The mixture is then set in a cool cellar to be stirred once a day for a month. The fish are finally pressed through a fine sieve to remove scales, bones, and spices and then packed into jars.

Pissaladière Niçoise

MAKES A 9- × 11-INCH PIE, SERVING 6 TO 8

*T*his unusual pie is often described as a Provençal pizza. True, the bread dough base is the same as is used in pizzas, but the strong-tasting anchovy-sardine paste (*pissala*) topping is pure Niçoise. You'll see squares of *pissaladière* in bakeshop windows and delis throughout eastern Provence, especially in Nice, where it's often sold right on the street. Accompanied by a green salad, *pissaladière* makes a great appetizer or lunch dish, and it reheats beautifully.

My French friends, when describing this pie, always emphasize a point made in Jacques Médicin's definitive book *La Cuisine du Comte de Nice,* that before baking, the onion layer must be exactly half as thick as the yeast dough or, if using a pastry base such as a pâte brisée, should be equally thick.

In the traditional recipe, the *pissala* is blended with a thick layer of long-cooked onions and spread generously over the dough. The pie is decorated with local black olives before baking. The pizza is served hot, warm, or best of all, at room temperature.

Included in this recipe is another tip, which I learned from the late cookbook author Mireille Johnson, who was born in Nice. For extra flavor, some of the reduced cooking liquid from the onions is added to the dough. So please prepare not only the pastry but the onions a day in advance.

PREFERRED CLAY POT:

A 3-quart earthenware or flameware casserole with a lid

If using an electric or ceramic stovetop, be sure to use a heat diffuser with the clay pot.

SUGGESTED CLAY ENVIRONMENT:

Double slabs of pizza stones or food-safe quarry tiles set on the upper and lower oven racks

3 pounds red onions, thinly sliced (about 9 cups)

¼ cup plus 2 tablespoons extra virgin olive oil

1 garlic clove, peeled

3 cloves

2 bay leaves

1 teaspoon herbes de Provence

Onion-Flavored Dough (recipe follows)

2 tablespoons anchovy paste

1½ teaspoons freshly ground black pepper

18 oil-cured anchovy fillets

18 small black Niçoise olives

½ cup semolina or whole-wheat flour for dusting

12 cherry or grape tomatoes

½ teaspoon sugar

1 One day in advance, prepare the onions and the onion-flavored dough. In an earthenware casserole, combine the sliced red onions with 2 tablespoons of the olive oil, the garlic stuck with the cloves, the

(continued)

bay leaves, and the herbes de Provence. Cover and cook over medium-low heat for 2 hours, or until the onions are meltingly soft and reduced in volume by two-thirds. Uncover, raise the heat to medium-high, and cook, stirring often, until the onions just begin to sizzle, about 5 minutes. Transfer the hot casserole to a wooden surface or folded kitchen towel to prevent cracking. Use a slotted spoon to transfer the onions to a storage container. Pick out and discard the garlic, cloves, and bay leaves. Reserve ½ cup of the oily cooking juices to use in the dough. Let the onion topping cool completely; cover and refrigerate until chilled. (The recipe can be made to this point up to a day in advance.)

2 Turn the chilled dough out onto a wooden board or other work surface and let stand at room temperature until doubled in size, about 1 hour. At the same time, preheat the stone- or tile-lined oven to 500°F for about 1 hour. Meanwhile, remove the browned onions from the refrigerator and gently press on them to express their liquid into a small bowl. Mix the anchovy paste, 2 tablespoons of the remaining olive oil, and pepper into this liquid. Fold in the onions and set aside at room temperature.

3 Rinse the anchovy fillets, place in a bowl of water, and soak for about 1 hour. Drain and pat dry. Pit the olives and soak them in a bowl of fresh water. Drain and pat dry.

4 Dust an 11- × 17-inch jelly roll pan with semolina flour. Place the dough in the center, sprinkle with more of the flour, and press out the dough into a rectangle about 6 by 10 inches. Cover with a cloth and let rest for 15 minutes. Press out the dough again to enlarge the rectangle, lifting and gently stretching it over your hands from time to time, until it fills the pan. Press the edges up into a ¾-inch ridge all around the pan.

5 Spread the onions over the dough to within ½ inch of the edge. Decorate the top with the anchovies, olives, and cherry tomatoes. Let stand at room temperature for 10 minutes. Dust the top with the sugar. Brush the remaining 2 tablespoons olive oil over the exposed edges of the dough.

6 Bake the pissaladière for 15 to 18 minutes, or until the dough is crisp and lightly browned. Cut into squares and serve hot, warm, or at room temperature.

Onion-Flavored Dough

This dough is designed especially for *pissaladière*, with its lush onion topping. It is best made one day before baking.

2¼ cups unbleached bread flour (11 ounces)

½ teaspoon rapid-rise dry yeast

1 teaspoon fine salt

½ cup oily onion juices from step 1 of the pissaladière

2 tablespoons extra virgin olive oil

1 In a food processor fitted with the plastic dough blade, combine the flour, yeast, and salt. Pulse briefly to mix.

2 Place the warm onion juices in a glass measuring cup. Add the olive oil and enough warm water to measure 1 cup. With the machine on, slowly add just enough of the liquid to the flour to form a dough. Continue to process for 15 to 20 seconds, or until the dough forms a smooth ball around the blade.

3 Turn the soft dough out onto a lightly floured board and knead gently into a tight, smooth ball. Pack the dough into a plastic or glass container, cover, and refrigerate overnight. The dough can be held in the refrigerator for up to 48 hours.

SOME MEDITERRANEAN FLAT BREADS

For me, cooking a thin flat round of dough on a clay saucer carries a spiritual connotation—grain grown in the earth cooked on slabs made of earth. It's all there: organic and inorganic—earth, fire, and water. The process goes back to Neolithic times, when wheat and barley grew naturally, were harvested, crushed, set on flat clay dishes atop piles of embers, and made into delicious, nourishing flat breads.

The Jewish unleavened matzo is probably the oldest of these ancient Mediterranean flat breads. With its simple combination of flour and water, this traditional Passover cracker must be assembled and set on hot clay in less than eighteen minutes so that, in accordance with religious tradition, the dough won't have time to ferment and start to rise. Today, one can still find Mediterranean bakers who cook their matzos on a layer of preheated tiles in their home ovens.

The Tunisian flat bread called *ftira* is also made with just flour and water, but it is left to ferment naturally overnight. Cooked on a hot clay dish called a *ghannaie* on top of the stove, it emerges soft and floppy, spotted with lovely black char marks. The tender bread is served with olive oil or wrapped around chopped black olives.

Another appealing flat bread is the round *piadina*, a white flour specialty of the Emilia-Romagna region of Italy, which resembles a Mexican flour tortilla. Baked on red clay disks called *teglias*, it's pierced as it cooks to deflate the air bubbles and keep it flat. *Piadine* are served as soon as they're cooked, stuffed with local salumi and/or cheese.

Moroccan Country Bread

MAKES 6 FLAT BREADS

*M*atloua is one of my favorite leavened Moroccan flat breads—a tender, spongy round that goes perfectly with tagines, whether eaten Moroccan style (using the bread to grasp food from a communal dish) or simply used to mop up sauce from a plate. These rounds are also wonderful simply smeared with butter or *smen* (page 295) and consumed along with some wildflower honey and a glass of mint tea.

This recipe comes from my favorite riad in Marrakech, Dar Les Cigognes, an elegant eleven-room boutique hotel that takes its name from the storks whose nests can be seen along the fortifications of the royal palace opposite.

(continued)

Traditionally, this bread is baked slowly on a saucer shaped clay *tanjin* over embers, resulting in a soft, golden brown exterior and tender moist interior and giving off a subtle smoky aroma. If your stove has a lava stone grill, you can bake the rounds on a clay flowerpot saucer set over heated lava stones. You can also bake them over very low coals on your outdoor barbecue or on top of a gas stove in an earthenware skillet. Just before serving, use tongs to hold the bread directly over a gas range flame to char the edges ever so slightly. Or simply pop them into a toaster for a slight reheating and charring.

To store: Though this bread is best eaten fresh from the hot clay pan, it may be baked earlier in the day, wrapped in a cloth and plastic, and left in a cool place before reheating in the toaster.

PREFERRED CLAY POT:

A 12-inch terra-cotta clay flowerpot saucer, unglazed flat tagine, La Chamba skillet, or *comal*

1 cup stone-ground whole-wheat flour (5½ ounces), plus more for kneading

1 cup semolina or pasta flour (5½ ounces), plus more for shaping

1 teaspoon granulated sugar

1 teaspoon salt

1 teaspoon rapid-rise yeast

1 tablespoon extra virgin olive oil

1 Combine the flours, sugar, salt, and yeast in the bowl of an electric mixer. Add the olive oil and use the paddle on low speed to mix to a gritty consistency. Gradually add up to 1 cup warm water as you knead the dough on low speed for 3 to 4 minutes. Let the dough rest for 5 minutes. Turn the machine to medium-low speed and knead the dough for 5 minutes, or until it is spongy, soft, and tacky to the touch. Cover the dough and let rest for 10 minutes.

2 Turn out the dough onto a floured work surface, dust lightly with whole-wheat flour, and knead until smooth and elastic, about 3 minutes. Gather into a ball, cover with a kitchen towel, and let stand at room temperature for 10 minutes.

3 Divide the dough into 6 balls. Using your palms, gently flatten each ball of dough into a 4- or 5-inch round. Dust with semolina flour, cover with a heavy cloth, and let stand for 30 minutes.

4 Poke one of the rounds with your finger to see if it remains deeply indented. If so, prick each round with a toothpick 8 or 9 times to release any gas.

5 Set the clay saucer over medium heat for ten minutes. Place half of the rounds of dough on the hot dry skillet and cook, uncovered, for 6 to 8 minutes, turning each once or twice, until nicely charred with black spots and golden brown on both sides. Stack the cooked breads while cooking the remaining rounds. Serve hot or warm or reheat the breads in a toaster.

NOTE TO THE COOK: The best flour for making Mediterranean flat breads is stone-ground whole-wheat flour such as Indian 100 percent whole-wheat flour (atta) with 12 percent protein, Bob's Red Mill, Arrowhead Mills, or King Arthur's 100 percent stone-ground whole (hard) wheat flour. If using a less finely ground flour, reduce the water by 2 to 3 tablespoons.

Moroccan Speckled Flat Bread

MAKES 8 ROUNDS (7 INCHES ACROSS)

Rafih Benjelloun, chef-owner of the Imperial Fez restaurant in Atlanta, Georgia, taught me this particular version of a smoky charred Moroccan bread called *melloui* from his hometown of Fez. Homemade *melloui* speckled with lots of black spots, he told me, is made by baking the bread on top of the stove on a hot clay saucer called a *ferrah*. The bread can also be purchased on the street, where, spread with butter and honey, it's enjoyed as a snack.

The bread is especially popular during the month of Ramadan, when it's served at nightfall as an accompaniment to spicy *harira* soup.

> **PREFERRED CLAY POT:**
>
> **A 12-inch unglazed terra-cotta saucer, flat-bottomed tagine, or La Chamba skillet**
>
> **If using an electric or ceramic stovetop, be sure to use a heat diffuser with the clay pot.**

2 cups stone-ground whole-wheat flour or fine semolina (11 ounces)

1 cup all-purpose flour (5 ounces)

2 teaspoons salt

½ cup extra virgin olive oil

1 In a mixing bowl, combine the flours, salt, and 2 tablespoons of the oil. Use your fingertips to mix to a gritty consistency. Gradually add up to 1½ cups warm water. Knead the dough until it becomes elastic and smooth, about 10 minutes. Work in additional warm water as described in the Note (page 260).

2 Divide the dough into 8 equal balls, coat each with 2 teaspoons of the remaining olive oil, and flatten gently. Place them side by side on a large cold work surface, such as a marble, plastic, or glass slab, or on a countertop. Cover with a sheet of plastic and a kitchen towel and let rest for at least 45 minutes.

3 Use your fingertips to flatten a piece of dough into a 9- by 7-inch rectangle. Fold one-third of the dough toward the middle, then the other part on top like a letter, making a triple-layered square of dough. Flatten again and repeat the folding; cover the square of dough and set aside. Repeat with the remaining balls of dough. Cover them all loosely with a kitchen towel and let stand for at least 30 minutes.

4 Set the clay saucer over medium heat. Remove one square of dough and use your fingertips to flatten and reshape the dough into a thin square or round. Using your fingertips, tap indents all over the top side of the dough, especially over any thick edges.

5 Place the dough on the hot dry saucer and cook, uncovered, for 4 to 5 minutes, turning it once or twice until nicely charred with black spots and golden on both sides. At the same time, flatten and reshape a second ball of dough as directed in step 4 Don't rush the cooking; the breads are best when they still have a soft, crunchy crust but are moist and not doughy inside. Stack the cooked breads between sheets of parchment to hold them while you cook the remaining breads. Serve hot or warm, reheating the breads by flipping each one for an instant in a hot skillet.

(continued)

NOTE TO THE COOK: The best flour for making Mediterranean flat breads is stone-ground such as Indian 100 percent whole-wheat flour (atta) with 12 percent protein, Bob's Red Mill 100 percent stone-ground whole (hard) wheat flour, or King Arthur's stone-ground whole-wheat flour.

Moroccans have a special method that enables dough to absorb additional water, which makes an especially moist, tender bread. I call the method "knuckling." To add more water to a dough that is already saturated, you simply dip your knuckles into warm water and use them to press down on the dough while gradually working the water in. Don't hurry or get overly enthusiastic; you just want to add a few more tablespoons water while keeping the dough soft. If you hear squishy sounds, you're doing it right. If the dough gets too wet, simply switch to your ordinary kneading motion, which will tighten the dough, or add a low-gluten flour and begin to knuckle in a few more drops of water to loosen the dough again.

To make *melloui* a day in advance, flatten each square between two sheets of parchment; roll up and store in a sealed zipper bag in the refrigerator. Let return to room temperature before reheating, one by one, in a hot dry skillet.

Before cooking this particular bread, Fassi, or the people of Fez, brush the unglazed hot skillet with a thin coat of beaten egg yolk and then immediately wipe the pan clean with a cloth before the first bread is added. It isn't necessary to repeat with each round. The Fassi say the egg seals the pores in the unglazed clay, which keeps the bread from sticking. When making similar breads for spicy foods, they lightly wipe the cut side of a moist onion with oil or melted butter and then use it to quickly rub the heated pan.

OVEN-BAKED BREADS

The traditional Mediterranean hearth oven, whether made of clay, stone, or brick, has what is referred to as a "beehive shape"—a flat cooking surface surrounded by curved walls and a domed top. This design directs heat—whether ambient, radiant, or conductive—directly at the bread, ensuring great oven spring and a lovely airy texture. For me it's these qualities along with a smoky wood aroma that make for a great bread.

There are various ways to turn an ordinary home oven into a baker's oven:

✳ Line the upper and lower racks of the oven with large pizza stones, firebrick, or food-safe quarry tiles

✳ Lay two large FibraMent slabs on the racks

✳ Bake beneath a La Cloche stoneware domed baker (which is, in effect, a small beehive oven)

✳ Bake inside a Romertopf clay baker

✳ Bake underneath a heavy unglazed terra-cotta flowerpot set on a stoneware slab

Please see page xviii for more information on ways to create an oven environment.

With regard to baking in a clay-lined oven, I'd be remiss if I didn't discuss the energy implications. Successful baking requires heating up your oven slabs for up to a full hour before inserting your bread. You can determine exactly how long it takes to properly preheat by using an oven thermometer or—even better—a laser thermometer such as Ratek, which directs light onto the stone to obtain a reading. Or simply use an oven thermometer directly on the stone. By measuring, you may discover that your particular oven requires more or less time to preheat. There is a nice way to save energy at the other end of the baking process, though. Once properly heated, clay or stone will hold heat for a long time. Thus, once your oven has achieved the proper temperature and your bread has risen, you can reduce the temperature for the final fifteen minutes of baking; or if using FibraMent slabs, in many instances, you can turn it off completely. Also, after your bread baking is complete, you can do as Mediterranean cooks do after baking their bread in a wood-fired oven: slip in a pot of beans, a gratin, or even some vegetables to roast in the receding heat.

Eastern Mediterranean Flat Bread

MAKES 2 LOAVES, EACH SERVING 4

*H*ere's an excellent recipe for a traditional eastern Mediterranean bread that's typically baked in a wood-fired oven. It calls for stone-ground, whole-wheat flour as well as bread flour. When baked in a clay environment, this bread truly comes into its own. It makes a great accompaniment to *guvec, yiouvetsis,* soups, and salads—or break it up and use as an edible scoop with spreads and dips.

> **SUGGESTED CLAY ENVIRONMENT:**
> **Double slabs of pizza stones or food-safe quarry tiles set on the upper and lower oven racks**

1¼ teaspoons active dry yeast

4 cups unbleached bread flour, preferably King Arthur (1 pound 3 ounces)

½ cup stone-ground whole-wheat flour (2 ounces)

2 tablespoons extra virgin olive oil

4 teaspoon fine salt

Semolina or coarse cornmeal for dusting

1 A day before you plan to bake the bread, make a sponge: In a mixing bowl, combine ¼ teaspoon of the yeast with ½ cup lukewarm water and 1 cup of the bread flour. Mix until smooth. Cover and let stand for a few hours at room temperature; then refrigerate overnight. Remove from the refrigerator about 1 hour before using.

2 To make the bread: In an electric mixer fitted with a dough hook or in a food processor, combine the sponge, remaining 1 teaspoon yeast, the olive oil, remaining bread flour, whole-wheat flour, salt, and 1¼ cups warm water. If using an electric mixer, beat on low speed for 1 minute. If using a food processor, process for 5 seconds. If the dough is too stiff, add 1 tablespoon water and beat or pulse for a second or two. If it is still too stiff, repeat with 1 to 2 tablespoons water. When the dough is soft but still tacky, let it rest for 10 minutes; then mix on medium-low speed for 10 minutes or process for 20 seconds.

3 Turn the dough out onto a lightly floured work surface and knead until smooth and soft, about 2 minutes. Place the dough in a large oiled bowl, cover with plastic wrap, and let stand at room temperature until doubled in bulk, about 2 hours.

4 About 1 hour before baking, preheat the oven to 500°F. Punch down the dough and divide into 4 equal pieces. Dust a wooden board or other work surface lightly with semolina or cornmeal. Flatten each piece of dough into a 5-inch round and place on the board. Cover with a kitchen towel and let rise until puffy, about 30 minutes.

5 Place a bowl of water next to a floured work surface. Dip your hands in the water and quickly flatten two of the rounds into 7- by 9-inch ovals. Make 3 or 4 deep grooves with your fingertips down the length of each oval. Dust a wooden pizza peel with semolina. Place the 2 ovals on the peel, gently shake it forward and back to be sure the ovals are loose, and slip them onto the hot stone in the oven. Bake until crisp on the bottom, 7 to 9 minutes. Repeat with the remaining 2 ovals. Wrap in a kitchen towel to keep them warm while the second batch bakes. Serve the breads warm.

NOTES TO THE COOK:

※ The best flour for making Mediterranean flat breads is stone ground, such as Indian 100 percent whole-wheat flour (atta) with 12 percent protein, Bob's Red Mill 100 percent stone-ground whole (hard) wheat flour, or King Arthur's stone-ground whole-wheat flour.

※ If necessary, rotate the bread. Timing depends upon the size of the bread and the retained heat of the stones or tiles.

※ For a softer bread: Leave the oven door open during the latter half of the baking time.

Mîche

MAKES 1 LARGE ROUND LOAF

*T*his dense, round French bread is made with either rye or whole-wheat flour mixed with bread flour, and it results in a perfect all-around bread to accompany country pâtés and rillettes. When it turns a little stale, it's perfect for stuffing a chicken. Slices are good in thick soups too. For best results, begin this bread two days in advance.

> **SUGGESTED CLAY ENVIRONMENT:**
> **Double slabs of pizza stones or food-safe quarry tiles set on the upper and lower oven racks**

½ teaspoon active dry yeast

1 teaspoon sugar

3½ cups unbleached bread flour (1 pound 3 ounces)

2 teaspoons fine sea salt

½ cup whole-wheat or rye flour

Coarse semolina, whole-wheat flour, or cornmeal for dusting

1 Make a starter 1 to 2 days before you plan to bake the bread: In a bowl or 1-quart glass measuring cup, mix the yeast with the sugar, ½ cup of the bread flour, and ¾ cup lukewarm water. Cover and let stand at room temperature overnight.

2 The following morning, dump the starter into a mixing bowl. Add ¾ cup lukewarm water and the salt. Stir to blend well. Add the whole-wheat flour and the remaining 3 cups bread flour 1 cup at a time, mixing thoroughly with a wooden spoon and allowing each cup of flour to be absorbed before adding the next. (You can use an electric mixer with a dough hook set on low speed.) Scrape down the sides of the bowl from time to time. If the dough is tacky, add 1 to 2 tablespoons more flour. If the dough is dry, add 1 to 2 teaspoons more water. By hand, knead the dough for 20 minutes. If using a mixer, knead on low for 10 minutes; then turn out and knead by hand for 1 minute to achieve the proper consistency—a smooth and elastic dough that remains slightly soft.

(continued)

3 Lightly grease a mixing bowl. Place the dough in the bowl, cover with plastic wrap, and let rise in a warm, draft-free place until almost doubled in bulk, about 2 hours.

4 Transfer the bowl to the refrigerator and let the dough continue to rise at a slower pace for 5 to 6 hours or overnight, until doubled.

5 Turn the dough out onto a board, fold it onto itself, and press down to deflate. Rub plenty of flour into a linen or heavy cotton cloth and line a round 8-inch bread-rising basket, a floured 8-, 9-, or 10-inch shallow basket, or a greased shallow bowl. Turn the dough into whatever mold you are using, cover with overlapping cloth or another cloth, and set in a warm place to double in bulk, 2 to 4 hours. The dough is ready when you poke it gently with your finger and it doesn't spring back.

6 Rearrange the oven so the pizza stone is on the second-lowest rack of the oven. Preheat the oven to 450°F. Place an empty roasting pan on the lowest rack.

7 Bring a quart of water to a boil. Meanwhile, sprinkle the bottom of the ball of dough with a light coating of coarse semolina. Place a small wooden pizza peel or cookie sheet over the basket or bowl and invert so the dough turns out onto the sheet or peel, round side up. Gently shake the dough to check that it is not sticking. Carefully lift any part of the dough that might be sticking and sprinkle more semolina flour underneath. With a razor blade, thin-bladed knife, or scissors, slit the bread deeply in a crisscross or checkerboard pattern. Let relax

for a few minutes; then mist the top with 4 to 5 spurts from an atomizer filled with water. Slide the bread onto the hot pizza stone, jerking the pizza peel away. Carefully pour the boiling water into the empty pan on the lower shelf, close the oven door, and bake for 50 minutes, or until it sounds hollow when tapped on the bottom or the internal temperature measures 195°F. Remove from the oven and transfer the bread to a rack to cool. The loaf will keep well for 3 to 4 days wrapped in a kitchen towel in a resealable plastic bag at room temperature.

NOTE TO THE COOK: Bread baked in a La Cloche stoneware domed baker is an amazing stand-in for a brick oven. It produces extraordinary crusty bread. To bake this bread in a La Cloche domed baker, follow the directions with these changes:

In Step 5, lightly grease the bottom of the baker and turn the dough onto it. Cover with the dome and let rise.

In Step 6, place a rack in the bottom rack of the oven and preheat the oven to 500°F.

In Step 7, slash the top of the loaf as directed. Omit the water bath. Place La Cloche in the oven. Reduce oven heat to 400°F. After 40 minutes of baking, uncover the bread and bake until the crust is brown and crisp and the internal temperature registers 195°F. Be sure to use heavy oven mitts whenever handling the baker.

Carefully transfer the whole baker to a wooden surface or folded kitchen towel to prevent cracking. As soon as possible, with a wide spatula, transfer the loaf to a rack and let cool.

Brooklyn-Style Sicilian Semolina Bread

MAKES 2 LOAVES

This is similar to the semolina bread I grew up on, the bread my mother purchased from the Sicilian-American bakery in our Brooklyn neighborhood. Sicilian bread is made with a mixture of fine-ground semolina, extra fine-ground durum, and unbleached bread flours, which gives it a pale yellow color and unique nutty flavor. The color may remind you of brioche, but the bread contains no eggs or butter, just a few tablespoons of olive oil added for richness and elasticity.

> **SUGGESTED CLAY ENVIRONMENT:**
> Double slabs of FibraMent slabs, pizza stones, or food-safe quarry tiles set on the upper and lower oven racks

1 teaspoon rapid-rise yeast or 2 teaspoons active dry yeast

1 cup unbleached bread flour (4¾ ounces)

1¼ cups semolina or pasta flour (6¾ ounces)

1 cup plus 3 tablespoons finely ground durum flour, extra-fancy durum, or durum atta flour (5 ounces)

2 teaspoons fine sea salt

2 tablespoons extra virgin olive oil

Coarse semolina, cornmeal, or whole-wheat flour for handling the dough

1 tablespoon sesame seeds

1 The morning of the day you plan to bake the bread, combine a pinch of the rapid-rise yeast or ½ teaspoon of the active dry yeast with 1 cup warm water and the bread flour in a 4-quart bowl. Cover and let stand until doubled in volume, about 1 hour.

2 Scrape this sponge into a food processor fitted with the plastic dough blade. Add the semolina flour, 1 cup of the durum flour, the remaining yeast, the salt, and the olive oil. Pulse a few times to combine. With the machine on, slowly add ⅔ to ¾ cup warm water through the feed tube and process for 20 seconds, or until a smooth dough forms. Transfer the dough to an oiled bowl, turn to coat all over, cover with a kitchen towel, and let rise at room temperature for 2 hours, or until almost tripled in bulk.

3 Turn out the dough onto a floured work surface; punch it down and knead for 1 minute. Sprinkle a wooden bread peel with coarse semolina or flour. Divide the dough in half and shape each into a 10-inch-long loaf. Cover with a cloth and let rise until doubled in size, about 1 hour.

4 Place 3 racks in the oven: one on the bottom shelf for an empty roasting pan, a second on the rack just above for one of the pizza stones, and the last one on the upper rack. Preheat the oven to 475°F for 1 hour.

5 Make a glaze with 3 tablespoons flour and 7 to 8 tablespoons water and lightly brush the top of the loaves. Save the remainder. Sprinkle with the sesame seeds and use a pair of long scissors or a long sharp knife to slash the dough on a diagonal at 3-inch intervals. Gently shake the loaves on the peel to be sure they can slide easily. Throw 4 or 5 ice cubes into the roasting pan. Slide the loaves onto the hot stone, close the door, and bake for 25 minutes, or until the crust is golden and the internal temperature of the bread registers 205°F. Transfer the loaves to a wire rack, brush again with the flour-water glaze, and let cool before slicing.

(continued)

NOTES TO THE COOK:

⁕ If using a La Cloche stoneware domed baker, note the following changes: In Step 3, instead of the peel, lightly oil the bottom round of the baker, sprinkle a little semolina or cornmeal on top, and place the 2 loaves inside. Cover with the dome and let them rise for 45 minutes. In Step 4, simply set a pizza stone slab on the bottom rack of the oven and preheat to 475°F. In Step 5, omit the ice cubes and roasting pan. Cover the dough with the dome, and quickly place the entire baker in the oven. Bake for 30 minutes. Use heavy oven mitts to remove the dome cover. Bake the bread for 10 to 15 minutes longer, or until the top is golden brown and the internal temperature of the bread is 205°F.

⁕ This bread can be stored at room temperature, wrapped in parchment, for up to 4 days.

⁕ Once you have this bread on hand, you can use it to make delicious *croûtes* for fish soup. To make the *croûtes:* Brush a griddle with a little fresh extra virgin olive oil and set over medium heat. When the oil sizzles, add a few slices of the stale bread and grill, turning once, until golden brown, about 2 minutes per side. Drain on paper towels and sprinkle lightly with sea salt, cayenne pepper, and Mediterranean oregano while still hot. Repeat with the remaining slices. Let cool to room temperature before serving.

CERAMIC CONTAINERS FOR NO-KNEAD BREAD

The famous Jim Lahey/Mark Bittman no-knead bread recipe, which showed that it's possible to make great bread with an incredible crust, very little yeast, on your own timetable and without having to spend twenty or so minutes kneading the dough, turned many home cooks into bread makers. Published in the *New York Times* in 2006, it's one of those recipes that literally change the culinary scene with discussions on hundred of blogs in dozens of languages around the world. (In case you missed it, search the archives of the New York Times for the recipe.)

The recipe suggests baking the no-knead bread in a preheated covered pot. For one loaf Mark Bittman used an old Le Creuset enameled cast-iron pot and for another, a heavy ceramic pot. Shortly after the recipe was published, I began receiving requests from people who knew I was working on a clay pot book, asking which ceramic container I would recommend. My suggestions: a dry (unsoaked) Romertopf clay baker or a dry La Cloche stoneware domed baker. Set empty in a cold oven, turn the oven on, and follow the instructions as given by Lahey and Bittman in the recipe.

Island of Cyprus Olive Bread

MAKES A 1½-POUND LOAF

This excellent Mediterranean olive bread is found only in the Larnaca district of Cyprus, where it is baked in a beehive oven. Here I use either a Romertopf clay baker or a La Cloche stoneware domed baker as a substitute. The dough requires a great deal of olive oil, accounting for the belief that the women of Larnaca have beautiful hands from their kneading of it. You can try for beautiful hands by hand-kneading, or (as I do) knead the dough in a food processor.

This moist, chewy, and dense bread includes a special method called "knuckling," which enables the dough to absorb additional ingredients such as chopped olives and minced onions after the first kneading without overworking the dough.

You can slice this bread and make sandwiches with halloumi cheese, dip the slices into thick lentil or bean soup, or simply dip slices into more olive oil for a snack.

SUGGESTED CLAY POT:

A La Cloche stoneware domed baker or a large Romertopf clay baker

---

2 cups unbleached bread flour (9¾ ounces), sifted

¾ cup stone-ground whole-wheat flour (4 ounces)

1½ teaspoons rapid-rise yeast

½ teaspoon sugar

⅓ cup extra virgin olive oil, plus 1 to 2 tablespoons for coating

¾ cup finely chopped fresh cilantro

½ cup minced onion

½ cup oil-cured black olives (3 ounces), **pitted**

Coarse semolina or fine cornmeal for dusting

2 teaspoons sesame seeds

1 Sift the bread flour and whole-wheat flour into a large bowl. Add the yeast and sugar. Drizzle on the ⅓ cup olive oil and rub with your fingers until the mixture resembles fine crumbs. Gradually add up to ¾ cup warm water to make a soft ball of dough. Turn out onto a wooden board or other work surface and knead until smooth, about 10 minutes.

2 Spread the cilantro, onion, and olives over the dough. Dip your fingers and knuckles into a bowl of warm water and gently press to incorporate the ingredients into the dough. Place the dough in a clean oiled bowl; turn greased side up, cover with plastic wrap, and let stand in a warm place for about 45 minutes, until puffy.

3 Turn the dough over, gently folding it in half to deflate; coat with more oil, cover the bowl with plastic wrap, and let stand until the dough has almost doubled in volume, about 45 minutes longer.

4 Transfer the dough to a work surface. With a lightly oiled hand, punch it down and shape into a round for the La Cloche domed baker or an oval for the Romertopf, being careful to tuck the dough under tightly so the loaf is very plump.

(continued)

5 To bake in the La Cloche domed baker: Lightly oil the bottom round and dust with a little semolina or cornmeal. Place the dough on the round and tuck the edges under to tighten the loaf. Cover with the dome and let it rise for 30 minutes. Meanwhile, set a rack on the bottom shelf of the oven and preheat to 475°F. Uncover the dough and use a sharp knife to slash the risen dough on a diagonal at 2-inch intervals. Brush the top of the dough with water and sprinkle with the sesame seeds. Lightly brush the inside of the dome with water; cover the dough and quickly place the entire baker in the oven. Bake for 50 minutes. Use heavy oven mitts to remove the cover and place on a wooden surface or folded kitchen towel to prevent cracking. Bake the bread for 10 minutes longer, or until the top is golden brown and the internal temperature registers 200°F. Transfer the bread to a wire rack and let cool for at least 4 hours before slicing.

6 To use the Romertopf: Soak the top and bottom in water for 15 minutes; drain and pat the inside dry. Lightly grease with oil and line the bottom with a sheet of nonstick parchment. Place the dough on the paper, tuck in the edges to form a smooth round, and let stand in a warm place for 30 minutes. Use a sharp knife to make 2 diagonal slashes on top. Dust with the sesame seeds. Cover and place in the center of a cold oven. Set the temperature at 500°F. Bake for 45 minutes. Remove the cover and continue to bake until the top is well browned and crusty, about 10 minutes. Transfer to a rack and let cool. The bread can be stored at room temperature, wrapped in parchment, for up to 4 days.

Thanks to Niki Lazaridou Moquist, a Cypriot now living in central California, for generously sharing this recipe.

Brioche Stuffed with Two Cheeses

This specialty bread from the town of St.-Affrique is called *le gatis*. A mixture of Cantal and Roquefort cheeses is baked in a brioche crust and served melting hot. I love the rustic quality of this dish, delicious with a green salad or as an accompaniment to fresh fruit. Serve it surrounded with slices of fresh pears and pineapple, green and black grapes, and small strawberries.

PREFERRED CLAY POT:

A 6- or 7-inch round or square stoneware, porcelain, or earthenware baking dish

SUGGESTED CLAY ENVIRONMENT:

Double slabs of pizza stones or food-safe quarry tiles set on the upper and lower oven racks

1 recipe Brioche Dough (recipe follows)

2 ounces Cantal cheese

1½ ounces Roquefort cheese, at room temperature

1 egg

1 teaspoon milk

1 teaspoon unsalted butter

1　Make the brioche dough up to 3 days in advance.

2　Shred the Cantal. Mash the Roquefort with a fork and blend with all but 2 tablespoons of the shredded cheese.

3　About 3 hours before serving, roll out half of the brioche dough on a cold, lightly floured work surface to make a 5- or 6—inch round or square. Butter the baking dish and place the brioche dough in it. Crumble the cheese blend evenly over the dough, leaving a ¾-inch margin all around.

4　Shape the remaining dough into small balls about 1¼ inches in diameter. Flatten each with your palm. Beat the egg with the milk to make a glaze. Brush the edges of the dough in the pan with some of the egg glaze. Arrange the flattened brioche rounds over the cheese side by side. Press the dough together around the rim of the dish only to seal the cheese around the edge. It does not matter if there is a little space between some of the rounds on the top; they will come together during the rising and baking. Cover loosely with buttered foil and set in a warm place for 2 hours, or until the dough is light and springy.

5　Preheat the oven to 425°F for 1 hour.

6　Brush the egg glaze over the brioche and scatter the reserved 2 tablespoons cheese on top. Place the brioche on the hot pizza stone and bake for 10 minutes. Lower the oven temperature to 350°F and bake for 10 minutes longer. Serve hot, directly from the baking dish.

Brioche Dough

MAKES 1¼ POUNDS DOUGH

3 tablespoons warm milk

1½ teaspoons active dry yeast

1⅔ cups unbleached bread flour, 8 ounces

3 large eggs at room temperature

3 tablespoons sugar

¾ teaspoon salt

10 tablespoons unsalted butter, melted but not hot

1 Place the milk and yeast in a food processor. Pulse to combine. Add ⅓ cup of the flour and 1 egg. Process for 2 to 3 seconds. Scrape down the sides of the bowl. Sprinkle the remaining flour over the mixture, but do not blend in. Cover and let stand for 1½ to 2 hours at room temperature.

2 Add the sugar, salt, and 2 remaining eggs to the mixture in the food processor. Process for 15 seconds. With the machine on, pour in the melted butter in a steady stream through the feed tube. Process for 20 seconds longer. If the machine stalls (this can happen if the butter is added too quickly), let the machine rest for 3 minutes. Meanwhile, check that the blade is not clogged.

3 Scrape the resulting soft dough into a lightly greased 3-quart bowl. Sprinkle the top lightly with the remaining 2 teaspoons flour to prevent a crust from forming. Cover tightly with plastic wrap. Let rise at room temperature for about 5 hours in warm weather or 6 hours in cold weather, or until the dough is light, spongy, and almost tripled in bulk. Refrigerate for 20 to 30 minutes.

4 Using a plastic scraper, deflate the dough by stirring it down. Turn out onto a lightly floured board. With floured hands, gently press the dough into a rectangle and then gently fold into thirds. Dust with flour. Wrap well and refrigerate overnight to allow the dough to ripen and firm up. If the dough rises, punch it down. (If well wrapped and weighted down, the dough will keep for up to 3 days in the refrigerator, or it can be frozen for 1 week but no longer. To defrost, thaw overnight in the refrigerator.)

Variation: Brioche Round Loaf

MAKES 1 LOAF

On the breakfast table this tall round brioche is a delight to the eye. Serve it sliced very thin and restacked, or if you want to keep it fresh for a couple of days, slice only as needed.

> **PREFERRED CLAY POT:**
>
> **A 6 or 7-inch round Le Creuset stoneware, or porcelain baking dish**
>
> **SUGGESTED CLAY ENVIRONMENT:**
>
> **Double slabs of pizza stones or food-safe quarry tiles set on the upper and lower oven racks**

1 recipe Brioche Dough, chilled overnight

2 tablespoons unsalted butter

1 Butter the bottom and sides of the baking dish and line the sides with buttered parchment paper. The paper should extend at least 2 inches above the upper edge of the mold.

2   On a floured surface, gently roll the dough into a fat cylinder. Place in the prepared mold and gently press the dough down so that it fits snugly. Cover loosely but air tight with buttered plastic wrap. Let rise in a warm place for about 3 hours.

3   Preheat the oven to 425°F. Place the prepared brioche on the baking stone and bake for 15 minutes. If browning too fast, cover with foil. Lower oven heat to 375° F and bake 25 minutes longer, or until the brioche starts to pull away from the sides of the paper. Test the brioche by inserting a long thin skewer into the center; if it comes out clean, the brioche is fully cooked. Let cool 10 minutes in the mold before removing. (The brioche can collapse if removed too soon.) To help loosen, tug gently on the paper. Cool the brioche, still wrapped in parchment paper, on a wire rack. The paper helps keep the crust soft.

Brioche Feuilletée

If you have worked with brioche and enjoyed it, this variation is guaranteed to enchant you. It makes the most delectable wrapping for strudels, juicy fruit tarts, and tortes. It also makes very light, thin galettes to be filled with either a dollop of crème fraîche or pastry cream.

To transform the above recipe for brioche dough into brioche *feuilletée,* roll out the dough to make an 8 × 12-inch rectangle. Cut ¼ pound softened unsalted butter into small pieces and cover ⅔ of the brioche dough with them. Fold the dough into thirds, beginning with the third not covered with butter. Chill until firm enough to roll out and fold into thirds again. Repeat a third time; then chill well before using.

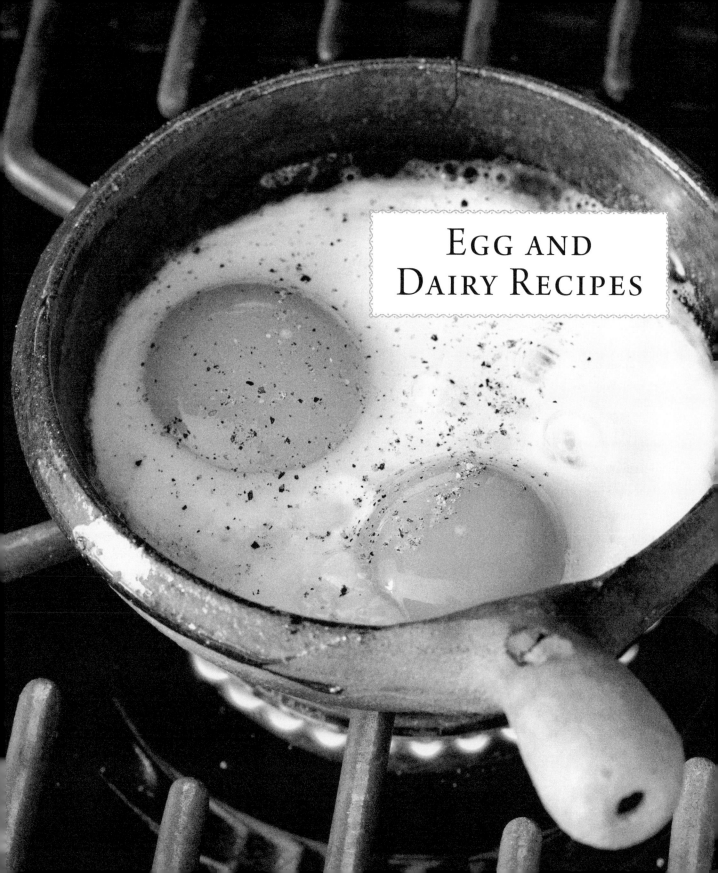

Egg and Dairy Recipes

Poached Eggs with Yogurt and Hot Red Pepper Sizzle

SERVES 2

Here's an unusual and delicious way to serve poached eggs, called *cilbir* in Turkey. Once you've poached your eggs, you set them in hot ceramic dishes to keep them warm, smother them with yogurt and then you devote full attention to preparing the last-minute sizzle of butter and hot red pepper. This sizzle heightens the flavor of the eggs and balances the richness of their garlic-yogurt toppings. Serve with hot toast.

> **PREFERRED CLAY POT:**
>
> 2 small cazuelitas, porcelain ramekins, or small gratin dishes

6 ounces sheep's, goat's, or cow's milk yogurt

1 garlic clove, peeled

½ teaspoon coarse salt

1 tablespoon white vinegar

Kosher salt

4 very fresh eggs at room temperature

4 tablespoons (½ stick) unsalted butter at room temperature

½ teaspoon Marash or Aleppo pepper

Pinch of sweet or hot paprika

1 Drain the yogurt in a sieve lined with a paper towel for 30 minutes, until thickened.

2 In a small bowl, mash the garlic to a paste with the salt. Add the yogurt and blend well. Set aside at room temperature.

3 About 20 minutes before serving, put 2 small cazuelitas in a wide saucepan of water to cover. Set over medium heat and slowly bring to a simmer. Carefully transfer the cazuelitas to a doubled kitchen towel to drain. Leave the pot of water on the stove.

4 Add the vinegar to the water and maintain at a simmer. One by one, break an egg onto a saucer and slip into the water. Cover the pot, turn off the heat, and poach the eggs until the whites are set but the yolks are still soft, about 2½ minutes.

5 Carefully remove the eggs with a slotted spatula and place 2 eggs in each warm cazuelita. Top each egg with one-quarter of the garlic yogurt.

6 Quickly melt the butter in a small conventional saucepan. Add the Marash pepper and paprika and stir; the butter will turn bright red. Drizzle the butter over each serving, leaving the paprika powder and pepper flakes behind in the saucepan. Serve at once.

Simple Spanish Fried Eggs

SERVES 1

*B*eing a clay pot collector, I was immediately attracted to a painting by Velázquez in which a solemn woman "of a certain age" is depicted poaching a pair of eggs in simmering olive oil in a deep cazuela while an equally solemn-looking boy waits nearby. British writer Tom Lubbock describes the painting thus: "Those eggs. . . are the only things that move. The bodies of the old woman and the boy are static. What looks like action is in fact a kind of mime. It is held as if for an old long-exposure camera. The woman, wooden spoon in hand, un-cracked eggs in the other, doesn't cook so much as demonstrate an act of cooking."

I like cooking eggs just that way—slowly in a clay skillet until the whites congeal around deep orange yolks. And with a nod to Velázquez, I like to give my fried eggs a Spanish accent by adding a pinch of sweet and smoky Spanish *pimentón de la Vera* just before serving.

You may ask: Why that paprika and not some other? Call me a food fanatic, but for me the depth and nuance of this particular Spanish paprika has no equal. It has a warm, rounded flavor produced by drying and smoking mature red peppers over oak fires, then stone-grinding them to a smooth powder almost like talc. And, like wine, surely it has to do with the soil in Spain's western region, Extremadura. You can grow peppers in your backyard, hang them from your window, and, when they're brittle-dry, grind them into powder, but no matter how carefully you do all this, your paprika just won't taste the same.

PREFERRED CLAY POT:

1 cazuelita or a 5-inch Spanish cazuela

Extra virgin olive oil

1 or 2 very fresh eggs

Sea salt and freshly ground black pepper

Pinches of pimentón de la Vera (smoked Spanish paprika)

1 Place a flat griddle or comal on the stovetop. Set the cazuelita or small cazuelita on top. Fill the cazuelita with ½ inch olive oil; turn the heat to medium and when the oil begins to simmer, carefully slip in the egg(s).

2 Cook, tilting the pan and frequently basting the egg(s) with the oil, until the whites begin to congeal, the edges turn crispy, and the yolk remains soft and tender, about 5 minutes. Carefully lift the egg (s) out onto a plate. Season with salt and pepper and a light dusting of pimentón de la Vera and serve at once.

LEBANESE FRIED EGGS

Kamal Mouzawak, founder of Slow Food Lebanon, who lives in Beirut, had a vision: He would bring small farmers and artisanal food producers from all over Lebanon to a farmers' market in Beirut. Despite vast social, political, and religious differences, he managed to bring his dream to life.

On a recent visit to the United States, Kamal came to my house for lunch, bringing along a large selection of red clay Lebanese pots. The one pot I fell most in love with was a small *meqleh*, a thick clay skillet with a handle used to fry a single egg at a time. The texture of an egg slow-fried in butter in this vessel was just perfect—the yolk properly runny, the white thick, glossy and firm. The egg also gained a superb earthy flavor.

In Lebanon there are all sizes of *meqlehs* in which eggs are cooked, sometimes along with shredded preserved lamb or slices of sausage spiced with Armenian chiles. A 4- or 5-inch cazuelita will make a fine substitute.

Scrambled Eggs with Bottarga

SERVES 4

There are so many Tunisian egg dishes that London-based Australian food writer Terry Durack has referred to Tunisian cuisine as "a study in eggnology." In a letter to me, Terry wrote: "[Eggs] turn up in most every course to thicken soups, to garnish salads and couscous, to lighten fish or meatballs, to fill crisp fried pastries. Big, aromatic dishes called *shashouka, tagine, tastira, leblebi,* and *ojja* are often used as backdrops to show off another way to cook an egg."

Ojja is a spicy scrambled egg dish somewhat similar to Basque *piperade* but with an unusual consistency achieved by cooking the egg yolks very slowly in sauce in an earthenware dish removed from the heat. In this version, taught to me by Chef Haouari Abderrazak, a few tablespoons of cream added to the eggs ensure they come out extra-creamy and mousselike. The garnish here is one of the great delicacies of the Mediterranean—pressed and dried grey mullet roe, sold here in the States as *bottarga di muggine* (see Sources). Smoked herring, not Tunisian but good all the same, can be nicely substituted.

PREFERRED CLAY POT:

A 10-inch Spanish cazuela or earthenware tagine

If using an electric or ceramic stovetop, be sure to use a heat diffuser with the clay pot.

¾ cup cured bottarga di muggine or smoked kipper herring (2¾ ounces)

¼ cup extra virgin olive oil

3 tablespoons tomato paste, preferably homemade (page 317), mixed with 2 tablespoons water

1 teaspoon ground caraway

1½ teaspoons crushed garlic

1 scallion, white part only, minced

1 teaspoon homemade harissa or hot red chili

¾ cup grated fresh tomato

½ cup finely diced fresh green chile, such as Anaheim or jalapeño

8 very fresh eggs

Salt and freshly ground black pepper

½ teaspoon fresh lemon juice

¼ cup heavy cream or crème fraîche

1 Soak the fish in a bowl of cold water for 20 minutes. Drain and cut into fine dice.

2 Slowly heat the olive oil in the cazuela over medium-low heat. Add the diluted tomato paste, raise the heat to medium, and cook, stirring, until it sizzles, about 10 minutes. Add the caraway, garlic, scallion, and harissa and cook, stirring, for 2 minutes. Add the grated tomato and diced chile and simmer until thick and well reduced, about 10 minutes.

3 Meanwhile, separate the eggs, dividing the yolks and whites between 2 bowls. Use a fork to lightly beat the egg whites. Stir the whites into the tomato-pepper mixture. Cook slowly over medium heat until they begin to congeal but the sauce remains loose, about 5 minutes.

4 Add the egg yolks, half of the fish, the lemon juice, and the cream. Cook, stirring gently to break up the yolks, until they turn creamy and form soft curds, about 1 minute.

5 Remove the cazuela from the heat, cover, and let stand for about 3 minutes. Season with salt and pepper to taste. Divide among 4 warmed ramekins or cazuelitas. Scatter the remaining fish on top and serve.

Scrambled Eggs with Argan Oil

SERVES 2 OR 3

Argan oil has a unique taste reminiscent of roasted nuts but more complex and pungent. It's long been popular for seasoning raw or cooked tomatoes, peppers, greens, and zucchini or infusing added flavor at the last minute into couscous, lentils, beans, and chickpeas. In the Souss region of Morocco, cooperatives run by women produce an oil extracted from the nuts of the argan tree, a plant unique to the region and famous for its attractiveness to goats, who literally climb up into its branches to feast on the nuts.

Argan oil is rarely used for cooking; rather, it is added raw to finished foods as a final fillip of flavor. The oil is traditionally blended with ground almonds to make a dip for bread, called *amlou*. And, as I learned from Moroccan restaurateur Fatema Hal, who includes such a recipe in her cookbook *Le Grande Livre de la Cuisine Marocaine,* it also makes a great medium in which to cook eggs.

You'll find argan oil at better food shops and Middle Eastern groceries or online. Keep argan oil in the refrigerator after opening.

When I scramble eggs in argan oil, I like to go "full Moroccan," cooking them in a *ferrah,* a round shallow unglazed clay dish usually used for baking bread. You can substitute a small Spanish cazuela or La Chamba skillet. When you cook this dish in a clay vessel, you gain an advantage similar to one you'd get using a double boiler: slow, steady, controlled heat, which produces moist, creamy scrambled eggs. A clay vessel, however, is not quite as slow as a double boiler; eggs that would take ten minutes to cook in a double boiler will cook in six minutes in clay.

Please be sure to remove your clay pan from the heat while the eggs are still a little underdone. The eggs will continue to cook slowly. When you're satisfied, remove them from the pan.

> **PREFERRED CLAY POT:**
>
> An 8- or 9-inch Spanish cazuela, La Chamba skillet, or a flameware skillet
>
> If using an electric or ceramic stovetop, be sure to use a heat diffuser with the clay pot.

4 or 6 very fresh eggs, at room temperature

3 tablespoons argan oil

Sea salt

Ground cumin, preferably Moroccan

1 In a mixing bowl, whisk the eggs together until well blended.

2 Gently warm the argan oil in the cazuela over medium-low heat. Add the beaten eggs and cook until set on the bottom and sides; then lift and fold over with a flat spatula. Gently stir to keep the eggs light and creamy.

3 Remove from the heat and continue cooking in the retained heat of the clay for 1 minute longer. Serve with a sprinkling of sea salt and tiny pinches of ground cumin to taste.

NOTE TO THE COOK: If your eggs are cold from the refrigerator, you can warm them to room temperature quickly by soaking them in a bowl of hot water for 5 minutes, changing the water once or twice.

Guvec with Eggs, Spinach, Spiced Beef, and Bulgur

SERVE 4

*H*ere's a variation on the classic combination of eggs and spinach, this one quite unique due to the addition of preserved spiced meat and bulgur.

Basturma (sometimes spelled *pastirma*) can be purchased at Middle Eastern groceries as well as mail-order sources in both lean and fatty versions. For this dish you can use either one. Accompany with warm pita bread.

> **PREFERRED CLAY POT:**
>
> **An 11- or 12-inch Spanish cazuela or straight-sided flameware skillet.**
>
> **If using an electric or ceramic stovetop, be sure to use a heat diffuser with the clay pot.**

1 pound baby spinach leaves, washed

¼ cup medium bulgur

3 ounces basturma, finely diced

2 tablespoons extra virgin olive oil

4 large fresh eggs

Salt and freshly ground black pepper

Pinch of Marash or Aleppo pepper

1 Place the wet spinach in the cazuela. Add ½ cup water, cover, and cook over medium heat until wilted, about 2 minutes. Uncover and cook the spinach for 1 to 2 minutes longer.

2 Stir in the bulgur and simmer for 10 minutes, stirring from time to time to ensure the bulgur is cooking evenly. Remove from the heat. Cover and let stand until all excess moisture has been absorbed by the bulgur.

3 Push the spinach and bulgur to one side and add the basturma and olive oil. Cook over medium heat until the meat begins to sizzle. Fold the basturma into the spinach.

4 Divide the spinach mixture into 4 little nests in the pot. Slip an egg into each indentation. Cover and cook until the whites are set but the yolks are still runny, about 5 minutes. Dust with salt, black pepper, and Marash or Aleppo pepper to taste and serve at once.

Provençal Upside-Down Omelet with Mushrooms, Croutons, and Lardons

SERVES 2 OR 3

*P*lease note: This is not the type of French fold-over omelet with a runny interior that we normally associate with the word. Rather, a Provençal omelet is firm like a frittata. It's also different in that it's as good cold as warm and is thus ideal for a picnic.

The mushroom filling for this delicious omelet recipe is best prepared in a clay pot with a glazed interior, such as a Chinese sandpot or other small casserole with cover. The mushrooms are wrapped in parchment and placed inside the pot, which is then covered and set to cook slowly for thirty minutes. This method intensifies the flavor of even the most ordinary cultivated mushrooms.

A typical Provençal cook will make her omelet in a metal skillet. Once the egg mixture is thickened throughout and well cooked on the bottom, she'll add her topping of choice—in this case a mixture of mushrooms, croutons, and slivered pancetta. Then the entire omelet is flipped over, slipped back into the pan to lightly crisp the topping and sear it in, producing a lovely marbled crisp outer surface sandwiching the thin soft egg interior. Flipping the entire contents of a pan can be a tricky business; thus the invention of the *tourne omelette* or the *vire omelette*, a slightly concave glazed terra-cotta plate with a knob on the bottom side.

When it's time to flip, the cook grasps the knob with one hand, placing the plate directly over the omelet. Holding the skillet handle with her other hand, she skillfully turns plate and skillet together a full 180 degrees and then slips the turned omelet back into the skillet. It's a lot of fun to do this, quick and easy. And because the knob is wide and perfectly centered, the *tourne omelette* makes an attractive platter on which to serve the finished omelet at table.

A *tourne omelette* is a perfect example of a potter creating a utensil to fulfill a cook's need. Bernard Duplessy, author of *The French Country Table: Pottery & Faience of Provence,* calls this utensil "a venerable piece of pottery in and of itself that dates back to several centuries before Christ when it was used by the Greeks of Massalia [Marseilles]."

A few Provençal potters still make these plates (see Sources). I can't insist you spend a hundred-plus dollars to buy one, but I think you'll be pleased if you do. I love mine and use it to serve tarts and pizzas too. Of course, you can just as easily flip your Provençal omelet with the assistance of a footed ceramic fruit platter or a wide metal pot cover.

18 fresh firm white mushrooms, trimmed

2 slices stale French baguette

1 garlic clove, halved

2 tablespoons unsalted butter

3 ounces thinly sliced lean pancetta, slivered

5 large eggs

⅓ cup heavy cream or crème fraîche

Salt and freshly ground black pepper

1 Quickly rinse the mushrooms under running water; wipe dry with paper towels. Wrap in a sheet of parchment and place in the Chinese sandpot. Cover, set over low heat, and cook for 30 minutes. Remove from the heat; slice the mushrooms and set aside.

2 Meanwhile, rub the baguette with garlic and cut enough into small dice to make about ½ cup. Set a 9-inch conventional skillet over medium heat, melt the butter in it, add the pancetta, and toss to coat. Add the bread cubes to the skillet and cook, tossing, until golden brown, about 5 minutes. Add the mushrooms and cook, stirring, for 5 minutes longer.

3 In a mixing bowl, use a fork to quickly beat the eggs until well blended. Beat in the crème fraîche and a small pinch of salt and pepper. Pour the eggs into the hot skillet and, with one hand, shake the pan back and forth to keep the mixture from sticking while stirring with a fork in the other hand for 1 to 2 seconds.

4 Tilt the pan and lift the omelet at the edges to let the uncooked portion run beneath. As soon as the bottom appears to set, shake the pan to be sure the omelet slides around easily. Use a buttered tourne omelette, a footed cake plate, or flat metal lid to flip the omelet. Place over the omelet and quickly invert to unmold. Slide the omelet back into the pan. Cook on the second side, about 2 minutes, shaking the skillet to keep the omelet moving. Slide onto the tourne omelet or a platter and serve at once.

With thanks to Master Potter Philippe Beltrando for sharing this recipe.

Provençal-Style Flat Omelet with Blue Cheese and Caramelized Onion

SERVES 3 OR 4

*H*ere's another Provençal omelet, this one topped with a mix of caramelized golden onions, cooked slowly in a cazuela with milk and blue cheese. You can make the topping in advance.

> **PREFERRED CLAY POT:**
>
> A 9-inch Spanish cazuela
>
> A *tourne omelette*, a 9-inch ceramic footed cake plate, or a flat metal pot lid
>
> If using an electric or ceramic stovetop, be sure to use a heat diffuser with the clay pot.

1 large onion, quartered lengthwise
    and thinly sliced

4½ tablespoons unsalted butter

¼ teaspoon salt

¼ teaspoon sugar

¼ teaspoon freshly ground black pepper

2 ounces creamy Roquefort cheese,
    cut into small pieces

½ cup milk

6 eggs

1 Put the onion, 2 tablespoons of the butter, the salt, and the sugar in the cazuela set over low heat. Cover and steam the onion for 45 minutes, until very soft. Season with the pepper.

2 Uncover, raise the heat to medium, and cook, stirring, until golden brown, 10 to 15 minutes. Add the Roquefort cheese and milk and cook until the mixture is very thick and creamy, about 10 minutes. (The recipe can be prepared to this point up to 2 days in advance and stored in the refrigerator.)

3 Beat the eggs lightly; strain into another bowl. Heat a 10-inch nonstick skillet over medium heat, add 2 more tablespoons of the butter, and swirl to coat the bottom and sides of the skillet. Add the onion mixture and reheat to sizzling. Quickly pour in the eggs and shake the skillet back and forth with one hand to keep the mixture from sticking while stirring with a fork in the other hand for 1 to 2 seconds. Tilt the pan and lift the omelet at the edges to let the uncooked portion run underneath. As soon as the bottom appears to be set and slightly browned, shake the pan to be sure the omelet slides around easily.

4 Use the rest of the butter to lightly grease a tourne omelette, footed cake plate, or flat metal lid. Place over the omelet and quickly invert to unmold. Slide the omelet back into the pan. Cook on the second side, about 2 minutes, shaking the skillet to keep the omelet moving. Slide onto a tourne omelette or a platter and serve at once.

Eggs on a Creamy Bed of Sorrel

SERVES 2

The secret to this flavorful sauce is not to overcook the sorrel leaves but to lightly steam them, ensuring they don't lose their fresh slightly bitter–sharp lemony flavor.

> **PREFERRED CLAY POTS:**
> 2 individual earthenware gratin dishes or cazuelitas; to substitute porcelain ramekins, see Note

2 tablespoons unsalted butter

2 ounces young sorrel leaves, shredded, 1½ cups

¼ cup heavy cream

¼ teaspoon salt

⅛ teaspoon freshly ground black pepper

¼ teaspoon freshly grated nutmeg

2 or 4 farm-fresh eggs

1 Butter the cazuelitas and place on a baking sheet in a cold oven; set the temperature at 350°F.

2 In a small nonreactive saucepan, cook the sorrel with 2 tablespoons of the cream until it melts, about 3 minutes. Season with the salt, pepper, and nutmeg.

3 Remove the baking sheet from the oven, divide the hot sorrel between the dishes, and top each with 1 or 2 eggs. Quickly spoon some of the remaining heavy cream over each yolk. Tent the dishes with a sheet of aluminum foil and return to the oven.

4 Bake for 12 to 15 minutes, until the whites are just firm and the yolks still runny. Serve at once.

NOTE TO THE COOK: To make this dish with porcelain ramekins: Bring a kettle of water to a boil. Arrange the ramekins in a deep baking pan. Place a dab of butter in each ramekin before adding the sorrel, egg, and a dab of cream. Pour boiling water into the baking pan to reach about halfway up the sides of the ramekins. Bake at 375°F for about 10 minutes. For firmer eggs, bake for another 1 to 2 minutes.

Baked Eggs with Ham and Caramelized Tomatoes

SERVES 4

In Spain and France, numerous egg dishes are presented as first courses, cooked and served in ramekins, individual gratin dishes, or custard cups. These vessels are filled and then set in hot water baths to be removed the moment the whites firm up but the yolks are still loose and runny.

In this wondrous Catalan dish, the eggs are set for cooking in a lovely rich ham and tomato sauce prepared in advance. Serve with crusty bread.

> **PREFERRED CLAY POTS:**
>
> A 9- or 10-inch Spanish cazuela
>
> 4 earthenware cazuelitas, 4 ounces each; to substitute stoneware or porcelain ramekins or custard cups, see Note.

1 pint cherry tomatoes

Extra virgin olive oil

½ cup chopped shallot

2 garlic cloves, sliced

Pinch of sugar

Salt and freshly ground black pepper

2 thin slices Serrano ham, slivered

4 eggs

¼ cup heavy cream

4 ounces Gruyère or Monterey Jack cheese, finely shredded (about 1 cup)

2 tablespoons slivered fresh tarragon leaves

1 About 1½ hours before serving, preheat the oven to 300°F. Cut each tomato in half and arrange cut side up in an oiled cazuela. Add the shallot, garlic, and sugar and season lightly with salt and pepper.

2 Bake for 1 hour, or until the tomatoes are lightly caramelized. Stir in the ham and continue to bake for 10 minutes and then remove from the oven.

3 Raise the oven temperature to 375°F. Divide the tomato mixture among the cazuelitas. Make a small well in each and break an egg into it; sprinkle with salt and pepper. Gently mix the cream and cheese and divide the mixture among the cazuelitas to cover each egg yolk.

4 Bake for 10 to 12 minutes, or until the egg whites are set. Dust with a little chopped tarragon and serve at once.

NOTE TO THE COOK: You can make this dish with ramekins or custard cups: Bring a kettle of water to the boil. Arrange the ramekins in a deep baking pan. Place a little olive oil in the bottom of each ramekin before adding the tomato mixture, eggs, and cream and cheese topping. Pour boiling water into the baking pan to reach about halfway up the sides of the ramekins. Bake at 375°F for about 10 minutes. For firmer eggs, bake for another 1 to 2 minutes.

Fig Teleme: Ancient Method

MAKES ABOUT ¾ CUP

Villagers living in Iskenderun in southeastern Turkey, near where the Tigris and Euphrates rivers flow toward Syria, still use fig tree sap as a curdling agent to make a soft white cheese, now called *Teleme*. This ancient method spread throughout the Middle East and even as far as Algeria. The great Greek philosopher Aristotle wrote about the technique, describing how adding the sap of an unripe fig to fresh goat's milk created a good white cheese.

When I learned about Turkish *Teleme* cheese, I was so intrigued I went out and bought a fig tree to see if I could make the cheese myself. The resulting cheese was appropriately mild, with a taste slightly redolent of sweetened coconut.

I present two ways to make *Teleme* cheese. Here I give the ancient method; in the following recipe, you'll find a modern chef's version.

If you have access to a fig tree, cut off a tender branch with just one unripe baby fig still attached. You don't want to detach the fig until you're actually making the cheese. Once your goat's milk is hot, break off the fig and allow just a few drops of milky liquid to drip into the milk and start the culturing process. I use the resulting mild cheese to stuff Swiss chard leaves and Italian cannelloni. Sweetened with just a touch of sugar, it is delightful with fresh fruit.

PREFERRED CLAY POT:

A 3-quart glazed or unglazed earthenware casserole

1 quart goat's milk

1 freshly cut fleshy 8- to 9-inch branch from a yellow fig tree with 1 slightly underripe yellow fig attached

1 Pour the milk into the earthenware casserole. Break off the fig and shake the white sap from the spot where the fruit was attached to the branch directly into the milk. There should be about 3 drops. Use a pair of scissors to cut the branch into 2 or 3 pieces on the bias and let them fall directly into the milk. Use the fig for some other purpose or discard. Slowly bring the milk to a boil over the lowest possible heat, stirring very often with a wooden spoon, about 30 minutes. There should be a great deal of evaporation, and the milk should separate into tiny curds.

2 Remove from the heat and let stand for 30 minutes.

3 Discard the pieces of fig branch and strain the curds and whey through a double thickness of dampened cheesecloth in a colander set over a bowl. When the curds are well drained, which can take anywhere from 5 to 15 minutes, wrap them in plastic wrap and refrigerate for up to 3 days.

Fig Teleme: Modern Chef's Version

SERVES 6

The brilliant Turkish chef, Musa Dağdeviren, whose name appears often in this book, devised a totally different modern way of making *Teleme* cheese using dried Turkish yellow figs. Musa cuts off and discards the tiny hard points of the dried figs, finely dices them, and reduces them to a paste in a food processor. With the processor still on, he slowly adds warm goat's milk so that the fig paste and milk bind together, a procedure similar to that used to make mayonnaise.

The fig-milk is then poured into clay ramekins and left to culture at room temperature; then it is chilled until served. This type of *Teleme* cheese, topped with toasted chopped walnuts, makes a delicious dessert.

Please note: When Musa was here in the United States he tried to make his *Teleme* cheese with domestic dried figs but wasn't all that satisfied with the flavor. Imported dried Turkish yellow figs are really the only way to go.

PREFERRED CLAY POT:
6 ceramic ramekins, 6 ounces each

1 quart fresh goat's milk

10 ounces imported dried Turkish yellow figs

1 In a large conventional saucepan, heat the milk to 112°F to 115°F.

2 Dice the figs; then chop them to a fine paste in a food processor or blender while slowly adding the warm milk. Do not strain, but simply fill the ramekins and let stand at room temperature for about 1½ hours.

3 Cover and refrigerate overnight. Serve the next day.

EARLY CHEESE MAKING

One of my great pleasures is making cheese and yogurt at home, perhaps because both involve enacting ancient processes in which milk and clay pots play essential roles. We sometimes forget how many different products can be made from milk—each with its own flavor, aroma, and texture.

One of the many amazing facts about cheese is the way it was discovered accidentally by nomads. Transporting fresh milk in bags made from the stomachs of animals, they found that the milk separated into curds and whey. What caused the milk to be transformed into what was essentially cheese was the action of rennet, an enzyme found in the stomach linings of ruminants. Once they realized the connection, these nomads began to make cheese intentionally.

There are other enzymes beside rennet that will coagulate milk. In some countries surrounding the Mediterranean, fresh fig sap and dried flower thistle are used for this purpose. Since most storage vessels at that time were made of clay, cheese making naturally led to the use of clay pots for holding and cooking milk and then storing cheese.

Mediterranean Thistle Flower Cheese

SERVES 4

The use of thistle flower as a cheese-making agent is a very old method, common throughout the western Mediterranean. In the Canary Islands, Aragon, and Catalonian Spain, ewe's milk is traditionally curdled by steeping a small satchel of dried flower thistles of wild cardoons (*Cynara cardunculus*) in the milk as it simmers. This produces a thick, firm, sweet-tasting cheese with wonderful herbal aromas.

In Morocco, the dried thistle flower of choice is the wild artichoke (*Cynara humulis*) called *qôq dyal afzan*. It makes a delicious pillowlike fresh cheese flavored with orange flower water. Called *rayeb* or *raipe,* this cheese, which is similar in texture to junket, is both prepared and stored in a clay jar called a *hallab*.

> **PREFERRED CLAY POT:**
>
> **A 3-quart earthenware casserole**
>
> **If using an electric or ceramic stovetop, be sure to use a heat diffuser with the clay pot.**

2 tablespoons dried thistle flowers (see Sources)

1 quart milk

2 tablespoons sugar

2 tablespoons orange flower water

1 Crush the thistle flowers to a coarse powder; there should be about 1 teaspoon. Wrap the thistle powder in a clean cloth, tie securely with white kitchen string, and set aside.

2 In the earthenware casserole, heat the milk to lukewarm (about 110°F). Add the cloth packet and swirl it around in the lukewarm milk, lift it out, and gently squeeze the packet to extract all the brown juices, letting them fall back into the milk; discard the packet.

3 Stir the sugar and orange flower water into the warm milk. Remove from the heat, cover, and set in a warm place for 1 to 1½ hours, until set.

4 To serve, divide the soft cheese among 4 custard cups. Serve cool or chilled as a snack.

EASTERN MEDITERRANEAN CLOTTED CREAM

Kaymak, a thick, rich clotted cream made from sheep or buffalo milk, is something like a combination of whipped cream and Italian mascarpone. I call it a true "guilty pleasure," because it is so fabulously rich that it evokes guilt and so marvelously good that it brings great pleasure.

Kaymak is eaten with fruit, spread on bread, used in place of butter when slow-cooking eggs, or simply gobbled up with a spoon. Samira Yogo Cholagh, a Chaldean Christian born in Iraq who now resides in the United States, told me that every Christmas she treats herself to a batch. Here's how she makes it:

She heats a quart of whole cow's milk in a heavy shallow pot; if she were back in the Middle East, she'd use sheep's milk. After bringing it to a boil, she reduces the heat to low and adds a quart of heavy cream. This blend of milk and cream is simmered for two hours. Then she turns off the heat and lets the pot sit undisturbed for seven hours before reheating the mixture, simmering it for thirty minutes, and letting it cool again. Finally, she chills the cream in the cooking vessel for two to three days. During refrigeration, the cream separates, and the *kaymak* rises to the top. When Samira is ready to serve it, she loosens this slab by running a knife along the edges and transfers the thick clotted cream to a plate, where it is accompanied by bread and honey or apricot or fig jam.

In the Turkish town of Ürgüp near Cappadocia, a pottery-making village in Central Anatolia, a local cook, Meryem Uresin described her method for making *kaymak:* "I soak a fresh unglazed *guvec* pot in water for a day to eliminate the new-clay odor. After draining the pot, I add a little sheep's milk and cook it until it boils. I let the milk simmer for half an hour, leave it to cool, and then add an equal amount of fresh milk. The cooked and uncooked milk are simmered together for another hour."

Meryem continues adding fresh milk to the milk she's already cooked and simmering it to reduce it until her *guvec* pot is filled, a procedure that takes about four days. These multiple warmings and coolings of cooked milk slowly perfect the *kaymak,* producing the luscious thick texture Turks adore. When her pot is filled, Meryem leaves it to rest overnight. The next morning, she spoons cream that has clotted along the sides of the pot to its center. At this point, when the cream is so thick it can literally be folded up, she uses her hands to transfer globs of it to a deep earthenware jug for storage.

If you don't feel ready to undertake either Samira's or Meryem's method, you can make some mock *kaymak* by folding ½ cup mascarpone into ½ cup heavy cream. Though it won't be the same, it may convey a bit of what *kaymak* is about.

Homemade Yogurt, Ohrid Style

SERVES 6

Throughout my childhood, my paternal grandmother regaled me with stories of the Balkans, where she was born. "Someday, Paulina, I hope you will go back to the old country. When you're there, you'll eat wonderful, wonderful food. And be sure and taste the yogurt. I think it's the best in the world."

In the 1960s, during my beatnik days, I did visit the region, spending a month in the Macedonian town of Ohrid near the Albanian border. My grandma Bertha did tend toward hyperbole, but I discovered there that she was right about the homemade yogurt: it was very good indeed.

I found a room in a private home, which cost me a dollar a night. The best part of living with the Kardrevski family was learning about their lifestyle. Among the many things my hostess taught me was how to make fresh sheep's milk yogurt. This recipe is my adaptation of her method. It employs small unglazed clay pots similar to the ones she used, and the yogurt comes out nearly as thick, creamy, and tasty as if it were made from sheep's milk.

PREFERRED CLAY POTS:

A 3-quart earthenware casserole

Six small earthenware bowls, preferably unglazed Pomaireware bowls, or ceramic ramekins

If using an electric or ceramic stovetop, be sure to use a heat diffuser with the clay pot.

---

1 quart whole or skim milk

¼ cup plain yogurt

1 In the earthenware casserole, bring the milk to a boil over medium heat. Reduce the heat slightly and simmer for 2 minutes. Remove from the heat and let the milk cool to lukewarm, about 110°F, or until a few drops of milk on the inside of the wrist feel warm.

2 Arrange the earthenware bowls or ramekins on a double layer of kitchen towels on a baking sheet. Stir the yogurt into the warm milk. Divide among 6 bowls or ramekins. Move the baking sheet to the warmest part of the kitchen. Cover with a sheet of paper towels and a kitchen towel and let stand to culture and set, which can take anywhere from 4 to 8 hours. Check after 4 hours by carefully tilting one of the containers to see whether the milk has thickened. If not, let stand for another 4 hours. When the yogurt is done, refrigerate and use within 1 week.

CATALAN TUPI CHEESE

According to legend, the delicious, salty, strong Catalan cheese, *tupi*, was, like so many cheeses, created by accident. And, it should be noted, a two-handled clay pot (called a *tupi*) played a vital role in its creation.

When Pyrenees peasants made their popular goat's cheese, *serrat*, there was often a good deal of leftover curds. The story goes that a particular shepherd mixed them with anise liqueur and fresh cow or sheep's milk cheese and then packed the mixture into a *tupi*, covered the clay pot with a cloth, and secured it with string to protect the contents. Opening the pot several months later, he discovered a strong-smelling and marvelously flavored cheese, which he called *tupi* after the pot in which it had fermented.

Though *tupi* is strong, it can be tamed by being mixed with honey or fig jam or combined with butter and spreading it on grilled bread lightly rubbed with garlic. It's available through www.anhmarket.com. And if you opt to go totally Catalan, you'll want to accompany it with some dried fig puree and a glass of cold sparkling *cava*.

CARAMELIZED MILK ICE CREAM AND YOGURT AS PREPARED IN ANTAKYA

Here's some "cutting edge" culinary news from Turkey, thanks to my friend Ayfer Ünsal, who writes a cooking column every other month for the Turkish food magazine *Sofra*. Well, maybe not quite "cutting edge," since the source of Ayfer's research, villagers in the Mediterranean coastal town of Antakya, claim their method for making burned milk for ice cream and yogurt goes back thousands of years!

Here's how it's done: A shepherd heats stones in a wood fire and then transfers some of these very hot stones to a pot filled with simmering milk. The hot stones cause the milk to boil and impart a special burnt flavor, enhanced as the first batch of stones is replaced several times by new sets of freshly heated stones. This caramelized milk is then churned in a torpedo-shaped unglazed earthenware casserole, after which it's used as the base for an extraordinary-tasting ice cream or yogurt.

Yogurt with Grape Molasses, Tahini, and Sautéed Nuts

SERVES 6

This sweet yogurt dessert snack bears the unlikely name *karga beyni*, literally "crow's brains" on account of its look—individual domes of yogurt crowned with various embellishments such as walnuts, hazelnuts, pistachios, figs, raisins, dried white mulberries, and drizzles of tahini and grape molasses. Grape molasses, also called *pekmez*, and dried white mulberries can be found at Middle Eastern stores.

PREFERRED CLAY VESSEL

A 10-inch Spanish cazuela

6 small ceramic custard cups, cazuelitas, or ramekins, 6 ounces each

If using an electric or ceramic stovetop, be sure to use a heat diffuser with the clay pot.

---

3 cups goat's milk yogurt

¼ teaspoon coriander seeds

5 allspice berries

1 small Ceylon cinnamon stick

½ cup shelled walnuts

9 tablespoons unsalted butter

¼ cup dried white mulberries, sour cherries, or diced Turkish dried yellow figs

¼ cup golden raisins

2 tablespoons peeled and chopped hazelnuts

5 tablespoons tahini

5 tablespoons pekmez (grape molasses) or Italian saba, sapa, or any unfermented grape syrup

2 tablespoons shelled and chopped pistachios

1 Drain the yogurt in a sieve lined with a paper coffee filter or a double layer of cheesecloth until thick, about 2 hours.

2 At the same time, soak the coriander seeds, allspice berries, and cinnamon stick in ¼ cup hot water.

3 In a medium conventional skillet, toast the walnuts over medium heat, stirring constantly, until fragrant and golden, 2 to 3 minutes. Transfer to a dish and let cool slightly. Chop the walnuts.

4 Set the cazuela over medium heat. Add 6 tablespoons of the butter, half of the toasted walnuts, the mulberries, golden raisins, pistachios, and hazelnuts. Cook, gently shaking the cazuela from time to time, until the nuts turn brown around the edges, about 20 minutes. Immediately stir in 3 tablespoons of the tahini and 3 tablespoons of the grape molasses. Turn off the heat.

5 Spoon half of the thickened yogurt into the custard cups. Cover with the nut and raisin mixture and top with the remaining yogurt.

6 Strain the spices, reserving their soaking water and discarding the whole spices. Add the spice water to the cazuela. Warm gently over low heat, scraping up any flavorings stuck to the bottom of the pan. Stir in the remaining 2 tablespoons grape molasses and 2 tablespoons tahini and bring to a boil. Drizzle this hot mixture over each serving of yogurt. Add the remaining 3 tablespoons butter to the cazuela, tilting the pot so it melts quickly, and spoon it sizzling on top. Garnish with the pistachios and the remaining toasted walnuts and serve at once.

With thanks to Musa Dağdeviren for sharing this recipe.

MOROCCAN SMEN

We know about foods that taste better when aged: wine, vinegar, some of the finest steaks. But few know the glories of aged butter better than Moroccans. They call it *smen* and use the condiment to add depth of flavor to soups, couscous, tagines, cured meats, and many local types of flat bread. Its nutty quality and pungent saltiness, the result of culturing, bear little relation to ordinary butter. Some Moroccan home cooks will spread *smen* thinly on warm semolina flat bread and serve it with a dollop of orange flower honey and a glass of mint tea as a snack.

Smen is similar to Middle Eastern *samneh* and Indian *ghee* in that all are created by churning fresh cream into butter, clarifying it, and then storing it. But Moroccan cooks go a step further by culturing or fermenting the butter *before* clarifying to develop a complex flavor and intense aroma. Methods differ a bit from region to region, resulting in slight differences in taste. There are herbal and nonherbal varieties made from fresh cow, goat, or sheep's milk, which, depending on local custom, is cultured with buttermilk, mildly soured cream, or yogurt to provide the proper bacterial culture and flavor. Once fermented, the milk is churned into butter and then aged for several days before clarification lest its unique flavor be lost.

After clarifying, the *smen* is packed into a clay jar, stored in a root cellar or buried in the ground, and aged for anywhere from one month to several years. (In my recipe, I age the *smen* for one month and then refrigerate and use it within a year.) A tiny bit of *smen* added to a bowl of freshly steamed couscous along with plenty of fresh butter will endow the couscous with an extra dimension of flavor.

My friend Mourad Lahlou, chef-owner of Aziza, San Francisco's much-acclaimed Moroccan restaurant, makes his own *smen*. He tells me that many families in his hometown of Marrakech still age their *smen* for a year before using it in small amounts to flavor special dishes. After so much aging, *smen* acquires an arresting intensity with hints of almonds and a subtle blue cheese flavor.

"A teaspoon of that kind of aged *smen* added to some fresh butter is all you need to perfume two pounds of couscous," he says.

A final note: It's unfortunate that *smen* is often translated into French as *beurre rance* meaning "rancid butter." In fact, if you don't make it properly, it can oxidize and taste "off." But if you follow my directions carefully, you'll end up with good *smen*, a great condiment to flavor your North African dishes.

Herbal Smen

MAKES ABOUT ⅔ CUP

$\mathcal{I}$ first tasted herbal *smen* in late spring of 1969 while traveling in Berber country in southern Morocco. There my host family treated me to some grilled flat bread hot off a clay griddle smeared with the family *smen,* a dense, straw-colored substance that had the richness of butter and the taste of a subtle mix of salt and local herbs.

The herbs, my host explained, were regional varieties of wild thyme, short bush oregano, and a local savory called *azukni,* known for its pleasant herbal tang and ability to inhibit bacterial growth in preserved butter. These dried herbs were boiled, strained, cooled, and worked into the just-churned butter. Then the butter was kneaded to remove every trace of moisture. This may sound easy, but, in fact, it requires much hard work. Often, in Moroccan villages, I've seen Moroccan women knead butter via a laborious process of knuckling and pressing, working to remove every drop of moisture lest it cause the butter to turn. (See my procedure below, using a food processor to "wash" and remove moisture from the butter.)

"This is new *smen,*" my hostess explained as she scooped out some of the dense butter from an earthenware crock. "It takes about a month to develop flavor. With time, the flavor grows stronger and stronger, and as it does, I use less and less in my cooking."

Herbal *smen* is called for in very small quantities in many recipes in this book, and this version will add extra flavor. Use it, for example, in egg dishes, Marrakech-Style Veal Tangia (page 155), preserved lamb, lentil dishes, and Moroccan Harira (page 42).

> **PREFERRED CLAY VESSEL:**
> 1 small earthenware crock with lid

1 tablespoon plus 1 teaspoon Mediterranean oregano

1 tablespoon sea salt

1 pint organic heavy cream

1 In a small saucepan, simmer the oregano and sea salt in 2 cups water for 15 minutes. Remove from the heat and let cool completely. Strain through a cheesecloth-lined sieve into a bowl. Freeze for 30 minutes, until ice cold but not frozen.

2 Meanwhile, pour the cream into a food processor. Process for 10 to 20 seconds, or until the cream seizes up, thickens, and throws off liquid. Pulse until the butter separates completely from the liquid, which is what we call buttermilk. Immediately pour off all the buttermilk and reserve for some other purpose. (You can freeze it and use for flavoring couscous.)

3 Pour ¼ cup of the ice-cold oregano-scented water into the butter and pulse once or twice; pour off and discard the water. Repeat two more times with equal amounts of the remaining oregano water. Now add

(continued)

½ cup fresh cold water and pulse again. Place the butter on a clean piece of parchment or freezer paper and use your knuckles to knead until no water is expressed.

4   Tightly pack the butter into a sterile and dry earthenware crock or dark glass jar; do not use metal. Cover tightly and store in a dark cool place for about 1 month before using. Once it has been opened, store in the refrigerator, where it will keep for 1 to 2 months longer.

NOTES TO THE COOK:

✳ Organic or raw cream is essential for this recipe because it contains live organisms that will facilitate the fermenting process and yield a nutty *smen*.

✳ Because this *smen* is only lightly salted, it cannot be stored as long as most other versions.

USING THE FOOD PROCESSOR TO CHURN AND WASH BUTTER FOR *SMEN*

In North Africa in the old days butter was churned by packing milk into an animal skin bag and shaking the bag vigorously. When the proper glopping sound was heard, chunks of butter were removed by hand and the remaining liquid, a type of buttermilk, was cooled and served as a drink to accompany food. In today's kitchen this churning and washing of the butter is easily done in a food processor, though you will need to let it mature.

After the *smen* is made, it is matured for a month, after which it's best to refrigerate it for safe storage. Traditionally, *smen* is not kept in the refrigerator but is packed into earthenware jars, and it shouldn't spoil if all the moisture has been removed. If for some reason your *smen* develops a few white spots on the surface, simply scrape them away. But if it shows bubbles or gives off an odor of gas or yeast, you should throw it out. Once your *smen* has developed a lovely nutty aroma, you might consider refrigerating or freezing it for longer storage. Otherwise it will develop even deeper flavor, definitely an acquired taste.

My versions of *smen* are not nearly as strong as the "infamous *smen*" of Fez and Marrakech, where some wealthy families boast of having put up their *smen* for years.

Salted and Cooked Smen Made from Cultured Heavy Cream

MAKES ABOUT ½ CUP

Use a tablespoon of this *smen* along with plenty of fresh butter in a bowl of couscous. It is also good in *kdra* tagines (see page 92 for Chicken Kdra). Or spread it thin on warm semolina bread and serve with a dollop of orange flower honey and a glass of sweet mint tea.

Note: You need to prepare this version of *smen* about one month in advance. It keeps for up to a year.

PREFERRED CLAY VESSEL:

1 small earthenware crock with lid

1 pint organic heavy cream

2 tablespoons whole-milk yogurt—sheep, cow, or goat

1½ teaspoons sea salt, preferably Maldon

1 In a small bowl, combine the cream and yogurt and let stand overnight at room temperature to culture.

2 Put the cultured cream into a food processor and whip for 10 to 20 seconds, or until the cream seizes and throws off liquid. Switch to pulsing and continue until the butter separates from the liquid. Pour off all the liquid buttermilk and reserve for some other purpose. (You can freeze it and use to moisten couscous.)

3 Now wash the butter by adding about 3 tablespoons ice-cold water to the processor and pulsing 2 or 3 times. Pour off and discard the liquid. Repeat twice with ½ cup ice-cold water. The water should run clear. If it doesn't, repeat one more time. Place the butter on a parchment paper–lined work surface. Sprinkle on the salt and knead until well blended. Divide into 6 equal parts. Press each part into a ¼-inch round and arrange side by side on a dry, clean cloth in a large bowl. Cover with another cloth, and let ripen in a cool dark place for 2 to 3 days.

4 To clarify the butter, place it in a small heavy saucepan and set over very low heat. Allow the butter to melt slowly without stirring and without browning. Remove the foam as it appears on the surface. When the butter is golden and clear, remove it from the heat and let stand until cool. Carefully spoon the butter through a double layer of dampened cheesecloth set over a bowl, leaving any white sediment at the bottom of the pan behind. To prevent the *smen* from turning rancid, strain again through clean cheesecloth. The smen must be absolutely clear. Discard any solids. Pour the butter into a sterile and dry container, preferably earthenware. Cover tightly and store in a dark place at room temperature for 1 month before opening. Store in a cool cupboard or the refrigerator after opening.

Salted and Cooked Smen Made from Store-Bought Butter

MAKES ABOUT ½ CUP

Though this version of smen doesn't have the depth of flavor and aroma of the previous two recipes, it is easier to make and far more economical.

8 ounces (2 sticks) organic unsalted butter, cut into 12 chunks

2 ounces coarse sea salt (about 7 tablespoons)

1 Knead the butter with the salt until well combined. Divide into 8 flat patties. Stack in an earthenware or dark glass container, cover, and store in a cupboard for 2 to 3 weeks to develop flavor.

2 Clarify the butter as directed in the preceding recipe. Spoon the cleared butter into a sterile and dry earthenware or glass container. When the butter is cool, seal and store in the cupboard for 1 month before using.

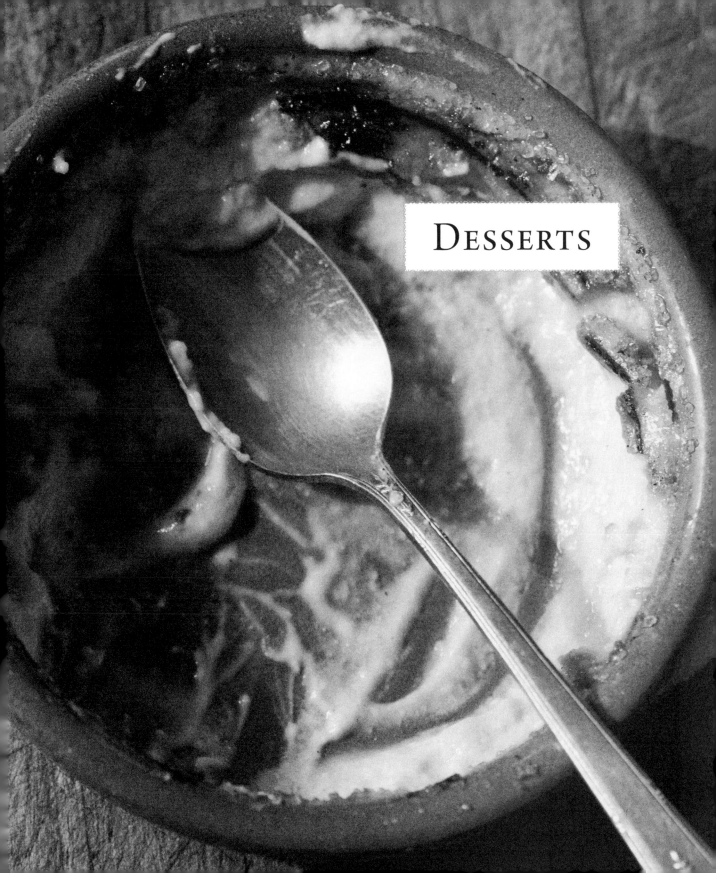

DESSERTS

Crèma Catalana as Prepared in the Nineteenth Century

SERVES 6

One of the most famous of all Spanish Catalan desserts, *crema catalana* is a simple stovetop-cooked custard served in shallow terra-cotta cazuelitas. A very hot salamander (a small kitchen iron with a long handle) is used to sear the top, forming a glassy, paper-thin crust that imparts a delicious burnt sugar taste and a wonderful smoky aroma.

In this version, which dates back more than a hundred years, a luxurious creaminess and depth of flavor are created through the extra step of baking the custards in a slow oven after the stovetop cooking. (David Kinch, chef-owner of the celebrated Manresa restaurant in Los Gatos, California, who worked previously at the Catalan restaurant Sent Sovi, confirmed to me that, in fact, some old Catalan culinary texts suggest this type of dual cooking.)

Interestingly, this second step brings the recipe close to the famous *crème brûlée*, but there are two main differences: *Crema catalana* is not baked in a bain-marie or water bath; it's made with a mixture of milk and cream, which makes it lighter than the French version, which is usually made entirely of heavy cream.

You can purchase cazuelitas along with a salamander or branding iron from www.tienda.com or www.spanishtable.com. See the Notes for tips on how to use the salamander and also how to finish the dish with a kitchen blowtorch or a gas broiler.

PREFERRED CLAY POTS:

A 3-quart glazed or unglazed earthenware or ceramic flameware saucepan or casserole

6 earthenware cazuelitas or very shallow porcelain or stoneware baking dishes, 6 ounces each, and about 5 inches in diameter

If using an electric or ceramic stovetop, be sure to use a heat diffuser with the clay pot.

1 quart whole milk

1 piece (2 inches) vanilla bean, split lengthwise

1 long strip lemon zest

½ cup egg yolks (7 or 8 yolks)

¼ cup plus 3 tablespoons granulated sugar

2 tablespoons cornstarch

6 tablespoons turbinado sugar

1 Pour the milk into the earthenware saucepan and set over low heat. Scrape the seeds from the vanilla bean into the milk and throw in the pod as well. Add the lemon zest, raise the heat to medium-low, and cook until bubbles appear around the rim of the pan. Transfer the hot saucepan to a wooden surface or folded kitchen towel to prevent cracking and let the flavorings steep in the milk for about 20 minutes.

2 Preheat the oven to 210°F. Reheat the milk over medium heat until hot but not boiling. Scoop out and discard the flavorings.

3 In a mixing bowl, combine the egg yolks, granulated sugar, and cornstarch. Beat until smooth, creamy, and pale in color, 2 to 3 minutes. Gradually whisk in about 1 cup of the hot milk. Scrape the egg yolk mixture into the remaining milk in the saucepan and cook over low heat, stirring, until the custard is creamy and thick enough to coat a wooden spoon thickly. Do not allow to boil.

4 Arrange the cazuelitas on a jelly roll pan. Ladle the custard into them, dividing it evenly. Bake for 1 to 1¼ hours, or until the custard is set around the edges but still slightly jiggly in the center. Let cool, then cover each little dish with plastic wrap and refrigerate for up to 2 days.

5 About 20 minutes before serving, remove the cazuelitas from the refrigerator and discard their plastic covers. Use a paper towel to gently blot away any surface moisture on top of each. Sprinkle 1 tablespoon of the turbinado sugar evenly over each custard. Caramelize in any of the three ways described in the Notes, and serve at once.

NOTES TO THE COOK:

✳ I purchase Tahitian vanilla beans online and keep them covered in white rum in a glass jar. The vanilla retains flavor, and the rum acquires a lovely aroma useful for flavoring cakes at some other time.

✳ To caramelize using an iron salamander: Place the salamander over a high flame on a gas stovetop, on the coil of an electric burner set to high, or on a flat glass-topped electric stove. Heat for at least 5 minutes. Working on one *crema* at a time, apply the hot round portion directly to the sugar and hold until sizzling and smoking. The moment you lift the salamander, the sugar topping will turn glassy. Wipe the salamander with a damp cloth; then return it to reheat for a few minutes before glazing the next *crema*. The *cremas* will retain their glassy crust for about 20 minutes, so you should have enough time to finish them all off. To clean your salamander, let it cool down completely, rinse under hot water, and scrub with a pumice stone until smooth; then rinse again and dry thoroughly.

✳ To caramelize using a kitchen blowtorch: Follow the manufacturer's instructions for igniting your blowtorch. Hold it about 3 inches above the sugar topping so the end of the flame just touches the sugar. Use a slow rotating movement, allowing the flame to "lick" the entire surface evenly until glazed and dark brown.

✳ To caramelize using a gas broiler: Preheat the broiler. Set the well-chilled custards about 5 inches below the flame and broil until the sugar surface turns deep brown. Using an electric broiler to caramelize is not recommended since by the time the sugar has glazed, the custards will lose their chill.

Turkish Stovetop Rice Pudding

SERVES 6

Ayfer Ünsal, who taught me this delicious rice pudding, is a wonderful cook, a modern Turkish woman, and the author of four books on Turkish cooking. She explained to me that a Turkish rice pudding may be cooked either in the oven or directly over heat on the stovetop. Either way, it's always in a clay pot, which gives the pudding a wonderful texture and flavor. Her stovetop version produces lovely golden brown bits that, when scooped and scraped up from the bottom, provide shots of creamy rich flavor.

I've known for a while that milk can help prime clay pots, whether glazed or unglazed, and, in fact, make them stronger. Several commercial producers, including Emile Henry and La Chamba, recommend milk curing before first use. And French potter Philippe Beltrando suggests cooking milk in his glazed earthenware pots for their maiden voyage in the kitchen. The idea is that casein, a milk protein that is not soluble in water, acts like a glue to seal tiny pores or cracks in the clay. This milk "patching" also works well if you need to repair a leaky Chinese sandpot.

When visiting the village of Sorkun in central Anatolia, Turkey, where unglazed casseroles have been made for centuries, I was told that an initial cooking of rice will also season and strengthen a clay pot. Thus it occurred to me that making Turkish rice pudding, which involves cooking both milk and rice, would be an ideal way to break in a new pot or reinforce an old one.

> **PREFERRED CLAY POTS:**
>
> A 3-quart glazed or unglazed earthenware, or flameware saucepan, or Turkish *guvec*
>
> 6 earthenware or stoneware ramekins, 6 ounces each
>
> If using an electric or ceramic stovetop, be sure to use a heat diffuser with the clay pot.

1 quart whole milk

⅓ cup Arborio, Baldo, or Carnaroli rice

3½ tablespoons plus ½ teaspoon sugar

2 small pieces mastic

⅛ teaspoon ground ginger

⅛ teaspoon freshly grated nutmeg

1 egg yolk

1 tablespoon all-purpose flour

1 tablespoon rosewater

2 teaspoons vanilla extract

¼ teaspoon salt

1 Place the milk in the earthenware casserole and set over medium-low heat. Bring to a boil, stirring from time to time to prevent a skin from forming on the bottom, about 10 minutes.

2 Meanwhile, rinse the rice in a sieve under cold running water until it runs clear. Add the drained rice to the simmering milk and continue to cook, partially covered, for 50 minutes, scraping up the tasty milky rice solids that gather on the bottom and sides of the pot.

3 Add ½ cup of hot water and continue to cook, uncovered, until the rice swells, about 5 minutes. Stir in 3½ tablespoons of the sugar and continue to cook for 50 minutes, scraping down the creamy golden rice solids that gather on the sides of the pot, or until the mixture is thick enough to coat a spoon.

4 Preheat the oven to 400°F. Crush the mastic with the remaining ½ teaspoon sugar, the ginger, and the nutmeg.

5 In a small bowl, whisk together the egg yolk, flour, and 2 tablespoons cold water until smooth. Stir 1 cup of the hot milky rice into the egg yolk mixture. Blend in the mastic mixture, rosewater, vanilla, and salt. Stir back into the pot with the rest of the rice.

6 Arrange the ramekins in a shallow baking pan and add enough hot water to reach ½ inch up the sides. Spoon the pudding into the ramekins and transfer to the center of the oven for about 5 minutes to heat through. Then turn on the broiler and broil the custards about 5 inches from the heat for about 10 minutes, until browned on top. If necessary, move the ramekins around to brown them evenly. Let cool, then refrigerate until chilled and thickened, at least 6 hours and up to 3 days.

Oven-Baked Budino di Riso

SERVES 6

Screenwriter Kathy Gori's family originally came from Lucca in Tuscany, which may account for the origins of her baked rice pudding. At my suggestion, Kathy tried out her family's rice pudding recipe in a clay casserole. She used a large, Korean black glazed earthenware pot which is very wide and heavy and holds heat very well. (I use either an Emile Henry FlameTop or a La Chamba casserole.)

Kathy's conclusion: her rice pudding tasted even better! Just what I wanted to hear!

What I love about Kathy's recipe is the combination of floral waters and the flavor of the milk solids that gather on the sides and bottom of the pot in the form of lightly caramelized tidbits. These solids, which are scraped down and around every twenty minutes or so for four hours, endow this pudding with its extraordinary texture and flavor.

Be sure to do the scraping with a heatproof silicone paddle. If you want, as a final step, you can pack the pudding into small ramekins, dust the tops with light brown sugar, and run them under the broiler to crisp.

This dessert is good warm and even better at room temperature.

PREFERRED CLAY POT:
A deep glazed or unglazed earthenware or flameware casserole

(continued)

2 tablespoons unsalted butter

6 cups milk

¼ cup plus 2 tablespoons granulated sugar

Pinch of salt

¾ teaspoon vanilla extract

⅓ cup Arborio rice

½ cup golden raisins

½ cup coarsely chopped pistachios

2 tablespoons rosewater, or 1 tablespoon each rosewater and Indian kewra water, or 1 tablespoon rosewater and 3 to 4 pesticide-free rose geranium leaves (see Note)

1 Use all the butter to liberally coat the inside of the earthenware casserole. Add the milk, sugar, salt, vanilla, and rice and mix with a wooden spoon. Transfer the casserole to the center of the oven, set the temperature at 350°F, and bake for 4 hours, stirring and scraping the bottom and sides with a wooden spoon every

20 minutes, until the pudding is thick and creamy, with lots of golden brown pieces of milky skin throughout.

2 While the rice pudding is baking, soak the golden raisins in a small bowl of warm water until very soft, about 1 hour. Drain well.

3 Remove the rice pudding from the oven and set the hot casserole on a wooden surface or folded kitchen towel to prevent cracking. Stir in the raisins, chopped pistachios, and rosewater. Serve the pudding warm or at room temperature.

Notes to the Cook:

❋ If using rose geranium leaves, rub 3 or 4 between the palms of your hands to develop their fragrance. Soak in a small amount of water for 3 to 4 minutes; discard the leaves, and use the scented water.

❋ A Korean black glazed earthenware casserole called a *jeel geu leut* (item no. 2897) can be purchased from www.koamart.com.

Turkish Caramelized Milk Pudding

SERVES 6

Paris has its cafés, Rome its wine bars, and Turkey its milk pudding houses. That's right: milk pudding! These establishments are called *muhallebici,* and unlike Turkish coffeehouses, which cater primarily to men, pudding houses are family friendly, welcoming women and children, and provide an excellent place to eat a light meal at any time of the day.

The huge variety of Turkish milk puddings includes bowls of sweetened milk seasoned with coconut or ground pistachios, ice cream made from wild orchids flavored with resinous mastic, caramel milk creams, rice puddings, starch wafers softened in sweetened milk and rosewater, and milk puddings blended with pistachios and almonds. One of my favorites is a thick milk pudding coated with a black caramelized skin called *kazan dibi,* which literally means "bottom of the pot."

The ebony skin is created by the slow caramelization of powdered sugar and butter on an unglazed clay pan on top of the stove. Many cooks substitute a metal pan and use ordinary granulated sugar. This results in a nice caramel brown skin, but the black coating can be achieved only on unglazed clay.

When done, the pudding is thick and supple. To serve, it is cut into wide strips; each strip is folded in half, skin side out, and presented simply and elegantly on a plate.

PREFERRED CLAY POTS:

A 10-inch La Chamba rimmed *comal* or other unglazed, shallow earthenware pan

A 3-quart glazed or unglazed earthenware or flameware casserole

If using an electric or ceramic stovetop, be sure to use a heat diffuser with the clay pots.

---

1 tablespoon unsalted butter

3 tablespoons confectioners' sugar

1 quart milk

½ cup granulated sugar

1 piece mastic, wrapped and tied in a small piece of cheesecloth

Pinch of salt

3 tablespoons cornstarch

¼ cup plus 3 tablespoons rice flour

1 tablespoon rosewater, or more to taste

1 Butter the comal. Sift the confectioners' sugar over the butter in a fine, even layer. Set aside in a cool place. (If using a metal pan, refrigerate for 1 hour after coating.)

2 Put 3½ cups of the milk, the granulated sugar, mastic, and salt in a 3-quart earthenware casserole and set over low heat. Slowly bring to a boil, stirring to dissolve the sugar.

3 Blend the cornstarch, rice flour, and remaining ½ cup milk until smooth. Gradually stir in about 1 cup of the hot milk. Blend this mixture into the remaining milk in the casserole and cook over low heat, stirring constantly, until it just comes to a boil and thickens enough to coat the spoon, about 10 minutes.

4 Remove and discard the mastic. Stir in the rosewater. Keep hot over very low heat.

5 Set the prepared comal over medium-low heat. When the comal is hot and the sugar is beginning to brown, quickly spread a thin layer of the batter over the hot pan. Immediately lift the pan and tilt gently to cover in a thin, even sheet. Cook, shifting the pan for even browning on the bottom, until you smell a slight burnt aroma, about 10 minutes. Immediately ladle the remaining milk pudding on top and tilt to even it out. Remove the pan from the heat and let stand until cool. Cover and refrigerate overnight.

6 The following day, slip a thin spatula under the pudding to loosen it. Divide into 6 long strips 1½ inches wide. One by one, lift out the strips and place on individual serving dishes, folding the custard over so that at least part of the caramelized crust is on top. Serve chilled.

Clafoutis with Prunes, Armagnac, and Candied Violets

SERVES 6

Clafoutis (sometimes spelled *clafouti*) is a shallow baked custard studded with fruit and is high on my list of wonderful quick-and-easy desserts. This one, from Gascon chef Dominique Toulousy, is exceptionally good, combining touches of Gascony (prunes and Armagnac) with a taste of Toulouse (candied violets). Dominique takes this simple dessert to a higher level by brushing a jelly of candied violets over the custard in the gratin and decorating it with candied violets. If you can't find the jelly, Dominique's wife, Maryse, tells me that strained apricot jelly will make a fine substitute.

Clafoutis is best eaten warm the same day it is baked, so I suggest you begin this dessert three to four hours before you plan to serve it.

> **PREFERRED CLAY POTS:**
> A 10-inch stoneware or ovenproof porcelain straight-sided baking dish suitable for use in an oven heated to 425°F

1 tablespoon unsalted butter at room temperature

½ cup plus 2 tablespoons all-purpose flour

12 prunes, preferably Agen, pitted and coarsely slivered

2 cups whole milk

1 vanilla bean, split lengthwise

3 eggs

2 egg yolks

7 tablespoons clarified butter, melted

7 tablespoons plus 1 teaspoon sugar

Pinch of salt

2½ tablespoons Armagnac or cognac

3 tablespoons candied violet jelly or strained apricot jam (see Notes)

12 candied violets for decoration (see Notes)

1 Preheat the oven to 425°F. Use the softened butter to grease the baking dish. Dust with 2 tablespoons of the flour and tap out any excess. Scatter the slivered prunes over the bottom of the dish.

2 Slowly bring the milk with the vanilla bean to a boil in a medium nonreactive saucepan. Meanwhile, in a large mixing bowl, whisk together the whole eggs, egg yolks, melted clarified butter, remaining ½ cup flour, 7 tablespoons of the sugar, and the salt until well combined. Add the Armagnac. Gradually beat in the boiling milk in a thin stream. Pour the custard over the slivered prunes in the baking dish.

3 Bake for 20 minutes. Transfer the hot dish to a wooden surface or folded kitchen towel to prevent cracking. Quickly warm the violet jelly with 1 tablespoon water until melted. Scatter the remaining 1 teaspoon sugar over the top. Brush the clafoutis with the jelly and decorate with the candied violets. Let stand for about 1 hour before serving.

NOTES TO THE COOK

✳ Candied violets from Candiflor, the Toulouse firm that has been making them for a couple hundred years, are available at upscale food shops.

✳ Candied violet jelly is sold by Hediard in Paris, and I've seen it turn up on the website www.thefrenchybee.com.

Raspberry Rhubarb Flan

SERVES 4

This flan from rural France is homey and comforting and makes an ideal ending to a hearty meal. In this recipe, fresh rose geranium leaves flavor a fine combination of rhubarb and raspberries.

> **PREFERRED CLAY POT:**
>
> **An 8-inch stoneware pie plate suitable for use in an oven heated to 400°F**

1 pound fresh tender rhubarb

½ cup plus 1 tablespoon sugar

2 tablespoons unsalted butter

1 cup fresh raspberries

¾ cup all-purpose flour

⅛ teaspoon freshly grated nutmeg

3 large eggs

1¼ cups whole milk

1 teaspoon vanilla extract

Pinch of salt

3 or 4 rose geranium leaves (optional; see Note)

1 A day in advance, trim the rhubarb, removing the greenish top of the stems and any leaves. If the rhubarb is late season, old, or thick, pull off the outer strings as you would for celery. Cut the rhubarb into 1-inch dice. You should have about 2 cups. Toss the rhubarb with 3 tablespoons of the sugar, cover, and let stand at room temperature overnight.

2 The following day, strain the rhubarb in a sieve set over a stainless-steel or enameled cast-iron saucepan to catch the juices; press to extract as much liquid as possible. Set over high heat and boil until the juices are reduced to about 3 tablespoons. Add this syrup to the rhubarb and toss to mix. (Very thin rhubarb stems might not produce any juice; just continue to the next step.)

3 Set the oven rack on the lowest shelf and preheat the oven to 400°F. Use all the butter to generously grease the pie plate. Add the raspberries to the rhubarb and fold to mix. Scrape the fruit and all the juices into the baking dish, spreading them out gently in an even layer.

4 In a mixing bowl, combine the flour, ¼ cup of the remaining sugar, and the nutmeg; whisk to blend. Add the eggs one at a time, stirring vigorously with a wooden spoon, always in the same direction, until each egg is incorporated and the mixture is smooth before adding the next. Gradually stir in the milk; mix in the vanilla and salt. Strain the batter over the fruit.

5 Set the dish in the preheated oven and bake for 45 minutes, or until the flan is firm and the top is lightly puffed and golden brown. Sprinkle the remaining 2 tablespoons sugar on top and serve while warm.

NOTE TO THE COOK: If you have a pesticide-free rose geranium plant in your garden, use a few leaves to perfume this flan. Rub the leaves in your palm and add along with the milk and vanilla in Step 4. Let the batter stand for 3 to 4 minutes before straining; then continue the recipe as directed.

Dried Plum and Almond Bread Pudding with Dandelion Jelly

SERVES 6

I found this homey dessert in a regional French cookbook called *Recettes Paysannes en Lozère*, a compendium of specialties from the Languedoc Roussillon region of southern France. The local name for the dish is *coupétade*, a reference to its vaselike shape, resembling an upside-down cupola, due to the shape of the clay vessel in which it is baked.

The original recipe called for glazing with a jelly made from dried dandelion blossoms. I had no trouble finding such a jelly on the Internet through the Amish mail order source Lehman's (see Sources). The taste is delicate, with some bitter and some fruity tones. I've also had fine results glazing this pudding with chestnut honey. Serve plain or with a dollop of crème fraîche.

Note: Besides being cooked in a clay vessel, this dessert requires a clay oven environment. Due to the even heat of a clay oven, the custard stiffens very slowly, staying soft and luscious, while the bread topping cooks to a lovely crustiness. In France, it would be baked in a brick-lined oven. If you have one, so much the better. Otherwise, use one of the clay oven adaptations suggested below.

> **PREFERRED CLAY POT:**
> A 5- or 6-cup earthenware or stoneware baking dish, preferably with fluted sides suitable for use in an oven heated to 425°F
>
> **SUGGESTED OVEN ENVIRONMENT:**
> Double slabs of pizza stones or food-safe quarry tiles set on the upper and lower oven racks

3 tablespoons unsalted butter

¾ cup pitted prunes (dried plums)

¼ cup golden raisins

¼ cup dried tart cherries soaked in warm water for 5 minutes and drained

8 ounces sliced stale dense sourdough bread, crusts removed

2 cups whole milk

½ vanilla bean, split lengthwise

4 eggs

⅓ cup sugar

2 tablespoons dandelion jelly or mild chestnut honey

3 tablespoons coarsely chopped blanched almonds

1 Grease the earthenware baking dish with 1 tablespoon of the butter. Scatter the prunes, raisins, and dried cherries over the bottom of the dish. Break up the stale bread into chunks and distribute on top.

2 In a small conventional saucepan, slowly warm the milk with the vanilla bean over medium-low heat until bubbles appear around the rim of the pan. Remove the vanilla bean; pat it dry and save for some other purpose.

3 In a mixing bowl, beat the eggs with the sugar until slightly thickened and pale yellow. Slowly whisk in the warm milk and beat until well blended. Pour over the bread and set a flat dish directly over the bread; weight it with a heavy pot for about 15 minutes to keep the bread submerged and allow it to soak up the custard.

4 Meanwhile, preheat the oven to 375°F. Melt the remaining 2 tablespoons butter with the jelly until liquid and smooth. Remove from the heat.

5 Stir the pudding gently to mix the bread and dried fruits; this is best done with your hands. Press down to make it compact. Brush the top of the pudding with the melted butter and jelly and sprinkle the chopped almonds on top.

6 Place the baking dish in the preheated oven. Raise the temperature to 425°F and bake for 45 minutes, or until the pudding is puffed and nicely browned. Serve warm or at room temperature.

Corsican Cheesecake

SERVES 4 TO 6

I based this recipe on a cultured and robust cheesecake served at the La Villa restaurant in Calvi on the island of Corsica. Corsicans most often bake their cheesecake in the receding heat of an outdoor stone oven. I substitute two slabs of stoneware, preheated in a hot oven for at least forty-five minutes before baking.

The popular sheep's milk ricotta called *brocciu* is richer and denser than our cow's milk ricotta. For this cheesecake to be successful, either make your own ricotta from milk and cream (see below) or use a very rich whole-milk ricotta from the store. I'm indebted to chef Daniel Patterson of the superb San Francisco restaurant Coi, for the notion of adding heavy cream to whole-milk ricotta to thicken and enrich it.

> **PREFERRED CLAY POT:**
>
> A 10-inch stoneware pie plate suitable for use in an oven heated to 450°F
>
> **SUGGESTED OVEN ENVIRONMENT:**
>
> Double slabs of pizza stones or food-safe quarry tiles set on the upper and lower racks of the oven

1 pound rich ricotta cheese, preferably homemade (recipe follows)

1 tablespoon unsalted butter at room temperature

4 large eggs

½ cup sugar

2 teaspoons grated lemon zest

½ teaspoon vanilla extract

Pinch of salt

2 tablespoons eau-de-vie de pore, eau-de-vie de Mirabelle, or dark rum, such as Myers

(continued)

1 If you are making your own ricotta, prepare it up to 5 days in advance. Remove it from the refrigerator about 2 hours before you plan to serve dessert.

2 Preheat the oven to 450°F. Butter the pie plate.

3 In a blender or food processor, combine the eggs and sugar. Process until light and creamy, about 20 seconds. Add the ricotta, lemon zest, vanilla, and salt. Blend until smooth and thick. Pour into the pie plate.

4 Bake for 20 minutes, or until well browned on top. Turn off the oven and, without opening the door, let the cake finish baking in the receding heat for 20 minutes.

5 Immediately sprinkle the eau-de-vie over the top of the cake, and let it cool for about 30 minutes before cutting it into wedges while still warm.

Homemade Ricotta

MAKES ABOUT 2 CUPS

2 quarts whole milk

1 cup heavy cream

3½ tablespoons fresh lemon juice

¼ teaspoon salt

1 In a 3-quart saucepan set over medium heat, combine the milk and cream. Bring to 190°F. Stir in the lemon juice and bring just to a simmer. Add the salt and cook for another minute; remove from the heat. Let stand without disturbing until you see small white particles floating on the surface of the liquid, about 2 minutes. Partially cover and let stand at room temperature for 10 minutes longer.

2 Line a colander with a double layer of dampened fine cheesecloth and set over a large bowl or in the sink. Carefully strain the contents of the saucepan. Let drain at room temperature for 2 hours. Do not touch the ricotta or break up the curds. Discard the whey or use as suggested in the Note. Unmold the ricotta into a container, cover tightly, and refrigerate for up to 5 days.

NOTE TO THE COOK: Whey has a lovely nutty tang and good acidity. It can be used to cook vegetables or be added to bread doughs or pie crusts.

Greek Semolina and Yogurt Cake

SERVES 8 OR 9

This delicate cake has a light crumb, delicate flavor, and crisp bottom crust due to the even insulation of a clay baking dish. Traditionally it is decorated like baklava, with diamond-shaped scoring and a whole almond in the center of each section. Serve warm or at room temperature.

> **PREFERRED CLAY POT:**
>
> A 10- or 11-inch round Spanish cazuela, tagine, or straight-sided flameware baking dish

1 cup whole-milk yogurt

½ teaspoon vanilla extract

½ teaspoon baking soda

1½ cups coarse semolina

¾ plus ⅔ cup sugar

½ teaspoon baking powder

3 tablespoons unsalted butter, melted and cooled slightly

18 to 24 blanched almonds, halved

½ lemon, preferably organic

1 In a small bowl, whisk together the yogurt, vanilla, and baking soda. Let stand for 10 minutes.

2 In a medium bowl, combine the semolina with ¾ cup of the sugar and the baking powder. Slowly stir in the yogurt mixture until blended.

3 Brush the cazuela with 1 tablespoon of the melted butter. Pour in the batter and tilt the pan to spread evenly; do not pat down. Let stand at room temperature for 1 to 2 hours to allow the semolina to absorb moisture and expand.

4 Use a thin-bladed knife to score small diamonds or squares on top; cut only about ¼ inch deep. Place an almond half in the middle of each square.

5 Preheat the oven to 375°F. Bake the cake in the top third of the oven for 25 to 30 minutes, or until golden brown.

6 Meanwhile, in a small conventional saucepan, combine the remaining ⅔ cup sugar with ½ cup water and the lemon half. Bring to a boil, stirring to dissolve the sugar. Continue to boil slowly for 5 minutes, or until reduced to about ½ cup. Strain the lemon syrup, discarding the lemon.

7 Transfer the hot cazuela to a wooden surface or folded kitchen towel to prevent cracking. Immediately run a knife along the scored lines to open them up. Brush the cake with the remaining 2 tablespoons melted butter; then drizzle the hot lemon syrup over the top. Cover and let stand at room temperature until the syrup is completely absorbed.

Oven-Baked Apple, Black Cherry, and Walnut Crisp

SERVES 4 TO 6

This unique and flavorful apple crisp from the Spanish region of Aragon utilizes a popular regional combination of the local *verde donecella* apples, similar to our Granny Smiths or pippins, along with walnuts and tart-sweet Morello cherry jam. I like to cook and present this dessert in individual earthenware cazuelitas or small gratin dishes, which allow me to glaze the tops with a salamander after baking. See notes on this method at the end of the recipe for Crèma Catalana on page 298.

PREFERRED CLAY POT:

4 to 6 cazuelitas, 5 or 6 ounces each

8 tablespoons (1 stick) unsalted butter

2 pounds tart green apples, such as Granny Smith, pippin, or greening

2 tablespoons fresh lemon juice

2 tablespoons confectioners' sugar

Pinch of ground cinnamon

1 cup coarsely chopped walnuts (6 ounces)

¼ cup all-purpose flour

½ cup packed light brown sugar

Pinch of salt

2 tablespoons Morello or black cherry jelly or jam

1 Preheat the oven to 375°F. Use 2 tablespoons of the butter to grease 4 to 6 cazuelitas.

2 Peel, core, and thickly slice the apples. Toss with the lemon juice. Combine the confectioners' sugar, cinnamon, and ⅓ cup of the chopped walnuts and add to the apples. Toss to mix. Divide the apples among the cazuelitas.

3 Dice the remaining 6 tablespoons butter and place in a medium bowl. Add the flour, brown sugar, and salt. Pinch and rub quickly with your fingertips to blend the dry ingredients with the butter until the mixture is the consistency of fine cornmeal. Stir in the remaining chopped walnuts and the cherry jelly. Spread over the apples.

4 Place the cazuelitas on a baking sheet and set in the preheated oven. Immediately raise the temperature to 450°F. Cover with a sheet of foil and bake for 30 minutes. Uncover and continue to bake until the apples are soft and the topping is nicely browned, about 10 minutes longer. Serve warm.

Roasted Peach Gratin

SERVES 4 TO 6

This gratin of peaches should be made at the peak of the season, when peaches are ripe and unblemished. Some cooks use raw peaches, but I'm of the school that believes poaching them first, even briefly, accentuates their delicate taste. This dessert is best eaten the moment it's ready. It can be held for a short time, however, in a low oven with the oven door left slightly ajar. Serve garnished with whipped cream or crème fraîche.

> **PREFERRED CLAY POT:**
>
> A 10- or 12-inch high-quality round or oval stoneware or flameware baking dish suitable for use in a 500°F oven

6 large yellow peaches—firm, ripe, and unblemished

1½ cups granulated sugar

4 to 5 tablespoons fresh lemon juice

8 tablespoons (1 stick) unsalted butter, at room temperature

6 tablespoons superfine sugar

2 eggs yolks

½ teaspoon pure vanilla extract

¼ cup black currant jelly

1 To peel the peaches, use the tip of a small knife to make very shallow crisscross slits through the skin on one side of each peach. Drop into a pot of boiling water, cook for about 30 seconds, remove with a strainer, and immerse in cold water. The skins will slip right off.

2 In a large nonreactive saucepan, combine the granulated sugar, 1 quart water, and 3 tablespoons of the lemon juice. Bring to a boil, stirring to dissolve the sugar. Reduce the heat to a simmer and add half the peaches at a time. Slip them into the syrup, cover with a circle of parchment or a small clean cloth to keep them submerged, and poach for 5 minutes. Remove the peaches with a slotted strainer and let cool slightly. Return the syrup to a simmer and repeat with the remaining peaches. Cut each peach in half and remove the pits. Drain, cut sides down, on a cake rack over paper towels.

3 In a mixing bowl with an electric beater or a wooden spoon, cream 7 tablespoons of the butter with the superfine sugar until fluffy. Gradually work in the egg yolks, one at a time, with a wooden spoon. Stir in the vanilla. Cover and refrigerate until you are ready to assemble the dish.

4 About 1 hour before serving, preheat the oven to 400°F. Use the remaining 1 tablespoon butter to grease the baking dish. Pat the poached peaches dry with paper towels. Arrange them cut side down in the baking dish. Scatter the butter-and-egg mixture between the fruit. Set the dish in the oven and raise the temperature to 500°F. Bake for 10 minutes, or until the butter mixture begins to set.

5 Warm the jelly over low heat until it melts. Stir in the remaining 1 to 2 tablespoons lemon juice to taste. Drizzle the warm jelly over the peaches and continue baking for about 3 minutes, until the gratin is glazed. Remove from the oven and let stand until warm, about 20 minutes, before serving.

NOTE TO THE COOK: Save the poaching syrup from step 2 for compotes or sangría, or use it to make a sorbet.

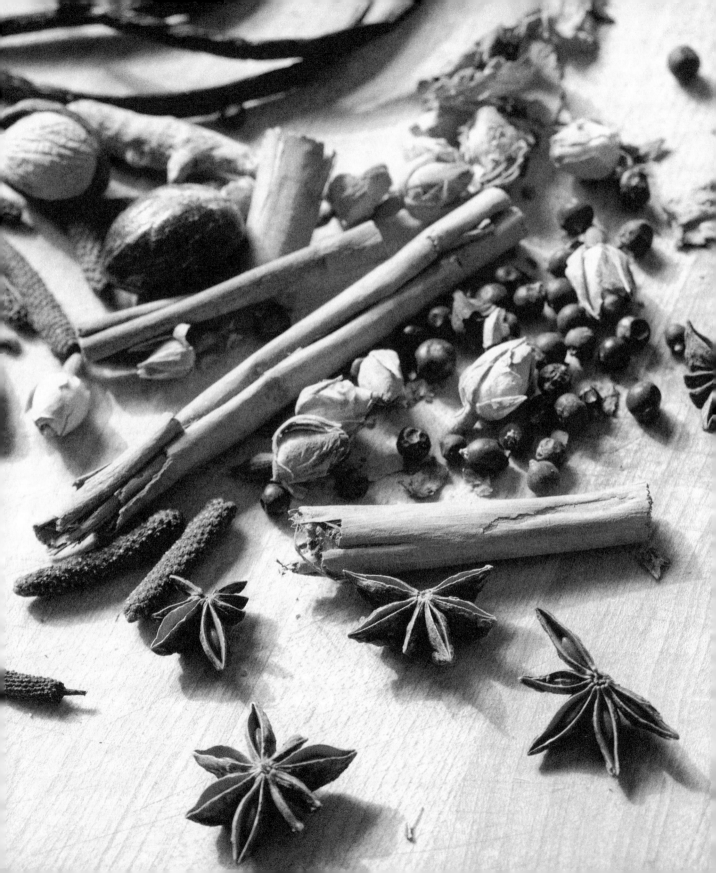

Appendices

MAKING YOUR OWN WINE VINEGAR WITH A CERAMIC CROCK AND A "MOTHER"

Good, simple red wine vinegar, the mainstay of numerous vinegar-based dishes in this book, is rarely found. Commercial manufacturers make it too fast and on the cheap. If you want to make a truly delicious *poulet au vinaigre* (page 103) or a mildly tart sauté of chicken livers with vinegar and onions (page 107), you're far better off using a homemade vinegar than one from the store. Also, making your own is fun.

So what makes homemade vinegar so special? Simply put, it's crisper, subtler, and better balanced, with a bright quality that enhances food. Used to deglaze a pan for a sauce, it yields far better results than commercial vinegar. Great wine vinegar coaxes out layers of flavor, creating a more seductive dish.

The process is easy, and very little kitchen work is required. Perhaps the most important component is patience. Good red wine vinegar takes time to develop—roughly from six to ten weeks. And time is what the commercial manufacturers don't have; that's one reason their products are inferior.

Here's the chemistry in a nutshell: If you leave leftover wine sitting around, sooner or later it will ferment and become vinegary. But that doesn't mean it will taste very good. Producing first-rate vinegar requires control. For this you'll need a starter or vinegar culture called a *mother,* which contains a harmless bacterium, acetobacter, which converts the alcohol in the wine to a mild vinegar.

A vinegar mother is a fascinating thing to see: a smooth, gelatinous layer or leathery, grayish veil that sits atop the wine inside the vinegar crock. It must not be disturbed while doing its work. Eventually this layer of mother becomes quite heavy and falls to the bottom, and another layer develops, taking its place on top. The bottom layers then stack up over time, creating an expired blob of useless mothers. Eventually this expanding blob must be removed lest it take over the crock.

Basically, there are three ways to obtain a good mother:

1 Get one from a friend, use it to inoculate your wine, and let it grow.

2 Buy one from a reliable source; I've included an address on page 314.

3 Make your own.

One thing you absolutely should *not* do is add commercial pasteurized vinegar to wine in an attempt to replicate a mother; this won't work because pasteurization has killed the mother in the bottle.

I purchased an excellent vinegar mother from Mark Larrow, owner of Beer and Winemaking Supplies in Northampton, Massachusetts (www.beer-winemaking.com). I was surprised by the way it looked: just a clear vermillion liquid in a bottle. When I asked Mark why it didn't come in blob form, he told me, "The traditional lumpy vinegar mother is what I call a visual security blanket. It's nice, but you don't really need it. You need the unfiltered liquid it lives in. Just follow the instructions on my bottle, and your mother will come to life."

How to Make Vinegar in a Crock

You will need a one-gallon ceramic crock with a spigot at the bottom. It should be glazed inside and out to preserve the taste of the vinegar and be thick enough to keep the temperature constant through the year. Emile Henry and Clay Coyote are two good brands, but there are others available all over the Internet. Just make sure the spigot is made of cork and soak it in hot water for a few hours before inserting it into the crock. Put in the spigot; then add water to check that there are no leaks.

To make red wine vinegar with 8 fluid ounces of commercial "mother of vinegar" or the same volume of a friend's mother: Combine the mother with 16 ounces (2 cups) red wine, preferably organic, and 8 ounces (1 cup) filtered water or spring water.

Air is needed for the conversion of alcohol to vinegar, so do not place a ceramic cover on your crock. Instead, cover the crock with a double layer of cheesecloth and fasten it with a rubber band. Be sure to add water at the start of the process, because if the mixture is too acidic, it may turn too fast, and then the mother will shut down.

Let the crock stand in a dark and warm (70°F to 90°F) place for 1 to 2 weeks; then gradually, over a period of another 1 to 2 weeks, start adding leftover red wine to feed the mother until the crock is two-thirds full. Let stand for 1½ to 2 months longer, until the vinegar is ready to use.

You'll be able to tell because the crock will emit a crisp, sharp vinegar aroma, and a visible mother in the shape of a thin veil will cover the top. Do not disturb, because if you break this layer, the mother may sink to the bottom and die from loss of oxygen. To avoid breaking the mother when feeding the vinegar, gently push it to one side while slowly adding leftover wine. If it does break, don't worry: A new mother will form.

To bottle your vinegar: Drain nearly all the vinegar off via the spigot, straining it through a plastic funnel lined with a paper coffee filter, into sterile bottles. The paper filter removes most of the active bacteria. The vinegar remaining in the crock (about 1 cup) is alive with active bacterial culture and can then be mixed with additional red wine and water to start the process again. By the way, the reason I don't address white wine vinegar here is that it can take up to a year to create a vigorous mother.

Your vinegar will continue to mellow in the bottle. You can use some of it at once, but please note that it will improve significantly with age. If you intend to age your vinegar for longer than 3 to 4 months, I recommend you do this: Pasteurizing the vinegar by heating it in a stainless-steel pot to 150°F to 155°F and holding it at that temperature for 20 to 30 minutes; do not allow it to come anywhere near a boil. Let cool; then pour into sterile bottles, seal the tops, and store in a cool, dry place.

Note: I don't recommend using homemade vinegar for pickling, as particular pickles require various specific amounts of acidity. If you wish to pickle, you must test for acidity with a titration kit available at home wine-making shops.

When Bad Things Happen to a Good Mother

Sooner or later you will have more mother than vinegar in your crock, and the fallen mother will start to rot and damage your cork spigot. To prevent this, reach into the crock with clean hands, pull out the clumps of dead mother, and discard.

Avoid using metal utensils, as they can easily corrode as well as damage the flavor of the vinegar.

Temperatures that are too low (below 60°F) or too high (over 90°F) will kill the mother. You'll know because the existing mother will sink to the bottom and no new film will form.

Cleanliness is paramount, or the mother may become polluted by other, less-friendly bacteria. If your vinegar begins to smell like furniture polish, this is a sign of pollution. Toss everything out, sterilize the crock, and start over.

Do not add sherry, sweet wine, or corked wine to the mixture as they will damage the mother.

Chlorinated water and/or well water with a lot of minerals should be filtered before being used to make vinegar because they will adversely affect the flavor.

Moroccan Spice Mixture: La Kama

There's a sweet spot in my food memory for *La Kama* spices, the favorite tagine seasoning mix in Tangier, where I lived on and off for seven years.

La Kama spices are similar to the more famous *ras el hanout* (which literally means means "top of the shop") in that its formula varies from cook to cook. Some *ras el hanout* mixtures contain as many as fifty different spices, others just ten or twelve. A good La Kama mixture may be made with just five, as shown here. You can increase the amount as you wish; simply maintain the same proportions.

1 tablespoon ground ginger

1 tablespoon ground turmeric

1 tablespoon finely ground black pepper

2 teaspoons ground Ceylon or Mexican cinnamon

2 teaspoons ground cubeb berries (optional; see Note)

1 teaspoon freshly grated nutmeg

1 Combine the ginger, turmeric, black pepper, cinnamon, cubeb berries, and nutmeg and transfer to a small jar with a tight-fitting lid. Store in a dark place and use within 6 months.

NOTE TO THE COOK: Cubeb berries are also known as *cubeb pepper* or *tailed pepper*. They have a peppery, aromatic, and bitter flavor that binds well with the spices in the La Kama mixture. You can purchase the dried berries at www.Kalustyans.com. Crush the berries to a powder in a mortar.

Homemade Tomato Paste

MAKES 1 CUP

Inspired by the Sicilian *strattu,* a tomato extract using sun-dried tomatoes, I make this intense, very flavorful concentrate, which I use in place of tomato paste.

> **PREFERRED CLAY POT:**
>
> **An 8-inch Spanish cazuela or a 2-quart Chinese sandpot**
>
> **If using an electric or ceramic stovetop, be sure to use a heat diffuser with the clay pots.**

1 small jar (6 to 8 ounces) sun-dried tomatoes packed in olive oil

1 can (6 ounces) tomato paste

1 can (14 ounces) whole plum tomatoes

½ teaspoon salt

Extra virgin olive oil

1 In a food processor or blender, combine the sun-dried tomatoes with the oil from the jar, the tomato paste, tomatoes with their juices, salt, and 2 tablespoons water. Puree until smooth.

2 Scrape into the cazuela and set over medium-low heat. Cook slowly, stirring often, until the tomato mixture reduces to a thick jam, about 30 minutes.

3 Scrape the tomato paste into a clean jar. Cover with ¼ inch of olive oil and the lid and store in the refrigerator. This paste keeps well for up to 2 months.

Preserved Lemons

Mustapha's jarred preserved lemons are excellent and available from www.chefshop.com. You can make your own with a mix of thin skinned lemons and thick skinned Eurekas, this produces thick lemon rind that will stand up in cooking, and thin rind for garnishing salads.

2 large organic lemons

⅓ cup coarse salt

½ cup fresh lemon juice

Extra virgin olive oil

Scrub the lemons and dry well. Cut each into 8 wedges. Toss them with the salt and place in a 1-cup capacity glass jar. Pour in the lemon juice. Close the jar tightly and let the lemons ripen at room temperature for 7 days, shaking the jar each day to distribute the salt and juice. To store, add olive oil to cover and store in a cool place or refrigerate for up to 1 year. Rinse lemons before using.

NOTE: It's possible that a white lacy growth will appear in your preserving jar as the lemons mature on your shelf. Don't worry about it—-simply discard it when you open the jar and rinse the lemons before use.

Food Sources

INGREDIENTS

Aleppo pepper: www.kalustyans.com;
www.zingermans.com

Almonds, fuzzy green: www.greenalmonds.com

Anchovies, salt-packed: www.chefshop.com;
www.formaggiokitchen.com

Flour: Indian stone-ground whole wheat (atta) and Nirav
Durum (atta), www.ishopindian.com

Argan oil: www.chefshop.com, www.exoticaoils.com

Basturma: www.haigsdelicacies.com, www.kalustyans.com

Beans, heirloom: www.ranchogordo.com

Beans, Greek fasolia gigantes:
www.greekolivewarehouse.com

Bottarga di muggine: www.manicaretti.com

Capers, salt-packed: www.tienda.com,
www.zingermans.com

Chestnut flour: www.chestnutsonline.com

Cinnamon sticks, Ceylon: www.kalustyans.com,
www.thespicehouse.com

Dandelion jelly: www.caneandreed.com/mrsmiller.htm

Eggplant, dried: www.tulumba.com

Flour: Italian-style; stone-ground whole wheat; semolina;
and extra fancy durum flour, www.kingarthurflour.com

Freekah (green wheat): www.kalustyans.com

Grape molasses, or unfermented syrup from grape must:
Turkish *pekmez,* www.tulumba.com; Italian *saba,*
www.zingermans.com

Lemons, preserved: www.chefshop.com

Linden flowers and leaves, dried: www.
mountainspiritherbals.com

Mhammas couscous from Tunisia: www.zingermans.com

Meats: Heritage pork and beef, www.dartagnan.com,
www.flyingpigsfarm.com, www.preferredmeats.com,
www.heritagefoodsusa.com

Mastic: www.kalustyans.com

Mulberries, dried: www.kalustyans.com

PAPRIKA AND PEPPER PASTES

Aleppo pepper: www.kalustyans.com

Cubeb Pepper Berries: www.kalustyans.com

Pepper paste Turkish sweet and hot: www.kalustyans.com

Peppers, piquillo: www.spanishtable.com, www.tienda.com

Piment d'espelette: www.spanishtable.com,
www.thespicehouse.com, www.tienda.com

Turkish Urfa pepper flakes and Turkish Marash red pepper flakes: www.zingermans.com, www.formaggiokitchen.com

Peppers, roasted Florina Peloponnese sweet pepper strips: www.hormelfoods.com

Spanish pimenton de la Vera (dulce): www.Spanishtable.com, thespicehouse.com, www.tienda.com

Plums, dried sour yellow: www.kalustyans.com

Pomegranate concentrate (molasses): www.kalustyans.com, www.tulumba.com

Poultry, chickens: 100% air-chilled or organic and free-range: www.dartagnan.com; www.preferredmeats.com

Ducks, duck fat, and game birds: www.dartagnan.com, www.preferred meats.com

Ramps or wild leeks: www.earthy.com

Rosebuds, dried, for cooking: www.kalustyans.com

Rosewater: www.kalustyans.com

Sausage, blood (black): www.tienda.com; www.spanishtable.com

Spices: www.chefshop.com, www.kalustyans.com, www.seasonedpioneers.com, www.spicehouse.com

Thistle flowers, dried: www.tagines.com

Tupi cheese: www.anhmarket.com

Verjus: www.chefshop.com

Vinegar mother: www.beer-winemaking.com

Violets, candied: India Tree, www.amazon.com

Clay Pot Sources

Recommended Stovetop Pots

GLAZED EARTHENWARE

Chinese sandpots: www.wokshop.com,
    www.gourmetsleuth.com

Casseroles, saucepans, skillets, and tagines of all sizes:
    www.bramcookware.com

Spanish cazuelas, cazuelitas, and ollas:
    www.spanishtable.com, www.tienda.com

French-Catalan Le Flambadou casseroles:
    www.lacfi.upcsites.com

Italian Vulcania umidieras and casseroles:
    www.bramcookware.com, www.frenchgardening.com

*Philippe Beltrando daubières, mortiers, and
    poêlon de terre:* www.frenchgardening.com

Philippe Bletrando's tourne omelette:
    www.barbotine.fr

Walter Potenza's "TerraWare": www.chefwalter.com

UNGLAZED EARTHENWARE

Chilean unglazed Pomaireware: www.kitchendance.com

Siglinda Scarpa's terra-cotta Pottery:
    www.siglindascarpa.com

Romertopf clay bakers: www.romertopfonline.com,
    www.fantes.com, www.surlatable.com

Turkish guvecs: www.tulumba.com

Italian mattone: www.surlatable.com

Diable (French potato devil):
    www.frenchgardening.com, www.poterie-marzat.com

UNGLAZED (MICACEOUS) CLAY POTS

*Colombian La Chamba casseroles, skillets, saucepans
    and tagines:*
    www.bramcookware.com, www.mytoque.com,
    www.gourmetsleuth.com

New Mexican micaceous clay bean pots:
    Felipe Ortega's micaceous utilitarian cookware,
    www.pasquals.com/galeria.html

Beth Foote's micaceous clay casseroles,
    contact: dancing4buddha@yahoo.com

GLAZED AND UNGLAZED EARTHENWARE TAGINES:

www.tagines.com, www.bramcookware.com,

www.surlatable.com, www.spanishtable.com

FLAMEWARE CLAY POTS:

*Casseroles, braziers, straight-sided skillets, saucepans,
    tagines, and pie plates:*
    www.claycoyote.com

Emile Henry flametop cookware:
    www.surlatable.com, www.williamssonoma.com

*High-end custom-made saucepans and casseroles
    by Bill Sax:* www.billsaxpottery.com

Recommended Stoneware Pots and Baking Dishes for the Oven

OVAL AND RECTANGULAR BAKING DISHES:

www.claycoyote.com, www.fantes.com,
    www.surlatable.com, www.williams-sonoma.com

Recommended Clay Baking Dishes for the Oven

ROUND, OVAL, AND RECTANGULAR BAKING DISHES:

Emile Henry and Le Creuset:
   www.williams-sonoma.com, www.surlatable.com

Claycoyote: www.claycoyote.com

EARTHENWARE AND STONEWARE PIE PLATES:

Unglazed earthenware pie plate: www.hesspottery.com

Large glazed earthenware French pie or tourte plate:
   www.frenchgardening.com

Glazed stoneware pie plate: www.claycoyote.com,
   www.surlatable.com, www.williams-sonoma.com

CHICKEN ROASTERS

Romertopf stoneware chicken roaster:
   www.surlatable.com, www.williams-sonoma.com

Vertical ceramic chicken cooker:
   www.EarlyMorningPottery.com

The French cocorico popularized by chef Michael Chiarello:
   www.napastyle.com

Stoneware BeerCan Roaster: www.claycoyote.com

MISCELLANEOUS:

Stoneware colander/steamer for couscous:
   www.claycoyote.com

Stoneware Vinegar crock: www.claycoyote.com

Building a Clay Oven Environment FibraMent
   (¾-inch-thick slabs): www.bakingstone.com

La Cloche stoneware domed baker:
   www.sassafrasenterprises.com, www.amazon.com

Catalan four-inch cast iron base salamander:
   www.fantes.com, www.spanishtable.com,
   www.tienda.com

Ceramic water-based nontoxic clay for wrapping a chicken:
   info@leslieceramics.com

Heat diffuser: Simmer Mat, www.amazon.com

Lead Check Tester: hardware stores or
   www.amazon.com

*Korean small black glazed earthenware crock for storing
   smen:* www.koamart.com, no. 2398

POTS FEATURED IN THIS BOOK

Page 1: Small glazed earthenware *guvec tepsisi** from Turkey. Source: www.tulumba.com. Use for dips, olives, rice puddings, and crema catalana.

Page 25: Three-quart flameware casserole. Source: www.claycoyote.com. Use for soups, stews, and beans.

Page 53: Unglazed earthenware *tagra* from Morocco. Source: www.tagines.com. Use for cooking fish, gratins, and baked noodle dishes.

Page 71: Unglazed earthenware tagine from southern Morocco. Source: www.tagines.com. Use for tagines, vegetable stews, and gratins.

Page 121: Flameware saucepan. Source: www.billsaxpottery.com

Page 182: Unglazed earthenware flowerpot saucer: Source: HomeDepot. Use for shaping meatballs, handling couscous, and kneading bread.

Page 207: Suzy Atkins stoneware tian. Source: www.poteriedudon.com. Use for gratins and tians.

Page 229: Micaceous clay casserole: Source: Beth Foote, dancing4buddha@yahoo.com

Page 251: Moroccan *tangia* pot. Source: www.berbertrading.com/pd_tangia.cfm. Use for stews, daubes, and beans.

Page 275: Unglazed earthenware *meqleh*. Source: unavailable in the United States. Substitute 4½-inch handled, glazed earthenware cazuela. Source: www.tienda.com. Use for eggs, crèma catalana, and Turkish rice pudding.

Page 299: Glazed earthenware cazuelitas. Sources: www.spanishtable.com and www.tienda.com. Use for crèma catalana and Turkish rice pudding.

Bibliography

Abdeni Massad, Barbara. *Inside the Street Corner Lebanese Bakery*. Lebanon: Alarm Editions, 2005.

Alexiadou, Vefa. *Greek Pastries and Desserts*. Salonika: Alexandou, 1995.

Bellakhdar, Jamal. *La Pharmacopée Marocaine Traditionnelle*. Paris: Ibis Press, 1997.

Bertolli, Paul. *Cooking by Hand*. New York: Clarkson Potter, 2003.

Béziat, Marc. *Recettes paysannes en Lozère*. Rodez, France: Du Curieux Eds Photogenie, 2003.

Chalmers, Irena. *Cooking in Clay*. Chapel Hill, NC: Potpourri Press, 1974.

Chanot-Bullier, C. Vielles Recettes de cuisine Provencale. Marseille: Editor Tacussel, 1972.

Downie, David. *Cooking the Roman Way: Authentic Recipes from the Home Cooks and Trattorias of Rome*. New York: William Morrow, 2002.

Duplessy, Bernard. *The French Country Table: Pottery & Faience of Provence*. New York: Harry N. Abrams, Inc., 2003.

Emel-Powell, Kay. *The Superstone Country Kitchen Stoneware Cookbook*. Evanston, IL: Sassafras Press, 1982.

Fletcher, Janet. "Bagna Cauda, Potent Mélange of Garlic, Anchovies and Olive Oil Brings Friends Rogether," *San Francisco Chronicle*, January 10, 1996.

Gedda, Guy. *Le Grand Livre de la Cuisine Provençale*. Neuilly-sur-Seine, France: Michel Lafon, 2000.

Hal, Fatema. *Le Grand Livre de la Cuisine Marocaine*. Paris: Hachette, 2005

Hawkins, Kathryn. *Clay Pot Cooking*. Edison, NJ: Chartwell Books, 1998.

Helou, Anissa. *Lebanese Cuisine*. New York: St. Martin's Griffin, 1998.

Heyraud, H. *La Cuisine à Nice*. Nice, France: Imprimerie Leo Barma, 1921.

Jacobi. Dana. *The Best of Clay Pot Cooking*. New York: William Morrow, 1995.

Konstantini, Klementine. *Traditions Culinaires de Tunisie: Les Recettes les Plus Appreciées de la Cuisine Tunisienne*. Tunis: Konstantini, 2001.

Kramer, Matt. *A Passion for Piedmont*. New York: William Morrow & Co., 1997.

Kummer, Corby. "Pesto by Hand: The Oldest—and Still the Best—Way to Make Most People's Favorite Pasta Sauce Need Not Be Laborious," *Atlantic Monthly*, August 1998.

Kummer, Corby, "The Rise of the Sardine," *Atlantic Monthly*, July/August 2007.

Lazari, Lucia Scodori. *Sapori, Colori della Cucina Salentina*, Lecce, Italy: Mario Congedo Editore, 1997.

Machlin, Edda Servi. *The Classic Cuisine of the Italian Jews*. New York: Dodd, Mead & Co., 1981.

Médecin, Jacques. *La Cuisine du Comté de Nice*. Paris: Éd. Julliard, 1972.

Mendel, Janet. *My Kitchen in Spain.* New York: William Morrow, 2002.

Meneau, Marc. *La Cuisine des Monastères.* Paris: Editions de la Martinière, 1999.

Muller, Claude. *Cuisine traditionnelle des Alpes.* Romagnat, France: DeBorée, 2007.

Parrish, Marlene. "Pot Cleaning Half Brain, Half Brawn," *Pittsburgh Post Gazette,* January 30, 2003.

Pillet, Marc. *Poteries Traditionnelles en France de 1980 à Nos Jours.* Vendin-le-Vieil, France: Editions la Revue de la céramique et du verre, 2007.

Potenza, Walter. "Master of Clay," *La Cucina Italiana* 3(5).

Roca, Joan y Brugués, Salvador. *La Cocina al Vacío.* Barcelona: Montagud Editores SA, 2003.

Romano, Guy-Stefan. *All About Clay Cookware (with recipes).* San Francisco: The Shields Press, 1976.

Rubel, William. *The Magic of Fire: Hearth Cooking: One Hundred Recipes for the Fireplace or Campfire.* Berkeley, California: Ten Speed Press, 2002.

Ruspoli, Mario. *Petit Bréviaire de la Cuisine Étrusque et Romaine.* Paris: M. Ruspoli, 1975.

Sales, Georgia MacLeod, and Grover Sales. *The Clay-Pot Cookbook.* New York: Atheneum, 1982.

Satin, Morton. *Death in the Pot: The History of Food Poisoning in History.* Amherst, NY: Prometheus Press, 2007.

Shapter, Jennie. *Clay-Pot Cooking.* London: Anness Publishing Ltd., 2003.

Tinayre, Marcelle (Marguerite Suzanne). *La France à Table 77* (March 1959). Paris: Rene Fleury.

Walter, Josie. *Pots in the Kitchen.* Wiltshire, UK: The Crowood Press Ltd., 2002.

Wildeisen, Annemarie. *Cuisson Douce de la Viande à Basse Temperature.* Berlin: Aarau/Electrolux SA, 1997.

Willard, Shirley. *Cooking in Clay Pots.* www.CookingwithShirley.com, 2002.

Willinger, Faith. *An Italian Food Lover: With Recipes from 254 of My Best Friends.* New York: Clarkson Potter, 2007.

Wolfert, Paula. *The Cooking of Southwest France,* 1st ed. New York: Dial Press 1983.

Wolfert, Paula. *Paula Wolfert's World of Food.* New York: HarperCollins, 1988.

Wolfert, Paula. *Mediterranean Grains and Greens.* New York: HarperCollins, 1998.

Wolfert, Paula. *Mediterranean Cooking.* New York: Times Books, 1975.

Toygar, Kamil and Berkok. *Nimet Ankara Mutfak Kulture ve Yemekleri.* Ankara: Vehbi Koç Vakfı, 1999.

Xiradakis, Jean-Pierre and Vincent Pousson. *La Cuisine de la Tupina.* Toulouse, France: Editions Milan, 2004.

Acknowledgments

And now for my thanks…

First, to my wonderful husband, Bill Bayer, who is also my best friend. A huge thank you to Ayfer Ünsal, Barbara Wilde, and editor Susan Wyler for their friendship, wisdom, and endless help in what has been the longest cookbook haul in my career.

I also want to thank the great team at John Wiley & Sons: my in-house editor Linda Ingroia, editorial assistant Cecily McAndrews, and senior production editor Jacqueline Beach, for their patience, effort, and encouragement. I offer very special thanks to copy editor Chris Benton, book designer Joel Avirom, proofreader Christine Gilmore, the hugely talented photographer Ed Anderson, and his food stylist, Jenny Martin-Wong.

A very special thank you to Dana Cowin, editor-in-chief of *Food and Wine* magazine, and also to my editors Tina Ujlaki and Emily Kaiser. Also many thanks to Marcia Kiesel, Grace Parisi, and Melissa Rubel for their continued and valuable support of my work.

For information and recipes on cooking in clay pots in Spain, I want to thank: culinary historians and cookbook authors Clara Maria G. de Amezua, Gerry Dawes, Lola Massieu, Janet Mendel, and the late Rudolf Grewe, chefs David Kinch, Maria Dolores Mejias, Magaret Nofre, and Carlos Posada.

For information and recipes on cooking in clay pots in France, I want to thank: cookbook author and home cook the late Mireille Johnson and the late Vivienne Foucart, chefs Dominique Bucaille, Eric Bouyssou, Pierre Etienne, Francis Garcia, Laurent Gras, Dominique Toulousy, and the late Jean-Louis Palladin.

For information and recipes on cooking in clay pots in Italy, I want to thank: chefs Loretta Keller, Carlo Middione, Donna Scala, Maria Sindoni, and Scott Warner, cookbook authors and home cooks Adam Balic, David Downie, Janet Fletcher, Judy Witts Francini, Kathy Gori, Lynne Rosetta Kasper, Alison Harris, Dana Jacobi, Vita Coppolo Poma, the late Mario Ruspoli, Morton Satin, Siglinda Scarpa, and Faith Willinger.

For information and recipes on cooking in clay pots in the Eastern Mediterranean, I wish to thank: chefs Musa Dağdeviren, Burak Epir, and Ilker Kaya, chef-owners Ahmet Kasibeyaz and Burhan Cadgas, cookbook authors Engin Akyn, Vefa Alexiadou, Samira Yogo Cholagh, Anissa Helou, Aglaia Kremezi, Mirsini Lamprini, and Gulsen Sozmer; Turkish government officials Mihaliccik Governor Mehmet Boztepe, and Eskishir and Nevsehir Ministries of Culture representatives Ms. Seyda Ceylan and Ms. Nilgun Hanim, Urgup's Mayor Bekir Odemis and Beypazari Mayor Mansur Yavaş. Food bloggers and home cooks Fethiye Akbulut, Bob Beer, Aydin Ayhan Guney, Filiz Hösukoğlu, Elena Kardrevski, Maviye Kayakiran, Kamal Mouzowak, Elie Nassar, Jale Robertson, Meryem Uresin, and Hatice Üslünyer.

For information and recipes on cooking in clay pots in North Africa, I want to thank: chefs Rafih Benjelloun, Abderrazak Haouari, Mourad Lahlou, and Farid Zadi. Many thanks to olive oil producer Abdelmajib Majoub, Robert Bergé, Fatema Hal, Eben Lenderking, and Joan Peterson.

I wish to thank the following testers for their careful attention to detail and for their insights: Jon and Barbara Beckmann, Abra Bennett, Judith Benton, Nancy Lang, Pat Miller, Lisa Lavagetto, Helena Sarin, Nancy Smith, Carolyn Tillie, Anne Wheeler, Kit Williams, and Donna Yee.

For general and specific information on cooking and serving in clay pots: Potters Philippe Beltrando, Terrie Wright Chrones, Beth Foote, Deborah Krasner, Betsy Price, Bill Sax, and Tom Wirt; chefs and cookbook authors Aliza Green, Sam Gugino, Jeremy Fox, Katharine Kagel, Sheilah Kaufman, Deborah Madison, Harold McGee, and Daphne Zepos.

Index

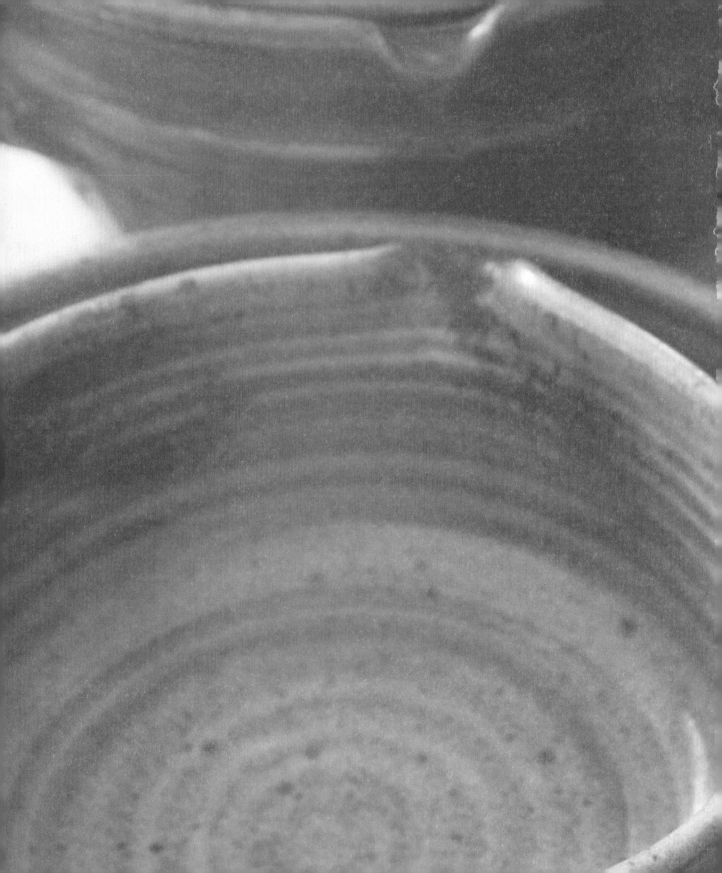